OSCE in
Fetal Medicine & Genetics

Disclaimer

All images in this work have been taken in accordance with the PCPNDT norms.

We are grateful to all our patients who have very graciously accorded their consent to the publication of the images of their scans/babies/reports in this publication.

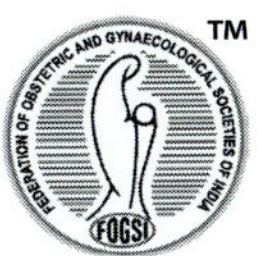

OSCE in
Fetal Medicine & Genetics

Editor-in-Chief

Jaydeep Tank
MD DNB FCPS FICOG FRCOG (Honoris Causa)
Obstetrician, Gynecologist, and IVF Consultant
Ashwini Maternity and Surgical Hospital
Center for Endoscopy and IVF
Mumbai, Maharashtra, India
President, FOGSI (2024–2025)
Chair, YGAA Committee, AOFOG
Project Lead, FOGSI-USAID Projects (2020–2024)

Editors

Seetha Ramamurthy Pal
MBBS DGO MD FRCOG
FICOG RCOG/RCR Diploma in Advanced Obstetric Ultrasound
Consultant
Department of Fetal Medicine and Obstetrics
Apollo Multispecialty Hospitals
Kolkata, West Bengal, India
Chairperson, Genetics and Fetal Medicine Committee, FOGSI (2023–2025)

Jaya Chawla
MBBS MS FICMCH
Fellow Maternal Fetal Medicine (AIIMS)
Professor
Department of Obstetrics and Gynecology
Atal Bihari Vajpayee Institute of Medical Sciences and
Dr RML Hospital, New Delhi, India
Executive Member, Genetics and Fetal Medicine Committee, FOGSI (2023–2025)

Forewords

Ashok Khurana **S Suresh**

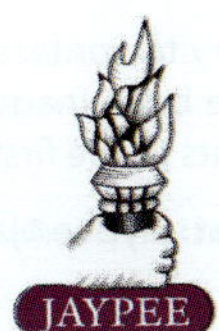

JAYPEE BROTHERS MEDICAL PUBLISHERS
The Health Sciences Publisher
New Delhi | London

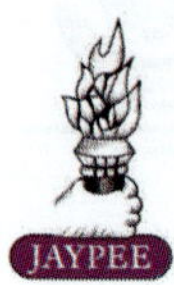

Jaypee Brothers Medical Publishers (P) Ltd

Headquarters
EMCA House, 23/23-B
Ansari Road, Daryaganj
New Delhi 110 002, India
Landline: +91-11-23272143, +91-11-23272703
+91-11-23282021, +91-11-23245672
e-mail: jaypee@jaypeebrothers.com

Corporate Office
4838/24, Ansari Road, Daryaganj
New Delhi 110 002, India
Phone: +91-11-43574357
Fax: +91-11-43574314
e-mail: jaypee@jaypeebrothers.com

Overseas Office
JP Medical Ltd.
83, Victoria Street, London
SW1H 0HW (UK)
Phone: +44-20 3170 8910
e-mail: info@jpmedpub.com

EU GPSR Authorised Representative
Logos Europe, 9 rue Nicolas Poussin
17000, La Rochelle, France
Phone: +33 (0) 6 67 93 73 78
e-mail: contact@logoseurope.eu

Website: www.jaypeebrothers.com
Website: www.jaypeedigital.com

Inquiries for bulk sales may be solicited at: jaypee@jaypeebrothers.com

OSCE in Fetal Medicine & Genetics

First Edition: **2026**

ISBN: 978-93-6616-897-5

Printed in India

Dedicated to

Our fetuses who have bestowed upon us
the inspiration to learn

Contributors

Akshatha Prabhu
MBBS MS (Obs & Gyne) MRCOG
Senior Consultant
Department of Fetal Medicine
Indraprastha Apollo Hospitals
New Delhi, India

Alok Varshney MD DNB (Radiodiagnosis)
Senior Consultant and Radiologist
Director, Central Diagnostics
New Delhi, India

Anita Kaul
MBBS MS (Obs & Gyne) FRCOG FICOG Diploma in Fetal Medicine (FMF-UK) Diploma in Advanced Obstetric Scanning (London)
Clinical Coordinator
Apollo Centre for Fetal Medicine
New Delhi, India
Director, Apollo Cradles Delhi-NCR

Apoorva Kulshreshtha
MBBS MD (Obs & Gyne)
Assistant Professor
Department of Obstetrics and Gynecology
Lady Hardinge Medical College
New Delhi, India

Arpit Jindal MBBS DNB (Radiodiagnosis)
Fellow in Advanced ObGyn Ultrasound
The Fetal Clinic
Puducherry, India

Bijoy K Balakrishnan MBBS MS
Head
FM Unit
CIMARKochi, Kerala, India

Chanchal MD FRCOG FICOG
Lead Consultant
Department of Fetal Medicine
Madhukar Rainbow Children's Hospital and BirthRight by Rainbow Hospitals
New Delhi, India

Chandra Kant Garg
MBBS DGO Fellowship in Fetal Medicine
Consultant
Department of Fetal Medicine
Jaipur Fetal Medicine and Research Centre
Jaipur, Rajasthan, India

Chinmayee Ratha
MS (Obs & Gyne) FRCOG (UK) FICOG FIMSA Diploma in Fetal Medicine (FMF-UK)
Director
Resolution Centre of Fetal Medicine and Research Institute, Hyderabad
Lead Consultant (Fetal Medicine)
KIMS Sunshine Hospitals, KIMS Cuddles, Hyderabad
Visiting Consultant
Arete Hospitals
Hyderabad, Telangana, India

Jaya Chawla
MS FICMCH Fellow Maternal Fetal Medicine (AIIMS)
Professor
Department of Obstetrics and Gynecology
Atal Bihari Vajpayee Institute of Medical Sciences and Dr Ram Manohar Lohia Hospital
New Delhi, India

K Aparna Sharma
MBBS DNB FICOG MNAMS Mastering in Maternal-Fetal Medicine (Barcelona)
Professor
Department of Obstetrics and Gynecology
All India Institute of Medical Sciences
New Delhi, India

K Manikandan
MBBS MD DNB MRCOG PDF-FM
Lead Consultant (Fetal Therapy)
The Fetal Clinic, Puducherry
Kovai Medical Center and Hospital
Coimbatore
Visiting Consultant, KEM Hospital, Pune
Visiting Professor
Department of Perinatology
Pondicherry Institute of Medical Sciences
Kalapet, Puducherry, India

Madhusudan Dey
MBBS MS (Obs & Gyne) Fetal Medicine
Commanding Officer
304 Field Hospital
Allahabad, Uttar Pradesh, India

Malathi Prasad
MBBS MD (Obs & Gyne) MRCOG (UK) DNB Diploma in Fetal Medicine (FMF Barcelona)
Director and Lead Consultant
Department of Fetal Medicine
Trichy Fetal Medicine and Fertility Centre
Tiruchirappalli, Tamil Nadu, India

Mandakini Pradhan
MBBS MD (Obs & Gyne, PGIMER, Chandigarh) DNB DM (Medical Genetics)
Professor and Head
Department of Obstetrics and Gynecology
Sanjay Gandhi Postgraduate Institute of Medical Sciences
Lucknow, Uttar Pradesh, India

Manisha Kumar
MS (Obs & Gyne) FICOG Expert in Fetal Medicine (Barcelona)
Director-Professor
Department of Obstetrics and Gynecology
Lady Hardinge Medical College
New Delhi, India

Megha Sharma
MBBS MS DNB Fellowship in Minimal Invasive Surgery PDCC
Consultant
Department of Fetal Medicine
Nidaan Heart and Fetal Medicine Center
Kota, Rajasthan, India

Navya KC
MBBS MD (OBG, PGIMER Chandigarh) DNB (OBG) Fellowship in Fetal Medicine & Fetal Invasives (FMF UK Accredited)
Senior and Lead Consultant
Department of Fetal Medicine and Fetal Therapy
Yashoda Hospital
Hyderabad, Telangana, India

Neha Gupta
MD DNB
Senior Consultant
Department of Fetal Medicine and Genetics
Kailash Hospital and Heart Institute
Noida, Uttar Pradesh, India

Nishigandha Mali
MBBS MS (Obs & Gyne) DNB ICOG Certification in Fetal Medicine
Consultant Fetal Sonologist
Department of Fetal Medicine
Nowrosjee Wadia Maternity Hospital
Mumbai, Maharashtra, India

Pooja Vaziraani
MBBS MD (Obs & Gyne) DNB FCPS DGO Fellowship in Fetal Medicine (Mediscan Fetal Care & Research, Chennai) International Master in Maternal-Fetal Medicine (University of BCN, BCNatal, Spain) Trained in Fetal Neurosonography Postgraduate in Fetal Cardiology (University of BCN, BCNatal, Spain)
Senior Fetal Medicine Consultant
Department of Fetal Medicine
Dr LH Hiranandani Hospital
Abipraay Centre for Advanced Fetal Medicine; and Nidan Fetal Medicine Centre
Mumbai, Maharashtra, India

Preeti Parekh Tomar
MBBS MD Fellowship in Fetal Medicine
Director and Lead Consultant
Department of Fetal Medicine
Aarohan Fetal Medicine Centre
Indore, Madhya Pradesh, India

Sakshi Yadav
MBBS MS (Obs & Gyne) DM Medical Genetics (AIIMS, New Delhi) Fellowship in Advanced Antenatal Ultrasonography (Mediscan, Chennai)
Clinical Geneticist
Care Diagnostic Centre, Zirakpur
Motherhood Chaitanya, Chandigarh
Faith Diagnostic and Fetal Centre
Mohali, Punjab, India

Sangeeta Yadav MBBS MD
Professor
Department of Maternal and Reproductive Health
Sanjay Gandhi Postgraduate Institute of Medical Sciences
Lucknow, Uttar Pradesh, India

Saswati Mukhopadhyay
MBBS DNB DrNB
Senior Consultant
Clinical Geneticist
Apollo Mutlispecialty Hospital, Kolkata
Visiting Consultant, Medical Geneticist, Institute of Post Graduate Medical Education and Research (IPGMER)
Kolkata, West Bengal, India

Saumya Srivastava
MBBS MS (Obs & Gyne) PDCC (Maternal and Fetal Medicine)
Consultant
Department of Fetal Medicine
Sansrishti Clinic
Hazaribagh, Jharkhand, India

Seetha Ramamurthy Pal
MBBS DGO MD FRCOG FICOG RCOG/RCR Diploma in Advanced Obstetric Ultrasound
Consultant
Department of Fetal Medicine and Obstetrics
Apollo Multispecialty Hospitals
Kolkata, West Bengal, India

Selvaraj Ravi Lakshmy MBBS
Director
Shri Lakshmi Clinic and Scan Centre
Krishnagiri, Tamil Nadu, India

Shruti Jain
MBBS MS (Obs & Gyne) DNB (Obs & Gyne) PDCC (Maternal and Fetal Medicine)
Consultant
Department of Fetal Medicine
Kailash Hospital and Neuro Institute
Noida, Uttar Pradesh, India

Sreelakshmi GN
KN MS DNB FICOG MRCOG (UK) Fellow in Medical Genetics
Consultant
Department of Fetal Medicine
Malnad Hitech Diagnostic Centre
Shivamogga, Karnataka, India

Sumitra Bachani
MD MNAMS Fellow Maternal Fetal Medicine (AIIMS, New Delhi) Expert in Fetal Medicine (BC Natal FMRC, Barcelona)
Professor, Senior Specialist, and Lead Faculty
Department of Obstetrics and Gynecology
Vardhman Mahavir Medical College and Safdarjung Hospital
New Delhi, India

Tulika Ranjan Joshi MBBS DNB
Consultant
Department of Fetal Medicine
Berlin Diagnostics and Day Care
Ranchi, Jharkhand, India

Vandana Bansal
MBBS MD DGO DNB MNAMS FICOG FRCOG (UK) FNB (High Risk Pregnancy and Perinatology)
Additional Professor
Department of Obstetrics and Gynecology
Head
Department of Ultrasound
Nowrosjee Wadia Maternity Hospital
Seth GS Medical College, Mumbai
Director, Surya Fetal Medicine Centre
Mumbai, Maharashtra, India

Vandana Chaddha
MBBS MS Certified Medical Geneticist, SGPGI Postdoctoral Fellowship Maternal Fetal Medicine (University of Toronto)
Director
Sattva Fetalkare Medicine
New Delhi, India

Vrunda Appannagari
MBBS DNB MRCOG
Consultant
Department of Fetal Medicine
Madhukar Rainbow Children's Hospital and BirthRight by Rainbow Hospitals
New Delhi, India

Message

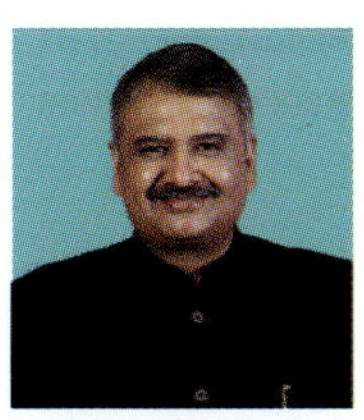

Fetal Medicine and Genetics is an ever-evolving subject. The growing interest in delving deeper into the enigmatic world of fetal abnormalities has encouraged the development of more insights into the genetic basis of these disorders and superior resolution has facilitated the process of not only earlier and more certain identification of these disorders but also the amelioration of some of them with appropriate interventions.

OSCE on this subject is an interesting concept that shares the clinically relevant insights in a more absorbable form for the enthusiastic readers. The question-answer format challenges the human mind to first attempt his own solutions and suggested reading at the end is inviting to scratch the surface—a little deeper in the hope of acquiring a better understanding of the scenario.

I would like to congratulate the Editors, Dr Seetha Ramamurthy Pal and Dr Jaya Chawla for the foresight in developing this concept into a book meticulously planned and elaborately illustrated. They have successfully accomplished the arduous task of bringing together a vast galaxy of experts in the field to share their precious experience amassed over years of painstaking practice and commitment to their craft.

I am sure it will be a collector's privilege.

Jaydeep Tank
MBBS MD DGO FCPS FICOG FRCOG
Consultant, Ashwini Maternity and Surgical Hospital
Centre for Endoscopy and IVF, Mumbai
President FOGSI (2024–25)
Chair, YGAA Committee, Asia Oceania Federation
of Obstetrics and Gynaecology (AOFOG)
Project Lead FOGSI, USAID Projects (2020–24)
Immediate Past Deputy Secretary, AOFOG
Secretary General FOGSI (2018–21)

Message

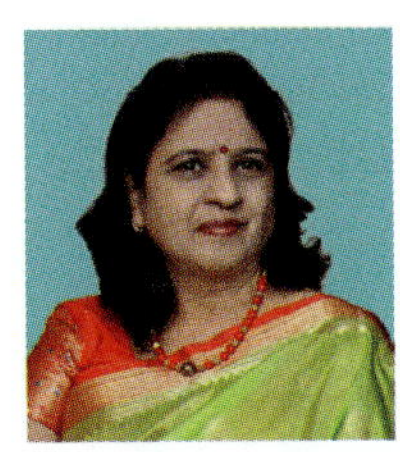

Both Fetal Medicine and Genetics are fields that have witnessed enormous growth in the last few years. This growth has paved the way for the development of insights into the genetic basis of disease on one hand and provided interventional solutions to fetal disorders on the other. This growth has also brought forth new opportunities for training young enthusiasts into these promising fields.

OSCE in Fetal Medicine and Genetics is an updated and meticulously compiled work that has brought stalwarts from across the country together to share their commendable work in the form of carefully crafted and illustrated questions and meticulously curated answers. The idea of inciting interest through these case-based discussions and leaving the interested reader with suggested reading to develop her understanding at her own pace without hindering the flow of the book is a commendable idea.

I personally congratulate the Editors, Dr Seetha Ramamurthy Pal and Dr Jaya Chawla for their exemplary planning and brilliant execution if this initiative which will benefit clinicians and students alike.

Madhuri A Patel
MBBS MD DGO FICOG
Hon. Clinical Associate, N Wadia Hospital, Mumbai
Hon. Consultant Police Hospital, Mumbai
Visiting Consultant
St Elizabeth's Hospitals, Mumbai
Former Professor and Head
Department of Obstetrics and Gynecology
ESIC-PGIMSR, MGMH, Mumbai
Secretary General, FOGSI
Editor-in-Chief
Journal of Obstetrics and Gynaecology of India (JOGI)
Joint Secretary, FOGSI - 2009
Committee Member, FIGO Preterm Birth

Message

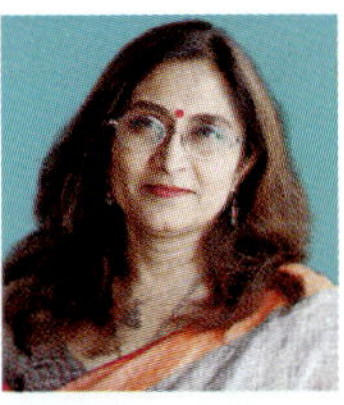

It is with great pride that we unveil the final edition of our book on *OSCE in Fetal Medicine and Genetics*—an invaluable resource meticulously refined to uphold the highest academic and clinical standards. This work stands as a testament to the dedication, expertise, and collaborative efforts of the Chairperson of the Genetics and Fetal Medicine Committee, the visionary leader Dr Seetha Ramamurthy Pal and Dr Jaya Chawla, National Coordinator, Genetics and Fetal Medicine Committee, FOGSI, under the dynamic leadership of FOGSI President, Dr Jaydeep Tank.

As the then Vice President of FOGSI overseeing this initiative, I am honored to see this endeavor reach its culmination, offering a structured and a comprehensive guide for practitioners and trainees alike. May this book serve as a beacon of knowledge, shaping the future of fetal medicine with precision and excellence.

Girija Wagh
MBBS MD FICOG DIP ENDO FICS
Professor, Department of Obstetrics and Gynecology
Bharathi Vidyapeeth Medical College Hospital, Pune
Senior Consultant (Gynecologist, Obstetrician and IVF Specialist)
Cloud Nine and Apollo Hospitals, Pune
Vice President, FOGSI 2024

Foreword

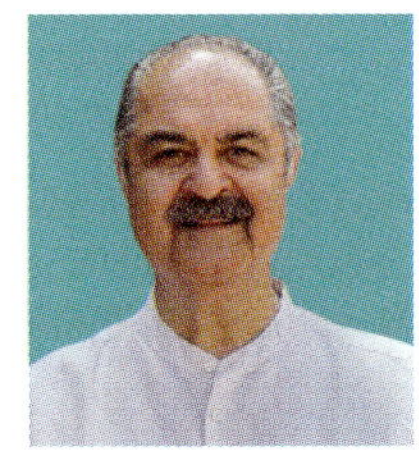

Learning and teaching are evolving at a rapid rate to adapt to changes in the perspective that potential beneficiaries have to their use. Conventional textbooks with chapters are giving way to subject-specific companion books, smartphones are replacing laptops as a preferred platform, and, even in conferences and continuing professional education programs, didactic teaching is sharing space with case-based teaching and case-based specialist panel discussions.

It is exciting, therefore, to see a text of Fetal Medicine which is case-based, well-illustrated and "chapterized". Excellent images, meticulous annotations, capsulized teaching points and well-researched references make this text "OSCE in Fetal Medicine and Genetics" unique, remarkably useful and a dream come true. The adage about one picture being worth a thousand words rings true as one leaf through the pages and case after case registers a lasting impression.

Each case has a high-quality image with relevant questions.... and answers! The references are appropriately pruned to recent review articles.

This treatise fulfills several needs within the realm of the practice of Fetal Medicine today. The first, and least, is a ready reference for those preparing for board examinations in the field. Far more importantly, it forms a brief but comprehensive ready reference for not only those in daily obstetric practice but for all practitioners of the multispecialty of fetal medicine: obstetricians, high-risk obstetricians, perinatologists, radiologists, geneticists, dysmorphologists, pediatricians, and pediatric surgeons.

The book includes an impressive authorship: two leading lights in the field today. Seetha Ramamurthy Pal and Jaya Chawla, being daily practitioners of the art and science of fetal medicine have indeed put together a book that is a must to possess. Their sensitivity to the optimal delivery of fetal healthcare is reflected in every page.

The text does not wander or deviate. It lights up the right path to opening minds to fetal needs. I congratulate them on this phenomenal achievement and encourage all practitioners in the realm of fetal, maternal and neonatal care to utilize this treasure on a daily basis.

Ashok Khurana MD
Professor
Mentor Emeritus, Society of Fetal Medicine
Chairman and Consultant in Reproductive Ultrasound
The Ultrasound Lab, New Delhi, India

Foreword

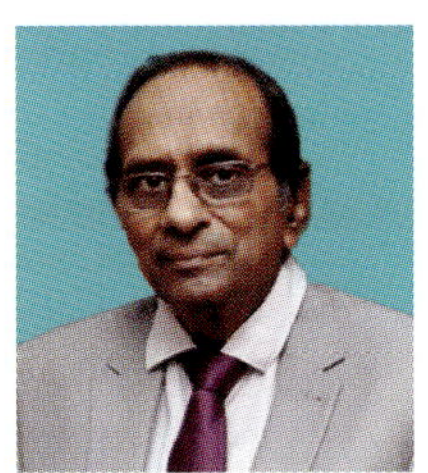

It is a privilege to contribute a foreword to this distinguished volume on the Objective Structured Clinical Examination (OSCE) in fetal medicine. As ultrasound has become an integral component of standard obstetric care, it is incumbent upon obstetricians and imaging specialists with an interest in this field to acquire a comprehensive understanding of fetal imaging, genetics, and pathology.

Fetal medicine has evolved into a highly specialized discipline, meriting recognition as a distinct subspecialty within obstetrics and radiology. In this context, the need for rigorous and objective methods of competency assessment is paramount. The Objective Structured Clinical Examination (OSCE) has emerged as a globally accepted evaluative framework, offering a structured and standardized approach to assessing clinical proficiency.

This book provides a meticulously organized and richly illustrated exploration of the breadth of fetal medicine. It is divided into six major sections encompassing 24 chapters, each of which addresses key domains including ultrasound imaging, fetal genetics, and pathology. The contributors have curated a wealth of clinically relevant cases, complemented by carefully constructed questions and high-quality imaging, thereby reflecting the complexities encountered in everyday clinical practice.

What distinguishes this volume is its utility as both an examination preparatory resource and a reference for practicing clinicians. The case-based, question-and-answer format is succinct yet thorough, and the inclusion of references at the end of each case enhances its value as a scholarly resource.

Another noteworthy feature is the book's flexible structure, which allows it to be read either sequentially or selectively, depending on the reader's needs. Each chapter stands alone in its comprehensiveness, enabling focused learning on specific topics while maintaining the integrity of the broader curriculum.

I commend the editors, Seetha Ramamurthy Pal and Jaya Chawla, for their vision and leadership in conceptualizing this project. Their efforts in assembling an accomplished team of contributors from across the country have resulted in a text that is both authoritative and accessible. This book will undoubtedly serve as an indispensable resource for postgraduate students, trainees, and practitioners of fetal medicine, both in India and internationally.

S Suresh
MBBS FRCOG (Hon) DSc (Hon)
Director MediScan Systems
Honorary Secretary Voluntary (CEO), Health Services, Chennai
Professor of Practice, Department of Medical Sciences, IIT Madras
Visiting Professor in Perinatology, SRMC, Chennai, Tamil Nadu, India
Visiting Professor in Perinatology, PSG Hospital, Coimbatore
Tamil Nadu, India

Preface

Objective structured clinical examination (OSCE) is a relatively new way of assessing a student's grasp over his subject. The format demands clarity of basic concepts as much as their application on clinically challenging situations which seldom present straight from the book. This new platform of assessment calls for an equally novel way of studying. Fetal Medicine and Genetics is an ever-evolving subject which is difficult to summarize in concise textbooks. Moreover, medical science, in general, is a field where hand holding by seniors and gaining insights from their extremely rich experience is key to success. Keeping this in mind, FOGSI's Genetics and Fetal Medicine Committee has invited stalwarts in the field of Genetics and Fetal Medicine from every nook and corner of the country to share their vast clinical experience of cases for the benefit of those who follow their legacy on the curve of learning.

The OSCE stations in this book have been consciously crafted in a manner that goes from basics to advanced on the area of interest. Pictorial stations help students assimilate the content better and have more recall value when such situations arise in clinical sojourn. Practical aspects such as cardinal rules of diagnosis, prognostic factors, further workup and tenets of counseling have been included in a crisp manner so as to keep the content relevant for everyday practice.

We sincerely hope that this initiative shall not only be well received by undergraduate, postgraduate and superspecialty students aspiring to sit for examinations but also practitioners of the Art of Fetal Medicine, Genetics, Obstetrics, Perinatology, Neonatology and Pediatric subspecialties alike. In medicine, and more so, in life, continuous follow-up and continuous learning, indeed go hand-in-hand.

Look forward to some great practical academics!

Jaydeep Tank
Seetha Ramamurthy Pal
Jaya Chawla

Acknowledgments

Blessed, in life, are those, that have the guiding light of their seniors to pave their way and the towering support of those they walk with, all at the same time. It cannot hold truer than when we begin to acknowledge the accomplished and gifted people who have come together for the genesis of this work, *OSCE in Fetal Medicine & Genetics.*

It is our pride and privilege to extend a word of humble gratitude to our dynamic President FOGSI, Dr Jaydeep Tank and Secretary General, Dr Madhuri Patel who have very graciously permitted and encouraged us in the creation of this book at every step of the process.

There are no words that can do justice to the commendable constellation of stalwarts in Fetal Medicine and Genetics who have agreed to lend their rich clinical experience, enviable collection of images and unparalleled academic prowess to this novel initiative. Uniquely crafted stations from their opulent collection, carefully collated over years of pain-staking follow-up of each and every clinical challenge, have made this work, the artwork it has turned out to be. We profusely thank our accomplished and endowed contributors for their generous and enlightening contribution.

This word of gratitude shall remain grossly shallow until we acknowledge the patient and silent contribution of all the families who have gone through the penance of bearing babies with fetal medicine and genetic concerns and facilitated our understanding of this enigmatic subject. We truly thank all of them with a genuine spirit of appreciation.

Lastly, this work would not have seen the light-of-the-day if our families and those of our contributors', would not have generously supported the proverbial burning of the midnight oil. So, we extend our heartfelt acknowledgments and profound gratefulness to each of our beloved family members for their patience and kind understanding.

Addendum

The Voluson Series of GE ultrasound equipment is armed with great resolution and state of the art technology to provide excellent 2D and 3D images that facilitate study of fetal anatomy in fine detail. Many of the images in this book are a testament to the same.

Contents

SECTION 1: First Trimester Evaluation

1. **Biochemical Screening for Aneuploidy** 3
Navya KC, Sreelakshmi GN

2. **Pre-eclampsia Screening** 22
Shruti Jain

3. **First Trimester Scan with Combined First Trimester Screening** 34
Chandra Kant Garg, Megha Sharma, Saumya Srivastava

4. **Non-invasive Prenatal Screening** 66
Sumitra Bachani, Sakshi Yadav

5. **Screening in Multifetal Gestations** 81
Seetha Ramamurthy Pal

SECTION 2: Organ Specific Anomalies

6. **Facial and Neck Abnormalities** 101
Selvaraj Ravi Lakshmy

7. **Abnormalities of Thorax** 119
Chanchal, Neha Gupta, Vrunda Appannagari

8. **Congenital Abnormalities of the Heart: Structural Defects and Arrhythmias** 136
Bijoy K Balakrishnan, Alok Varshney

9. **Congenital Abnormalities of the Gastrointestinal Tract and Abdominal Wall** 164
Tulika Ranjan Joshi

10. **Congenital Abnormalities of the Kidney and Urinary Tract** 181
Chinmayee Ratha

11. **Central and Peripheral Nervous System Abnormalities** 194
Akshatha Prabhu, Anita Kaul

12. **Skeletal Dysplasias** 213
Manisha Kumar, Apoorva Kulshreshtha

SECTION 3: Soft Markers

13. **Soft Markers** 225
Sangeeta Yadav

SECTION 4: Mixed Bag

14. Fetal Infections **239**
Vandana Bansal, Nishigandha Mali

15. Fetal Growth Restriction **255**
Madhusudan Dey, Seetha Ramamurthy Pal

16. Red Cell Isoimmunization **267**
Mandakini Pradhan

17. Hematological Disorders **277**
Saswati Mukhopadhyay

18. Nonimmune Hydrops Fetalis **291**
Jaya Chawla, K Aparna Sharma

SECTION 5: Fetal Interventions

19. Fetal Interventions in Singleton Pregnancies **313**
Vandana Chaddha

20. Fetal Interventions in Multifetal Gestations **331**
Vandana Chaddha

21. Medical Transplacental Therapy **350**
K Manikandan, Arpit Jindal

22. Prophylactic Interventions **365**
Preeti Parekh Tomar

SECTION 6: Completing the Jigsaw

23. Drugs and Radiation **375**
Malathi Prasad, Pooja Vaziraani

24. Fetal Autopsy **387**
Manisha Kumar

Index *405*

SECTION 1

First Trimester Evaluation

1. **Biochemical Screening for Aneuploidy**
   Navya KC, Sreelakshmi GN
2. **Pre-eclampsia Screening**
   Shruti Jain
3. **First Trimester Scan with Combined First Trimester Screening**
   Chandra Kant Garg, Megha Sharma, Saumya Srivastava
4. **Non-invasive Prenatal Screening**
   Sumitra Bachani, Sakshi Yadav
5. **Screening in Multifetal Gestations**
   Seetha Ramamurthy Pal

CHAPTER 1

Biochemical Screening for Aneuploidy

Navya KC, Sreelakshmi GN

STATION 1. **A 37-year-old software engineer primigravida with a history of primary infertility for 5 years with spontaneous conception at 12 weeks of gestation has come for nuchal translucency (NT) scan. Medical history is normal—body mass index (BMI) - 24, non-alcoholic, and non-smoker. She is very apprehensive about Down syndrome. She put forth her concern about screening tests and wanted to do what is best for her and her pregnancy. Her questions are given below.**

1. **What is an aneuploidy screening test?**
2. **What markers of aneuploidy are looked for at her gestation? What is the detection rate of Down with this information?**
3. **What is the sensitivity and false positive rate of screening test in detection of Down syndrome using (a) maternal age alone (b) maternal age + dual marker (c) combined first trimester screen and (d) maternal age + enhanced first trimester screen?**
4. **What are the best screening test options considering her age?**
5. **What are prerequisites to consider before double marker test?**

Ans.

1. Screening tests identify individuals broadly as high-risk or low-risk for major chromosomal aneuploidies T21, 18, 13, and sex chromosomes. Positive screening test result only places the patient in a high-risk group and does not in any way imply that fetus is affected.
2. Nuchal translucency scan is an ultrasound done when crown to rump length (CRL) is between 45 and 84 mm which falls between approximately 11–13 + 6 weeks of gestation. In this window period, specialist can confirm dating of pregnancy, looks for markers of Down syndrome such as size of NT, presence or absence of nasal bone, additionally ductus venosus (DV) and tricuspid regurgitation (TR) and also other structural abnormalities. Detection of Down syndrome with NT scan alone is 75–80% with maternal age risk.

3. Detection rate depends on parameters taken for risk assessment. See the table below.

Parameters	*Detection rate %*	*FPR %*
1. MA	30	5
2. MA + serum free beta-human chorionic gonadotropin (β-hCG) and placenta-associated plasma protein-A (PAPP-A)	60–70	5
3. MA + NT + serum free β-hCG and PAPP-A (combined test)	85–95	5
4. Combined test + nasal bone or ductus doppler or tricuspid flow [enhanced first trimester screening (FTS)]	93–96	2.5

4. Either combined or enhanced FTS done by a specialist (detection rate is 90–96%, FPR is 2.5–5%) or non-invasive prenatal screening (NIPS) (detection rate is 99.99%, false positive rate of 0.01%).
5. The following prerequisites are to be considered:
   - Parity
   - Correct age or preferably date of birth to be noted. Donor age in case of IVF pregnancy. Frozen embryos then date of freezing should be considered as maternal age.
   - Weight and height of patient (BMI)
   - Racial origin
   - Smoking status
   - Mode of conception
   - Date of last delivery (for interval from last pregnancy)
   - Whether there is history of hormone therapy
   - Diabetes on insulin: Yes/No
   - Previous history of pre-eclampsia or chronic hypertension, family history of PE.
   - Autoimmune disorders and SLE
   - Previous history of small baby
   - Previous history of spontaneous delivery between 16 and 30 weeks.
   - Period of gestation by CRL
   - NT centile as per gestational age

   Nasal bone, ductus venosus PI and tricuspid regurgitation are optional markers.

SUGGESTED READING

1. Nicolaides KH. Screening for fetal aneuploidies at 11 to 13 weeks. Prenat Diagn. 2011;31(1):7-15.

STATION 2. A 35-year-old second gravida with previous normal healthy child presents at 12 weeks of gestation, spontaneous conception. CFTS

showed NT 25th centile, high biochemical risk in double marker report though final risk is below >1:250. She is worried and is seeking your consultation. The reports are as follows:

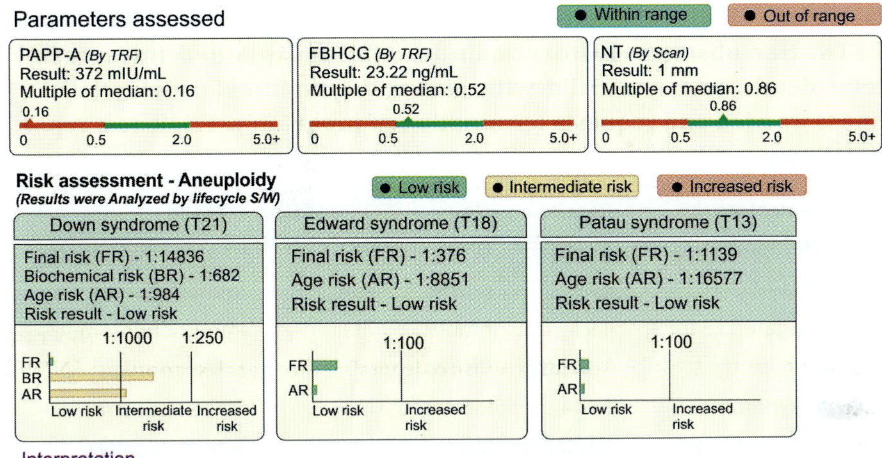

Parameters assessed — ● Within range ● Out of range

PAPP-A (By TRF)	FBHCG (By TRF)	NT (By Scan)
Result: 372 mIU/mL	Result: 23.22 ng/mL	Result: 1 mm
Multiple of median: 0.16	Multiple of median: 0.52	Multiple of median: 0.86

Risk assessment - Aneuploidy
(Results were Analyzed by lifecycle S/W)

● Low risk ● Intermediate risk ● Increased risk

Down syndrome (T21)	Edward syndrome (T18)	Patau syndrome (T13)
Final risk (FR) - 1:14836	Final risk (FR) - 1:376	Final risk (FR) - 1:1139
Biochemical risk (BR) - 1:682	Age risk (AR) - 1:8851	Age risk (AR) - 1:16577
Age risk (AR) - 1:984	Risk result - Low risk	Risk result - Low risk
Risk result - Low risk		

Interpretation

The first trimester screening for the given sample is found screen negative

1. **What is a priori risk for Down syndrome in this report?**
2. **What is the detection rate of DS if maternal age plus NT is used as a criterion?**
3. **What is biochemical risk and final risk in Double marker test report?**
4. **Does high biochemical risk in the background of a low CFTS warrant further testing?**

Ans.

1. Age risk is a priori risk based on maternal age alone. It is 1:984.
2. The detection rate for DS is 65–70% with this approach.
3. Biochemical risk is a priori risk which is re-calculated based on the MoM of the serum markers of the dual test namely, free β-hCG, and PAPP-A. Final risk incorporates the nuchal translucency centiles in addition to the above. Here, biochemical risk for Down is 1:682 and final risk is 1:14836.
4. No. The combined risk has the biochemical component (serum marker levels) already factored in.

SUGGESTED READING

1. Benn P, Borrell A, Chiu RW, Cuckle H, Dugoff L, Faas B, et al. Position statement from the Chromosome Abnormality Screening Committee on behalf of the Board of the International Society for Prenatal Diagnosis. Prenat Diagn. 2015; 35(8):725-34.
2. Nicolaides KH. Screening for fetal aneuploidies at 11 to 13 weeks. Prenat Diagn. 2011;31(1):7-15.

STATION 3. **A 35-year-old G3P2L1, consanguineous couple, spontaneous conception, was referred at 14 weeks of gestation for amniocentesis as her triple marker was high risk (1:144) for DS. Medical history is normal—BMI - 29, non-alcoholic, and non-smoker. She missed her CFTS. Her obstetric history includes one unexplained intrauterine fetal death, and one child with global developmental delay (GDD). She is worried and requests termination of pregnancy. Triple test report as follows:**

Biochemical results	*Result*	*Units*	*CORR. MoM*	*Method*
Alpha fetoprotein (AFP)	69.96	U/mL	1.51	Immunofluorometry
Free beta-hCG	64.9	ng/mL	7.78	Immunofluorometry
Unconjugated E3 (uE3)	4.91	nmol/L	0.71	Immunofluorometry
Disorder	*Risk ratio*	*Risk category*		*Screen result*
Down's syndrome	1:144	Increased		Screen positive
Edward's syndrome	1:100000	Low		Screen negative
Patau's syndrome	1:17900	Low		Screen negative

1. **What would be an ideal gestation to perform second trimester serum screening?**
2. **What would be an ideal test to perform second trimester serum screening?**
3. **Can triple marker be considered a valid second trimester screen test? Give reasons for your answer.**
4. **Patient has a previous child with global developmental delay. She is concerned, whether second trimester biochemical screen will answer her concern of risk of recurrence of GDD.**

Ans.

1. Second trimester screening is performed when the head circumference (HC) is between 101.0 and 172.0 mm (15–22 weeks).
2. Quadruple marker which includes the following hormones: hCG, inhibin, unconjugated estriol, and alpha-fetoprotein (AFP).
3. No. Triple marker is not a valid test in the present era as sensitivity and specificity of the test is below 70%.
4. Patient should be clearly counseled second trimester biochemistry reports will not predict the risk of developmental delay in the current pregnancy. Affected child should be evaluated in detail by a geneticist and further investigation advised as indicated.

SUGGESTED READING

1. American College of Obstetricians and Gynecologists' Committee on Practice Bulletins Obstetrics; Committee on Genetics; Society for Maternal-Fetal

Medicine. Screening for fetal chromosomal abnormalities: ACOG Practice Bulletin, No. 226. Obstet Gynecol. 2020;136(4):e48-e69.

2. NHS. Fetal Anomaly Screening Programme. Down's syndrome, Edwards' syndrome and Patau's syndrome screening Handbook for Laboratories, 2024.

STATION 4. A 27-year-old primigravida with spontaneous conception came to you at 14 weeks with high risk for trisomy 21 as shown in the report attached. Medical history is normal—BMI - 31, non-alcoholic, and non-smoker. She is concerned about the baby and was sent to you for counselling. The report is as follows:

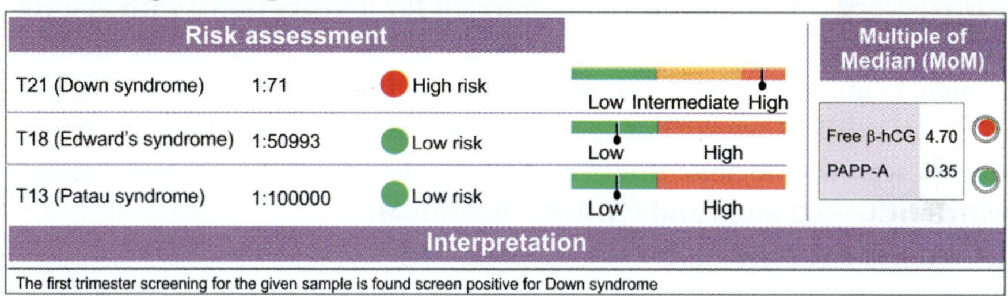

Risk assessment				Multiple of Median (MoM)	
T21 (Down syndrome)	1:71	High risk	Low Intermediate High	Free β-hCG	4.70
T18 (Edward's syndrome)	1:50993	Low risk	Low High	PAPP-A	0.35
T13 (Patau syndrome)	1:100000	Low risk	Low High		

Interpretation

The first trimester screening for the given sample is found screen positive for Down syndrome

1. **What is β-hCG?**
2. **What is the significance of this high or low β-hCG value in aneuploidy screening?**
3. **Is the value in the test could be falsely high? If yes what is the better next step?**
4. **Should she go for NIPS?**

Ans.

1. Human chorionic gonadotropin is a glycoprotein, largely produced by the syncytiotrophoblast cells and found abundantly in the blood and urine of pregnant women. It comprises two subunits, α and β. First-trimester screening tests use the *free β-hCG* value, while the quadruple test may use either *free* β-hCG or *total* β-hCG value, depending on the testing laboratory.
2. Serum free β-hCG in trisomy 21 is high whereas in trisomies 18 and 13 this is low.
3. Falsely raised β-hCG levels in euploid pregnancies—delay in shipping the sample, recent hCG injection, vanishing twin, partial moles, and hCG-secreting tumors.
4. No. Screening is ideally offered only once in pregnancy and high-risk screening result should be followed by confirmatory tests following invasive testing.

SUGGESTED READING

1. NHS. Fetal Anomaly Screening Programme. Down's syndrome, Edwards' syndrome and Patau's syndrome screening Handbook for Laboratories, 2024.

2. Spencer K, Liao AW, Skentou H, Cicero S, Nicolaides KH. Screening for triploidy by fetal nuchal translucency and maternal serum free beta-hCG and PAPP-A at 10-14 weeks of gestation. Prenat Diagn. 2000;20(6):495-9.
3. Spencer K, Ong C, Skentou H, Liao AW, Nicolaides KH. Screening for trisomy 13 by fetal nuchal translucency and maternal serum free beta-hCG and PAPP-A at 10-14 weeks of gestation. Prenat Diagn. 2000;20(5):411-6.
4. Spencer K, Tul N, Nicolaides KH. Maternal serum free beta-hCG and PAPP-A in fetal sex chromosome defects in the first trimester. Prenat Diagn. 2000;20(5): 390-4.

STATION 5. A woman, 33 years married for 5 years G3A2 with spontaneous conception, comes to you at 13 weeks of pregnancy. Medical history is normal—BMI – 24, non-alcoholic but she smokes two packets of cigars until 11 weeks but stopped when she realized she is pregnant. Her NT scan was normal. However dual test shows low risk for aneuploidies with β-hCG – 1.2 MoM and PAPP-A – 0.08 MoM.

1. **What is PAPP-A?**
2. **What disorders can be screened for using PAPP-A?**
3. **What factors can increase or decrease the serum levels of this marker?**
4. **In the absence of aneuploidy what are the other risks for pregnancy associated with a low PAPP-A?**

Ans.

1. Placenta-associated plasma protein-A (PAPP-A) is a large, glycosylated protein produced by the developing trophoblast. It is offered between 10 and 14 weeks.
2. Commonly used as a screening tool for trisomy 21, 18, 13, and triploidy, preeclampsia, fetal growth restriction.
3. The concentration of PAPP-A is influenced by the machine and reagents used, gestational age, maternal weight, ethnicity, smoking status, and method of conception. Serum PAPP-A is lower (defined as <0.4 MoM)—in trisomies 18 and 13 than in trisomy 21. In Black women the PAPP-A level is about 60% higher than in White women. In women who smoke and those conceiving by IVF serum PAPP-A is decreased.
4. Low PAPP-A levels are associated with an increased risk of preeclampsia and fetal growth restriction.

SUGGESTED READING

1. NHS. Fetal Anomaly Screening Programme. Down's syndrome, Edwards' syndrome and Patau's syndrome screening Handbook for Laboratories, 2024.

2. Spencer K, Liao AW, Skentou H, Cicero S, Nicolaides KH. Screening for triploidy by fetal nuchal translucency and maternal serum free beta-hCG and PAPP-A at 10-14 weeks of gestation. Prenat Diagn. 2000;20(6):495-9.
3. Spencer K, Ong C, Skentou H, Liao AW, Nicolaides KH. Screening for trisomy 13 by fetal nuchal translucency and maternal serum free beta-hCG and PAPP-A at 10-14 weeks of gestation. Prenat Diagn. 2000;20(5):411-6.
4. Spencer K, Tul N, Nicolaides KH. Maternal serum free beta-hCG and PAPP-A in fetal sex chromosome defects in the first trimester. Prenat Diagn. 2000;20(5): 390-4.

STATION 6.

1. **What is estriol?**
2. **Estriol is part of which tests for aneuploidy?**
3. **How does serum estriol vary with common aneuploidies?**
4. **What are additional disorders screened with estriol levels?**

Ans.

1. Estriol is the dominant estrogen during pregnancy which is secreted by the fetoplacental unit. Dehydroepiandrosterone sulfate (DHEAS) produced in fetal adrenals undergoes aromatization in the syncytiotrophoblasts to form estriol. Estriol levels continue to increase throughout pregnancy till term.
2. It is used in quadruple test to rule out aneuploidies.
3. Low unconjugated estriol (<0.25 MoM)—DS and trisomy 18 do not significantly change in T13.
4. Low unconjugated estriol—fetal growth restriction, fetal demise or loss, and large neural tube defects, such as anencephaly, fetal adrenal insufficiency, Smith-Lemli-Opitz syndrome, X-linked ichthyosis, and aromatase deficiency. High levels of uE3—fetal congenital adrenal hyperplasia and impending preterm birth.

SUGGESTED READING

1. NHS. Fetal Anomaly Screening Programme. Down's syndrome, Edwards' syndrome and Patau's syndrome screening Handbook for Laboratories, 2024.
2. Spencer K, Liao AW, Skentou H, Cicero S, Nicolaides KH. Screening for triploidy by fetal nuchal translucency and maternal serum free beta-hCG and PAPP-A at 10-14 weeks of gestation. Prenat Diagn. 2000;20(6):495-9.
3. Spencer K, Ong C, Skentou H, Liao AW, Nicolaides KH. Screening for trisomy 13 by fetal nuchal translucency and maternal serum free beta-hCG and PAPP-A at 10-14 weeks of gestation. Prenat Diagn. 2000;20(5):411-6.
4. Spencer K, Tul N, Nicolaides KH. Maternal serum free beta-hCG and PAPP-A in fetal sex chromosome defects in the first trimester. Prenat Diagn. 2000;20(5): 390-4.

STATION 7.

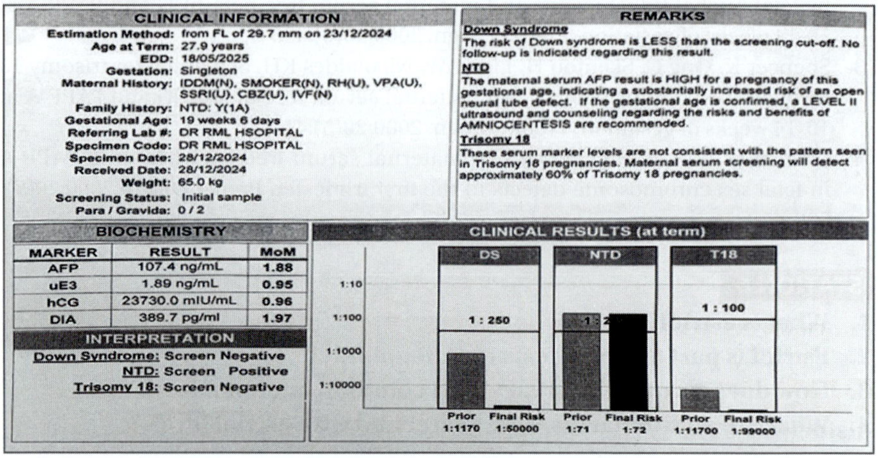

CLINICAL INFORMATION

Estimation Method: from FL of 29.7 mm on 23/12/2024
Age at Term: 27.9 years
EDD: 18/05/2025
Gestation: Singleton
Maternal History: IDDM(N), SMOKER(N), RH(U), VPA(U), SSRI(U), CBZ(U), IVF(N)
Family History: NTD: Y(1A)
Gestational Age: 19 weeks 6 days
Referring Lab #: DR RML HSOPITAL
Specimen Code: DR RML HSOPITAL
Specimen Date: 28/12/2024
Received Date: 28/12/2024
Weight: 65.0 kg
Screening Status: Initial sample
Para / Gravida: 0 / 2

REMARKS

Down Syndrome

The risk of Down syndrome is LESS than the screening cut-off. No follow-up is indicated regarding this result.

NTD

The maternal serum AFP result is HIGH for a pregnancy of this gestational age, indicating a substantially increased risk of an open neural tube defect. If the gestational age is confirmed, a LEVEL II ultrasound and counseling regarding the risks and benefits of AMNIOCENTESIS are recommended.

Trisomy 18

These serum marker levels are not consistent with the pattern seen in Trisomy 18 pregnancies. Maternal serum screening will detect approximately 60% of Trisomy 18 pregnancies.

BIOCHEMISTRY

MARKER	RESULT	MoM
AFP	107.4 ng/mL	1.88
uE3	1.89 ng/mL	0.95
hCG	23730.0 mIU/mL	0.96
DIA	389.7 pg/ml	1.97

INTERPRETATION

Down Syndrome: Screen Negative
NTD: Screen Positive
Trisomy 18: Screen Negative

CLINICAL RESULTS (at term)

1:10
1:100
1:1000
1:10000

DS: 1 : 250 — Prior 1:1170; Final Risk 1:50000
NTD: 1 : 2 — Prior 1:71; Final Risk 1:72
T18: 1 : 100 — Prior 1:11700; Final Risk 1:99000

Courtesy: Dr Jaya Chawla.

A 35-year-old G3A2, spontaneous conception, missed her combined first trimester screen. She had her first visit at 19 weeks, ultrasound was within normal limits with gestational age corresponding to 19 weeks and 6 days and her Quad test reveals a high AFP of 1.88 MoM with low risk for T21 (1:50000) and high risk for neural tube defects (NTD). She has been told that baby might have spina bifida and wants to terminate this pregnancy. She was sent to you for further management.

1. **What is AFP?**
2. **Where is AFP used in aneuploidy screening?**
3. **What is increase or decrease in AFP in aneuploidy screening define?**
4. **Does this pregnancy need termination?**

Ans.

1. Alpha-fetoprotein (AFP) is a glycoprotein is secreted by the yolk sac and the fetal liver, is the predominant protein in fetal plasma akin to albumin in post-natal life.
2. It is used in first trimester screening test in FTS-Quad test and second trimester triple test and quadruple test.
3. Raise in maternal serum alpha-fetoprotein (MSAFP)—multiple pregnancy, fetal demise, placental abnormalities, oligohydramnios, polyhydramnios secondary to open neural tube defects (ONTDs), abdominal wall defects, polycystic kidneys, esophageal atresia, duodenal atresia, teratoma, cystic hygroma, and hydrops. Low levels of MSAFP—in trisomy 21 and 18 and diabetes.
4. No. When the fetus is structurally normal, it is unlikely the fetus has spina bifida.

SUGGESTED READING

1. NHS. Fetal Anomaly Screening Programme. Down's syndrome, Edwards' syndrome and Patau's syndrome screening Handbook for Laboratories, 2024.
2. Spencer K, Liao AW, Skentou H, Cicero S, Nicolaides KH. Screening for triploidy by fetal nuchal translucency and maternal serum free beta-hCG and PAPP-A at 10-14 weeks of gestation. Prenat Diagn. 2000;20(6):495-9.
3. Spencer K, Ong C, Skentou H, Liao AW, Nicolaides KH. Screening for trisomy 13 by fetal nuchal translucency and maternal serum free beta-hCG and PAPP-A at 10-14 weeks of gestation. Prenat Diagn. 2000;20(5):411-6.
4. Spencer K, Tul N, Nicolaides KH. Maternal serum free beta-hCG and PAPP-A in fetal sex chromosome defects in the first trimester. Prenat Diagn. 2000;20(5): 390-4.

STATION 8. **A 34-year-old G5P2L1A1, spontaneous conception, with history of chronic hypertension for 5 years on anti-hypertensives came to you with previous obstetric history of intrauterine fetal death (IUFD) at 26 weeks in her first pregnancy and a fetal loss at 24 weeks in her 3rd pregnancy. Both were diagnosed to be due to severe preeclampsia. She is now at 11 + 6 weeks of gestation came for counseling. Her NT scan was normal. Bilateral uterine artery notching was present in her scan. Her CFTS report is as follows.**

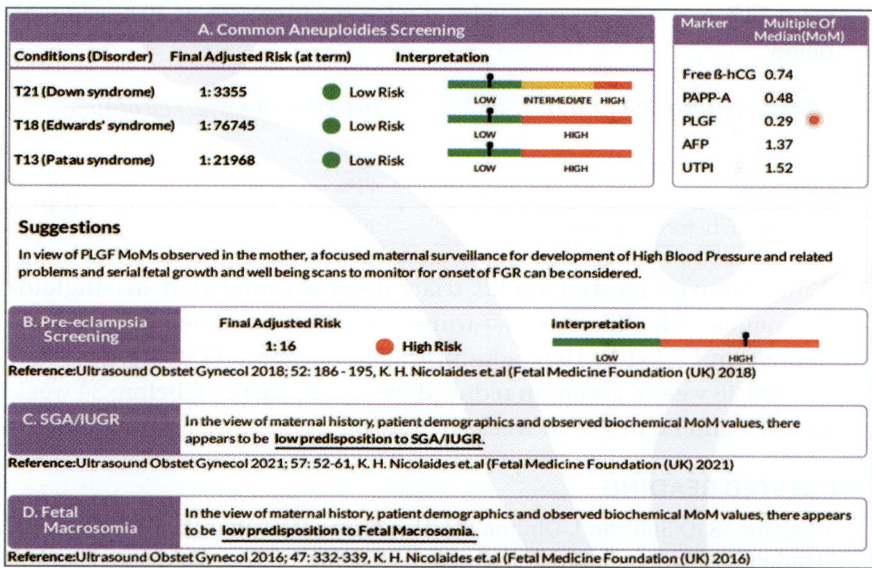

A. Common Aneuploidies Screening

Conditions (Disorder)	Final Adjusted Risk (at term)	Interpretation
T21 (Down syndrome)	1: 3355	Low Risk
T18 (Edwards' syndrome)	1: 76745	Low Risk
T13 (Patau syndrome)	1: 21968	Low Risk

Marker	Multiple Of Median(MoM)
Free ß-hCG	0.74
PAPP-A	0.48
PLGF	0.29
AFP	1.37
UTPI	1.52

Suggestions

In view of PLGF MoMs observed in the mother, a focused maternal surveillance for development of High Blood Pressure and related problems and serial fetal growth and well being scans to monitor for onset of FGR can be considered.

B. Pre-eclampsia Screening	Final Adjusted Risk	Interpretation
	1: 16	High Risk

Reference: Ultrasound Obstet Gynecol 2018; 52: 186 - 195, K. H. Nicolaides et.al (Fetal Medicine Foundation (UK) 2018)

C. SGA/IUGR: In the view of maternal history, patient demographics and observed biochemical MoM values, there appears to be low predisposition to SGA/IUGR.

Reference: Ultrasound Obstet Gynecol 2021; 57: 52-61, K. H. Nicolaides et.al (Fetal Medicine Foundation (UK) 2021)

D. Fetal Macrosomia: In the view of maternal history, patient demographics and observed biochemical MoM values, there appears to be low predisposition to Fetal Macrosomia..

Reference: Ultrasound Obstet Gynecol 2016; 47: 332-339, K. H. Nicolaides et.al (Fetal Medicine Foundation (UK) 2016)

1. **What maternal factors in history should be reviewed to assess the risk of preeclampsia in current pregnancy?**
2. **What are the biochemical markers to screen for preeclampsia?**
3. **What biophysical parameters are used in the algorithm for assessment of risk of preeclampsia?**
4. **How to interpret the risk of preeclampsia?**

5. What prophylaxis is available for high risk for PE identified on first trimester screen? By how much does it reduce the risk?

Ans.

1. Maternal age, parity, mode of conception, history of preeclampsia in a prior pregnancy, known history of chronic hypertension, diabetes, systemic lupus erythematosus (SLE), anti-phospholipid syndrome (APS).
2. Low levels of placental growth factor (PlGF) and PAPP-A and high soluble fms-like tyrosine kinase-1 (sFlt-1) are used as PE markers. sFlt-1/PlGF ratio also used in women who presented with suspected PE in second trimester. If this ratio >38 [positive predictive value (PPV) of 36.7%]—the risk for developing PE in the next 4 weeks is high [negative predictive value (NPV) of 97%].
3. Mean arterial pressure and mean uterine artery PI.
4. Combined screening model for PE including maternal history, maternal risk factors, mean arterial pressure (MAP), mean uterine artery pulsatility index (UtA-PI) and serum markers PAPP-A and PlGF. The software program converts each of these values into MoM and integrates them to arrive at a risk estimate. If it is >1:100 then it is considered as high risk for PE. The detection rates of preterm PE and term PE were 75% and 43%, respectively, at false-positive rate of 10%, see table below.

Preeclampsia (ASPRE 2017)	*Detection rate with FPR of 10%*
Preterm PE	75%
Term PE	43%
Severe PE before <34 weeks	90%

5. A randomized study (ASPRE trial) demonstrated that in singleton pregnancies identified by first-trimester screening as being at high-risk of preterm PE (>1 in 100), administration of aspirin (150 mg/day) from 12 until 36 weeks' gestation reduced the incidence of PE before 34 weeks by >80% and PE before 37 weeks by >60%.

SUGGESTED READING

1. Cerdeira AS, O'Sullivan J, Ohuma EO, Harrington D, Szafranski P, Black R, et al. Randomized interventional study on prediction of preeclampsia/eclampsia in women with suspected preeclampsia: INSPIRE. Hypertension. 2019;74(4):983-90.
2. Cerdeira AS, O'Sullivan J, Ohuma EO, James T, Papageorghiou AT, Knight M, et al. Ruling out preeclampsia in the next 4 weeks using a soluble fms-like tyrosine kinase 1/placental growth factor ratio ≤38: secondary analysis of the interventional study on prediction of preeclampsia/eclampsia in women with suspected preeclampsia. Am J Obstet Gynecol. 2022;226(3):443-5.

3. O'Gorman N, Wright D, Poon LC, Rolnik DL, Syngelaki A, Wright A, et al. Accuracy of competing-risks model in screening for preeclampsia by maternal factors and biomarkers at 11–13 weeks' gestation. Ultrasound Obstet Gynecol. 2017;49:751-5.
4. Rolnik DL, Wright D, Poon LCY, Syngelaki A, O'Gorman N, de Paco Matallana C, et al. ASPRE trial: performance of screening for preterm preeclampsia. Ultrasound Obstet Gynecol. 2017;50:492-5.

STATION 9. 42 years old primigravida, spontaneous conception, presents at 12 weeks of gestation. Medical history is normal. BMI – 26. Non-alcoholic and non-smoker. She is concerned of her age risk of trisomy 21, hence referred for screening.

1. **Can the patient be offered non-invasive prenatal screening to rule out trisomy 21 as a first line test?**
2. **Is USG necessary prior to offering NIPS?**
3. **What is the detection rate for trisomy 21 in low risk non-invasive prenatal testing (NIPT)?**
4. **Should NIPS be offered as a reflex screening test when the CFTS is low risk?**

Ans.

1. Yes, NIPS can be offered to all pregnant women as a first line screening test.
2. Yes, because structural abnormalities or raised NT or absent nasal bone are indicative of the need for invasive testing and preclude offering NIPS.
3. Low-risk NIPT has a detection rate of 99% with FPR of 0.1% for trisomy 21, 18, and 13 when the fetal fraction of >4%.
4. No, one should not offer serum screening test twice.

SUGGESTED READING

1. ACMG Practice Guideline. Non-invasive prenatal screening (NIPS) for fetal chromosome abnormalities in a general-risk population: An evidence-based clinical guideline of the American College of Medical Genetics and Genomics (ACMG). Genet Med. 2023;25:100336.
2. LeFevre NM, Sundermeyer RL. Fetal Aneuploidy: Screening and Diagnostic Testing. Am Fam Physician. 2020;101(8):481-8.
3. NHS. Screening for Down's syndrome, Edwards' syndrome and Patau's syndrome: NIPT, 2024.

STATION 10.

1. **What are second trimester aneuploidy markers?**
2. **How do second trimester biochemical markers differ in aneuploidies?**
3. **What is the source of inhibin?**
4. **What is the relevance of increase or decrease in inhibin?**

Ans.

1. Beta-human chorionic gonadotropin (both free and total), inhibin, estriol, and alpha fetoprotein are used as second trimester biochemical markers.
2. Beta-human chorionic gonadotropin increased in T21, but decreased in T18 and unchanged in T13.
   Inhibin increases in T21 and T13, does not change in 18.
   Estriol decreases in T21 and T18, does not change in 13.
   AFP decreases in T21 and T13, does not change in 18.
3. Inhibin A is initially secreted by the dominant follicle and the subsequently formed corpus luteum in the non-gravid state and ultimately by the placenta. Inhibin B is produced by the small antral follicles.
4. In DS, maternal serum levels of inhibin A remain unaltered until the 11th week of gestation but are significantly elevated at 15–18 weeks because of increased placental synthesis. Inhibin A is raised in trisomy 13 and 21, but not in trisomy 18.

SUGGESTED READING

1. American College of Obstetricians and Gynecologists' Committee on Practice Bulletins—Obstetrics; Committee on Genetics; Society for Maternal-Fetal Medicine. Screening for fetal chromosomal abnormalities: ACOG practice bulletin, number 226. Obstet Gynecol. 2020;136(4):e48-69.

STATION 11. **A 31-year-old primigravida, conceived spontaneously, non-consanguineously couple, medical history within normal limits. Nuchal scan done at 12 weeks was normal with normal NT. Combined FTS was low risk for aneuploidies. Her obstetrician offered her a quadruple marker test to be doubly sure. Quadruple marker—high risk for T21 (1 in 95) with following serum markers. She comes to you for further management. Quadruple report as follows:**

Specimen details

				Test Name	Conc.	Unit	Corr. Mom
Sample ID	: 2470000350	CRL	: 65.77 mm				
Collection Date	: 10/04/2024	CRL2	:	Free-ß-hCG	30.79	ng/mL	1.87
Scan Date	: 23/03/2024	BPD	:	AFP	23.07	ng/mL	0.70
GA at Coll Date	: 15 Weeks 3 Days	BPD2	:	uE3	03.31	nmol/L	1.18
GA at Scan Date	: 12 Weeks 6 Days	HC	:	Inhibin A	546.40	pg/mL	2.62
Received on	: 13/04/2024	HC2	:				

GA: Gestation Age | CRL: Crown Rump Length | BPD: Bi-parietal Diameter | HC: Head Circumference | free-ß-hCG: free-Beta Human Chorionic Gonadotropin
NT: Nuchal Translucency | PAPP-A: Pregnancy-associated Plasma Protein-A

Risk

Disorder: Down Syndrome				Result:	High Risk
Final risk:	1:95	Age risk:	1:970		
Cutoff	1:250	Risk type	Risk At Term		
Disorder: Edwards' Syndrome				**Result:**	**Low Risk**
Final risk:	1:100000	Age risk:	1:7400		
Cutoff	1:100	Risk type	Risk At Term		
Neural tube / Abdominal wall defect				**Result:**	**Low Risk**
Final risk:	-	Age risk:			
Cutoff	2.5	Risk type	Risk at Term		

1. **What is contingent or integrated or stepwise sequential screening?**
2. **What is the most commonly used screening method?**
3. **Which test should be offered in second trimester?**
4. **What is the consensus regarding the use of two screening methods in the same pregnancy?**

Ans.

1. *Integrated screening:* A blood sample is taken following the 11–13 + 6 weeks scan. Screening result is not calculated. Second blood sample is taken between 15 and 22 weeks. A statistical software calculates risk using maternal age, NT, (nasal bone optional), PAPP-A, β-hCG, AFP, unconjugated estriol, and inhibin A. Women who get a high-risk (screen-positive) result are offered invasive testing.
   Down syndrome DR = 90% for an FPR of 2.6% (risk cutoff, 1:245); DR = 85% for an FPR of 1.2% (risk cutoff, 1:120). Integrated screening without USG markers is no longer recommended.
   Sequential stepwise screening: Result of FTS is informed to the pregnant woman. All *low-risk* women undergo repeat blood sampling in the second trimester and the final risk is calculated using the integrated test. Down syndrome DR = 95% for a 5% FPR.
   Contingent screening: Result of FTS is informed to the woman. The risk is reported as high, low, or intermediate. Low risk no further testing. High risk patients undergo diagnostic CVS or amniocentesis. And all *intermediate-risk* women undergo repeat blood sampling and DS screening either through an integrated test (final risk is calculated by integrating first-trimester and second-trimester serum markers with maternal age and NT) or NIPT. The final risk is used to decide further management.
   Second trimester ultrasound markers were earlier used for contingent screening, but this is no longer recommended. Down syndrome DR = 88%–94% for a 5% FPR.
2. Combined FTS (MA + NT + PAPP-A + β-hCG; DR: 85-95% with FPR 5%) or enhanced FTS (combined test +NB or TR or DV; DR: 93–96% with FPR: 2.5%) or NIPT (detection rate is 99.99%, FFP of 0.01%).
3. Quadruple test (MA + serum free β-hCG + AFP + estriol + inhibin A; DR 70–75%, FPR 5%).
4. Independent serum screening should never be repeated in the second trimester when it has already been done in the first trimester. If screening is to be done in both trimesters, an integrated or contingent screening model should be followed.

SUGGESTED READING

1. American College of Obstetricians and Gynecologists' Committee on Practice Bulletins—Obstetrics; Committee on Genetics; Society for Maternal-Fetal Medicine. Screening for fetal chromosomal abnormalities: ACOG practice bulletin, number 226. Obstet Gynecol. 2020;136(4):e48-69.

2. Benn PA, Campbell WA, Zelop CM, Ingardia C, Egan JF. Stepwise sequential screening for fetal aneuploidy. Am J Obstet Gynecol. 2007;197(3):312.e1-5.
3. Wald NJ, Watt HC, Hackshaw AK. Integrated screening for Down's syndrome based on tests performed during the first and second trimesters. N Engl J Med. 1999;341(7):461-7.
4. Wright D, Bradbury I, Benn P, Cuckle H, Ritchie K. Contingent screening for Down syndrome is an efficient alternative to non-disclosure sequential screening. Prenat Diagn. 2004;24(10):762-6.

STATION 12. **A 26-year-old primigravida spontaneous conception at 15 weeks presents following FTS report. Her medical history was normal—BMI - 26, non-alcoholic, and non-smoker.**

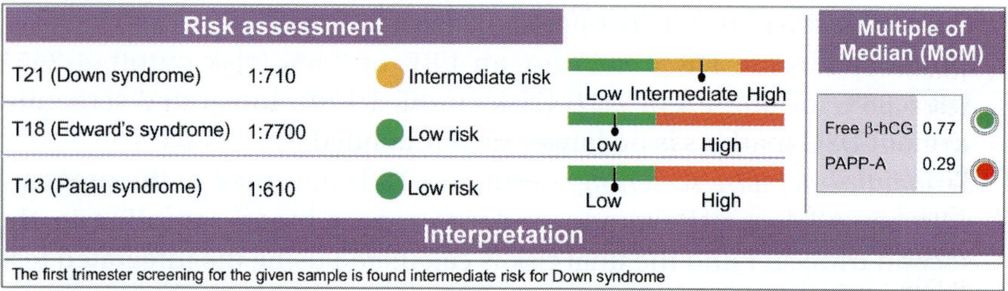

Risk assessment			
T21 (Down syndrome)	1:710	Intermediate risk	Low Intermediate High
T18 (Edward's syndrome)	1:7700	Low risk	Low High
T13 (Patau syndrome)	1:610	Low risk	Low High

Multiple of Median (MoM)	
Free β-hCG	0.77
PAPP-A	0.29

Interpretation

The first trimester screening for the given sample is found intermediate risk for Down syndrome

1. **What is intermediate risk for trisomy 21?**
2. **What are the preferred options after an intermediate risk report?**

Ans.

1. Generally, the risk between 1 in 250 to 1 in 1000 is considered as intermediate risk.
2. a. Genetic sonogram using CFTS risk as the a priori risk or
   b. NIPT or
   c. If the woman herself requests a confirmatory invasive test, her request must not be denied.

SUGGESTED READING

1. NHS. Screening for Down's syndrome, Edwards' syndrome and Patau's syndrome: NIPT, 2024.
2. LeFevre NM, Sundermeyer RL. Fetal Aneuploidy: Screening and Diagnostic Testing. Am Fam Physician. 2020;101(8):481-8.

STATION 13. **A 38-year-old primigravida with IVF conception with dichorionic diamniotic twin pregnancy with own embryos for DS screening. Medical history was normal—BMI - 26, non-alcoholic, and non-smoker.**

1. **Which screening test for aneuploidy can be offered to twin gestation in the first trimester**
2. **What is fetus specific risk and pregnancy specific risk?**

3. **Can a quadruple test be advised to a twin pregnancy?**
4. **What is the performance of NIPT in twin pregnancy?**

Ans.

1. Combined FTS (DR 75–80% while maintaining a 5% FPR) or NIPT
2. *Fetus-specific risk:* The risk of one particular fetus having DS done in DC twins. *Pregnancy-specific risk*—the risk of the pregnancy resulting in the birth of at least one child with DS in MC twins.
3. Ideally, should not be offered as the test has reduced sensitivity and specificity with high FPR (DR 50% with 8% FPR) in both DC or MC.
4. NIPT can be done with same sensitivity as in singletons.

SUGGESTED READING

1. Judah H, Gil MM, Syngelaki A, Galeva S, Jani J, Akolekar R, et al. Cell-free DNA testing of maternal blood in screening for trisomies in twin pregnancy: updated cohort study at 10-14 weeks and meta-analysis. Ultrasound Obstet Gynecol. 2021;58(2):178-89.
2. Khalil A, Archer R, Hutchinson V, Mousa HA, Johnstone ED, Cameron MJ, et al. Noninvasive prenatal screening in twin pregnancies with cell-free DNA using the IONA test: a prospective multicenter study. Am J Obstet Gynecol. 2021;225(1): 79.e1-79.e13.
3. NHS. Fetal Anomaly Screening Programme. Down's syndrome, Edwards' syndrome and Patau's syndrome screening Handbook for Laboratories, 2024.
4. Spencer K, Liao AW, Skentou H, Cicero S, Nicolaides KH. Screening for triploidy by fetal nuchal translucency and maternal serum free beta-hCG and PAPP-A at 10-14 weeks of gestation. Prenat Diagn. 2000;20(6):495-9.

STATION 14. **A 26-year-old primigravida, spontaneously conceived dichorionic diamniotic (DCDA) twins with a history of vanishing twin at 9 weeks, currently a singleton pregnancy. She had come at 12 weeks with first trimester screening report of combined FTS showing an intermediate risk for trisomy 21 risk – 1:432 with β-hCG 8.3 MoM, PAPP-A 0.71 MoM. USG showed a DCDA twins with dead fetus in situ. Other fetus was appropriate for gestational age (AGA). Medical history was normal—BMI - 27, non-alcoholic, and non-smoker.**

1. **What is the DS screening strategy with dead fetus in situ either vanishing or post reduction?**
2. **Can we offer serum screening test for DS in vanishing twin? Why?**
3. **Can we offer NIPS in vanishing twin?**
4. **What is the screening method used in higher order pregnancy (three or more)?**

Ans.

1. In vanishing twin with an empty gestational sac, the combined test can be used for screening because serum free β-hCG and PAPP-A are no

different from those in singleton pregnancy. Second sac has a detectable dead embryo—first-trimester screening should rely on maternal age and fetal NT alone.

2. No, serum screening either CFTS or NIPT should not be offered. In a vanishing twin, the placenta continues to function for a considerable time after fetal demise and produces serum markers. Since the markers secreted by the vanishing twin's placenta cannot be separately measured, serum screening becomes inaccurate.
3. Yes, at a later gestation when at least 14 weeks have elapsed since single fetal demise.
4. Only scan-based screening for higher order pregnancies using maternal age and NT.

SUGGESTED READING

1. Chaveeva P, Wright A, Syngelaki A, Konstantinidou L, Wright D, Nicolaides KH. First-trimester screening for trisomies in pregnancies with vanishing twin. Ultrasound Obstet Gynecol. 2020;55(3):326-31.
2. Huang T, Boucher K, Aul R, Rashid S, Meschino WS. First and second trimester maternal serum markers in pregnancies with a vanishing twin. Prenat Diagn. 2015;35(1):90-6.

STATION 15. A 37-year-old primigravida IVF conception with single embryo transfer. PGT-A is normal. Medical history was normal—BMI-28, non-alcoholic, and non-smoker. She presents at 12 weeks gestation for aneuploidy screening.

1. **Can one offer dual test after PGT-A testing?**
2. **Can NIPT be offered after PGT- A?**
3. **What would be the test of choice for aneuploidy after an IVF/PGT-A conception?**

Ans.

1. No since test results are inaccurate. PGT-A is a screening test with high sensitivity and high specificity, hence dual test should not be offered.
2. No. PGT-A and NIPT results reflect the chromosomal complement of the trophectoderm or placental cytotrophoblast respectively and not the inner cell mass which represents fetal chromosomes. Hence both are not diagnostic testing.
3. Invasive diagnostic testing preferably amniocentesis.

SUGGESTED READING

1. Dungan JS, Klugman S, Darilek S, Malinowski J, Akkari YMN, Monaghan KG, et al. Non-invasive prenatal screening (NIPS) for fetal chromosome abnormalities in a general-risk population: An evidence-based clinical guideline of the

American College of Medical Genetics and Genomics (ACMG). Genet Med. 2023;25:100336.
2. Grace MR, Hardisty E, Dotters-Katz SK, Vora NL, Kuller JA. Cell-free DNA screening: complexities and challenges of clinical implementation. Obstet Gynecol Surv. 2016;71(8):477-87.
3. LeFevre NM, Sundermeyer RL. Fetal Aneuploidy: Screening and Diagnostic Testing. Am Fam Physician. 2020;101(8):481-8.
4. NHS. Screening for Down's syndrome, Edwards' syndrome and Patau's syndrome: NIPT, 2024.

STATION 16.

1. **What is a priori risk for Down syndrome?**
2. **What is OAPR?**
3. **Please give the OAPR for Down syndrome in first and second trimester respectively?**
4. **What is likelihood ratio?**

Ans.

1. A priori risk is the baseline risk of having a baby with Down syndrome. It is initially based on the age of the mother (or the donor in case of a donor ovum IVF).
2. Odds of being affected with DS, given a positive risk (OAPR), higher the OAPR better is the test. It is used in patient counselling for invasive testing.
3. OAPR is 1:22 for combined FTS, 1:30 for quadruple test.
4. Likelihood ratio is a ratio that compares the probability of a test result in a patient with a disease to the probability of the same result in a patient without disease.

SUGGESTED READING

1. Agathokleous M, Chaveeva P, Poon LCY, Kosinski P, Nicolaides KH. Meta-analysis of second-trimester markers for trisomy 21. Ultrasound Obstet Gynecol. 2013;41:247-61.
2. Seyyed Kavoosi E, Younessi S, Farhud DD. Screening of Fetal Chromosome Aneuploidies in the First and Second Trimester of 125,170 Iranian Pregnant Women. Iran J Public Health. 2015;44(6):791-6.

STATION 17. **A 30-year-old primigravida has conceived on ovulation induction. Her 11–13 + 6 weeks scan shows dichorionic (DADC) twins with CRL of 46 mm and NT values 1 mm (17th centile), and CRL 45 mm and 2.4 mm (96th centile), respectively. Rest of the findings on ultrasound are within normal limits. She has undergone a combined FTS which is reported as follows, serum PAPP-A: 0.67 MoM, serum free β-hCG: 1.13 MoM. Fetus A DS screen negative which had normal NT (1.0 mm) – 1 in**

5,000, fetus B with increased NT (2.4 mm) – screen positive (1:90). She was anxious about the further course in her pregnancy and was referred to you.

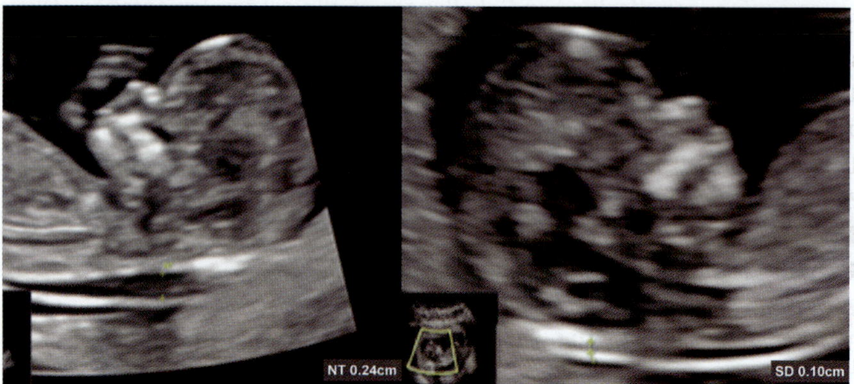

1. **Can we offer NIPT in this case?**
2. **Can we test only affected fetus?**
3. **What is the test of choice?**
4. **What is the option if one twin turned out to be trisomy 21?**

Ans.

1. Non-invasive prenatal testing is not recommended in DC twins with discordant findings, as the karyotypes can be discordant. The cell-free DNA (cfDNA) from the normal placenta can mask the cfDNA from the aneuploid placenta, as aneuploidy is associated with a reduced fetal fraction.
2. Dichorionic twins can be monozygotic if the embryo splits early. Hence, testing of both fetuses is recommended, even though only one fetus appears to be at high risk for aneuploidy.
3. Diagnostic CVS or amniocentesis.
4. Can continue the pregnancy if the couple wishes or can offer selective fetal reduction.

SUGGESTED READING

1. Committee on Practice Bulletins—Obstetrics, Committee on Genetics, Society for Maternal-Fetal Medicine. Practice bulletin no. 163: screening for fetal aneuploidy. Obstet Gynecol 2016;127:e123-37.
2. NHS. Fetal Anomaly Screening Programme. Down's syndrome, Edwards' syndrome and Patau's syndrome screening Handbook for Laboratories, 2024.
3. Zwingerman R, Langlois S. SOGC Committee Opinion No. 406: Prenatal testing after IVF with preimplantation genetic testing for aneuploidy. J Obstet Gynaecol Can. 2020;42(11):1437-43.e1.

STATION 18. **A 42-year-old primigravida, IVF conception with donor ovum. Medical history was normal—BMI - 38.5, non-alcoholic, and non-smoker. She was on regular daily hCG 5000 IU injections as a part of IVF treatment. Her NT scan at 12 weeks was normal. Her dual test β-hCG showed high MoM 9.9, low PAPP-A 0.01 MoM with high risk for T21 and T18. She declined invasive testing and opted for NIPT which was screen-positive for trisomy 21 and 13 with fetal fraction of 3.1%.**

1. **Does β-hCG injections impact the FTS?**
2. **Can we terminate the pregnancy based on NIPT report?**
3. **What are the odds of the fetus being trisomy 18 or 13 in this case?**
4. **What is the next step in this case?**

Ans.

1. Yes. Ideally FTS should not be offered within 2 weeks of administration of injection hCG.
2. No. NIPT is a screening test, not a diagnostic test. The fetal fraction is low (<4%). Low fetal fraction reduces performance of NIPT.
3. When the fetus is structurally normal, it is very unlikely if trisomy 18 or 13 are present. This can be a false-positive result.
4. Amniocentesis. CVS is not preferred in this case as there is a high likelihood of confined placental mosaicism.

SUGGESTED READING

1. Committee on Practice Bulletins—Obstetrics, Committee on Genetics, Society for Maternal-Fetal Medicine. Practice bulletin no. 163: screening for fetal aneuploidy. Obstet Gynecol 2016;127:e123-37.
2. NHS. Fetal Anomaly Screening Programme. Down's syndrome, Edwards' syndrome and Patau's syndrome screening Handbook for Laboratories, 2024.
3. Zwingerman R, Langlois S. SOGC Committee Opinion No. 406: Prenatal testing after IVF with preimplantation genetic testing for aneuploidy. J Obstet Gynaecol Can. 2020;42(11):1437-43.e1.

CHAPTER 2

Pre-eclampsia Screening

Shruti Jain

STATION 1. A 32-year-old primigravida, period of gestation (POG) 11 weeks with history of preeclampsia (PE) in sister's pregnancy, wants to understand about PE screening.

1. **At what gestation should screening for PE be performed?**
2. **What is the traditional approach for screening for PE based on National Institute for Health and Clinical Excellence (NICE) and the American College of Obstetricians and Gynecologists (ACOG) recommendations?**
3. **What is the prediction rate with NICE and ACOG recommendations for screening of PE?**
4. **What is a combined screening for PE and prediction rate?**

Ans.

1. 11–13 weeks
2. Traditional approach is based on identification of women at risk of PE depending on maternal factors. The NICE in the UK recommends the identification of the high-risk group on the basis of 10 factors from maternal characteristics and medical history. The ACOG recommends the use of aspirin in women with a history of PE in ≥2 pregnancies or history of PE with delivery <34 weeks.
3. The NICE guidelines for screening of PE identifies only about 40% of cases of preterm PE and 35% of term PE. The ACOG method identifies 5% of cases of preterm PE and 2% of term PE.
4. Combined screening for PE incorporates with maternal characters, meaning arterial pressure (MAP), uterine artery pulsatility index (PI) and PlGF (placental growth factor). The test has detection rates of 90% and 75% for the prediction of early and preterm PE, respectively, with a 10% false-positive rate.

SUGGESTED READING

1. Sotiriadis A, Hernandez-Andrade E, da Silva Costa F, Ghi T, Glanc P, Khalil A, et al. ISUOG Practice Guidelines: role of ultrasound in screening for and follow-up of pre-eclampsia. Ultrasound Obstet Gynecol. 2018;53:7-22.

2. Tan MY, Wright D, Syngelaki A, Akolekar R, Cicero S, Janga D, et al. Comparison of diagnostic accuracy of early screening for pre-eclampsia by NICE guidelines and a method combining maternal factors and biomarkers: results of SPREE. Ultrasound Obstet Gynecol. 2018;51(6):743-50.

STATION 2. **G2, previous one normal delivery has presented at 12 weeks and 4 days for first trimester combined screening for PE.**

1. **List four maternal characteristics and history-based factors that are associated with increased risk for PE.**
2. **Which three are the parameters which have a high risk of association?**
3. **Name the Indian risk scoring system that is available to assess the risk of PE based on maternal risk factors.**
4. **What is the sensitivity and specificity of PE based on the score in question 3 above?**

Ans.

1. Advancing maternal age, increasing weight, Afro-Caribbean and South Asian racial origin, medical history of chronic hypertension, diabetes mellitus and systemic lupus erythematosus or antiphospholipid syndrome, conception by in vitro fertilization and family history or personal history of PE.
2. Previous history of PE, chronic hypertension and antiphospholipid antibody syndrome have a very high association with development of PE.
3. Gestosis score
4. Sensitivity 85%; specificity 97%

SUGGESTED READING

1. Malone SL, Haj Yahya R, Kane SC. Reviewing Accuracy of First Trimester Screening for Preeclampsia Using Maternal Factors and Biomarkers. Int J Womens Health. 2022;14:1371-84.

STATION 3.

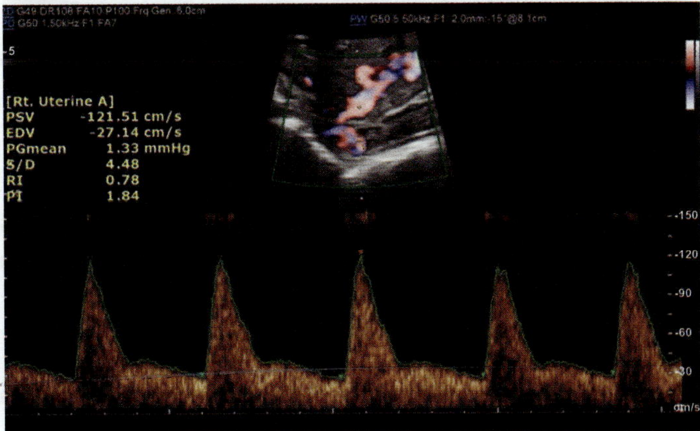

1. **Identify the Doppler waveform.**
2. **Which route is the preferred route for measuring uterine artery PI? Transabdominal or transvaginal or either of them can be used?**
3. **What are the criteria that should be fulfilled for interrogating the uterine artery?**
4. **When is the uterine artery Doppler considered abnormal?**

Ans.

1. This is uterine artery waveform.
2. Either transabdominal or transvaginal route can be used for measurement of uterine artery PI. For combined screening it is better to use transabdominal route because algorithm was defined using transabdominal route.
3. Sampling gate should be narrow (approximately 2 mm), angle of insonation <30°, peak systolic velocity should be >60 cm/s.
4. When it is >95th centile for the gestational age.

SUGGESTED READING

1. Sotiriadis A, Hernandez-Andrade E, da Silva Costa F, Ghi T, Glanc P, Khalil A, et al. ISUOG Practice Guidelines: Role of ultrasound in screening for and follow-up of pre-eclampsia. Ultrasound Obstet Gynecol. 2018;53:7-22.

STATION 4.

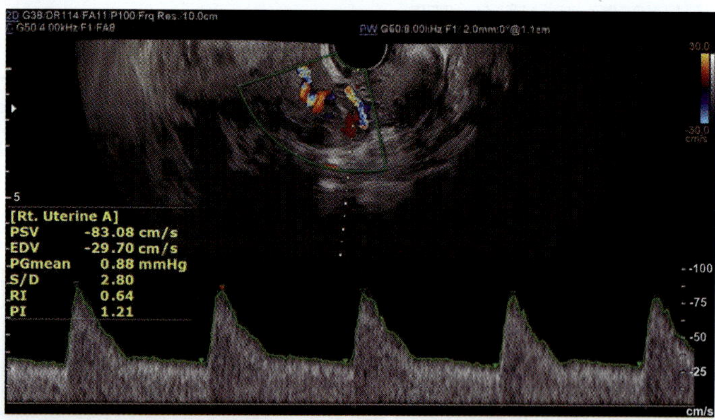

1. **Identify the waveform and the route.**
2. **What is the cut-off of mean uterine artery PI in the first trimester?**
3. **Is there any difference in value of uterine artery PI depending upon the route of measurement?**

Ans.

1. This is a uterine artery waveform measured by a transvaginal route.
2. 2.35
3. Uterine artery measurement by transvaginal route has higher PI.

SUGGESTED READING

1. Sotiriadis A, Hernandez-Andrade E, da Silva Costa F, Ghi T, Glanc P, Khalil A, et al. ISUOG Practice Guidelines: role of ultrasound in screening for and follow-up of pre-eclampsia. Ultrasound Obstet Gynecol. 2018;53:7-22.

STATION 5.

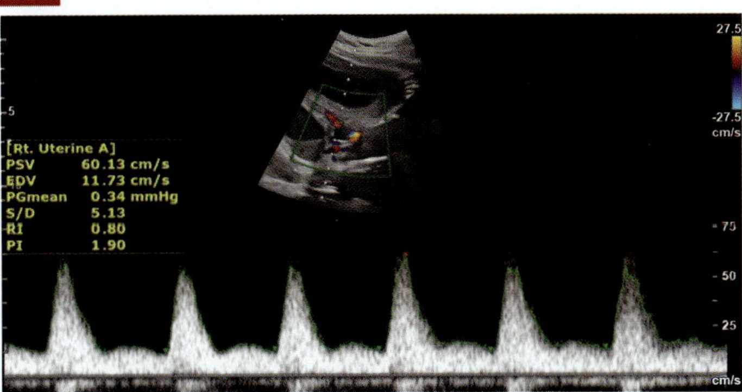

1. **Which Doppler velocimetry parameter should be used for assessing uterine artery? Is it PI or resistance index (RI) or systolic/diastolic (SD) ratio? Give reasons for your answer.**
2. **Can uterine artery notching be used to identify high risk pregnancy in case of normal mean uterine artery PI?**
3. **If one side uterine artery PI is high but mean is normal, should the uterine artery Doppler be considered raised?**

Ans.

1. Uterine artery PI should be used. Its advantage is that it includes in its calculation the averaged value of all maximum velocities during the cardiac cycle. That is why it does not approach infinity when there are absent or reversed diastolic values.
2. No.
3. Only mean uterine artery PI should be considered.

SUGGESTED READING

1. Sotiriadis A, Hernandez-Andrade E, da Silva Costa F, Ghi T, Glanc P, Khalil A, et al. ISUOG Practice Guidelines: role of ultrasound in screening for and follow-up of pre-eclampsia. Ultrasound Obstet Gynecol. 2018;53:7-22.

STATION 6.

1. **Which factors affect uterine artery PI measurement?**
2. **How can the efficiency of screening be increased in the presence of these factors?**
3. **Which free of charge software can be used to facilitate combined screening for PE in outpatient department (OPD) setting?**
4. **What is the sensitivity and specificity of raised uterine artery PI when used alone?**

Ans.

1. The uterine artery PI may be affected by maternal factors, including ethnic origin, body mass index (BMI) and previous PE.
2. It is always preferred to use combined screening with maternal factors, MAP, and serum analytes than value of uterine Doppler velocimetry alone.
3. Fetal Medicine Foundation (FMF) software for calculating risk for PE can be used which is freely available to use.
4. When used in isolation, the Ut-A PI in the first trimester has a sensitivity of 48% and specificity of 92% for the prediction of early-onset PE.

SUGGESTED READING

1. Sotiriadis A, Hernandez-Andrade E, da Silva Costa F, Ghi T, Glanc P, Khalil A, et al. ISUOG Practice Guidelines: role of ultrasound in screening for and follow-up of pre-eclampsia. Ultrasound Obstet Gynecol. 2018;53:7-22.

STATION 7.

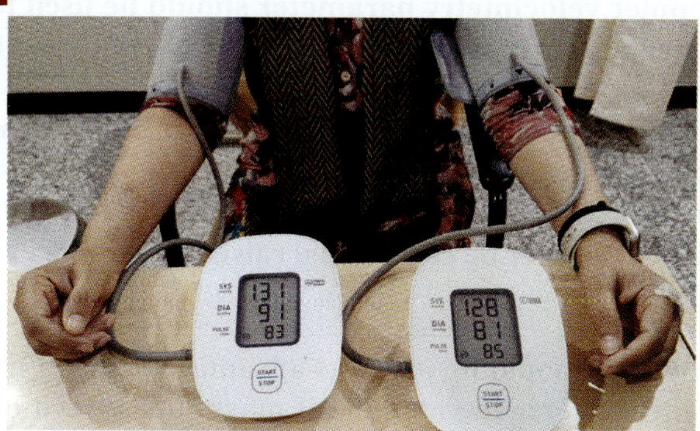

1. **How is MAP calculated?**
2. **Write three criteria for proper assessment of MAP.**
3. **Which is better predictor of PE—systolic blood pressure or diastolic blood pressure or MAP?**

Ans.

1. MAP = DP + 1/3(SP – DP) or MAP = DP + 1/3 (PP)
2. The recordings should be made by healthcare professionals who had received appropriate training on the use of these machines.
   - The women should be in a sitting position and their legs should not be crossed. Crossing the legs may raise the MAP.
   - The arms of the patient should be supported at the level of her heart. If the upper arm is below the level of the right atrium the MAP is overestimated and if the arm is above the level of the heart the MAP is underestimated. If the arm is held up by the patient without support the MAP is overestimated.

- A normal (22–32 cm) or large (33–42 cm) adult cuff should be used depending on the mid-arm circumference of the patient. If the cuff is too large the MAP is underestimated and if the cuff is too small the MAP is overestimated.
- After rest for 5 minutes, two measurements of MAP should be taken from each arm simultaneously and the average of the four should be considered in the assessment of risk.

3. Mean arterial pressure is a better predictor for PE than either systolic or diastolic blood pressure taken in the first and second trimesters.

SUGGESTED READING

1. Malone SL, Haj Yahya R, Kane SC. Reviewing Accuracy of First Trimester Screening for Preeclampsia Using Maternal Factors and Biomarkers. Int J Womens Health. 2022;14:1371-84.

STATION 8. A primigravida at 12 weeks is identified as high risk of PE based on combined screening. Her risk for PE is one in 37 for PE before 34 weeks.

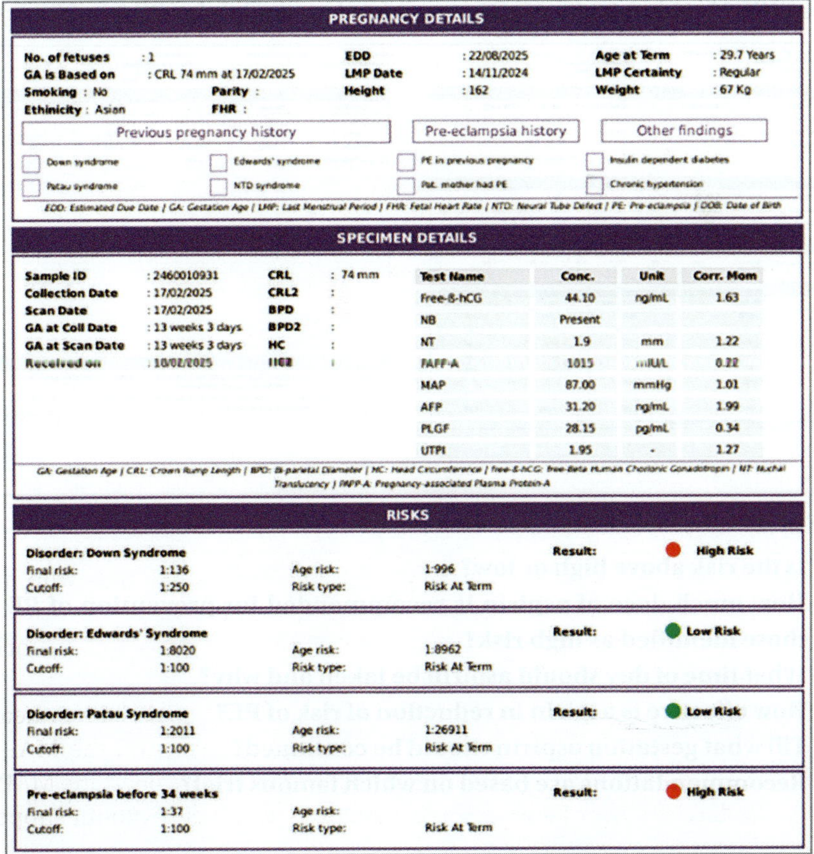

PREGNANCY DETAILS

No. of fetuses : 1 **EDD** : 22/08/2025 **Age at Term** : 29.7 Years
GA is Based on : CRL 74 mm at 17/02/2025 **LMP Date** : 14/11/2024 **LMP Certainty** : Regular
Smoking : No **Parity** : **Height** : 162 **Weight** : 67 Kg
Ethinicity : Asian **FHR** :

Previous pregnancy history		Pre-eclampsia history	Other findings
☐ Down syndrome	☐ Edwards' syndrome	☐ PE in previous pregnancy	☐ Insulin dependent diabetes
☐ Patau syndrome	☐ NTD syndrome	☐ Pat. mother had PE	☐ Chronic hypertension

EDD: Estimated Due Date | GA: Gestation Age | LMP: Last Menstrual Period | FHR: Fetal Heart Rate | NTD: Neural Tube Defect | PE: Pre-eclampsia | DOB: Date of Birth

SPECIMEN DETAILS

Sample ID : 2460010931 **CRL** : 74 mm
Collection Date : 17/02/2025 **CRL2** :
Scan Date : 17/02/2025 **BPD** :
GA at Coll Date : 13 weeks 3 days **BPD2** :
GA at Scan Date : 13 weeks 3 days **HC** :
Received on : 10/02/2025 **HC2** :

Test Name	Conc.	Unit	Corr. Mom
Free-ß-hCG	44.10	ng/mL	1.63
NB	Present		
NT	1.9	mm	1.22
PAPP-A	1015	mIU/L	0.22
MAP	87.00	mmHg	1.01
AFP	31.20	ng/mL	1.99
PLGF	28.15	pg/mL	0.34
UTPI	1.95	-	1.27

GA: Gestation Age | CRL: Crown Rump Length | BPD: Bi-parietal Diameter | HC: Head Circumference | free-ß-hCG: free-Beta Human Chorionic Gonadotropin | NT: Nuchal Translucency | PAPP-A: Pregnancy-associated Plasma Protein-A

RISKS

Disorder: Down Syndrome **Result:** High Risk
Final risk: 1:136 Age risk: 1:996
Cutoff: 1:250 Risk type: Risk At Term

Disorder: Edwards' Syndrome **Result:** Low Risk
Final risk: 1:8020 Age risk: 1:8962
Cutoff: 1:100 Risk type: Risk At Term

Disorder: Patau Syndrome **Result:** Low Risk
Final risk: 1:2011 Age risk: 1:26911
Cutoff: 1:100 Risk type: Risk At Term

Pre-eclampsia before 34 weeks **Result:** High Risk
Final risk: 1:37 Age risk:
Cutoff: 1:100 Risk type: Risk At Term

1. **Which biochemical marker is used in combined screening for PE?**
2. **How much is the improvement in detection rate for PE with addition of the marker in Question 1?**
3. **What is the cut off to consider a woman high risk for developing PE on combined screening in first trimester?**

Ans.

1. Placental growth factor
2. 7%
3. 1:100

SUGGESTED READING

1. Wright D, Tan MY, O'Gorman N, Syngelaki A, Nicolaides KH. Serum PlGF compared with PAPP-A in first trimester screening for preterm pre-eclampsia: Adjusting for the effect of aspirin treatment. BJOG. 2022;129(8):1308-17.

STATION 9. Primigravida at 12 weeks and 5 days, there is no maternal high-risk factor. Uterine artery PI is 1.2 multiples of the median (MoM). Her PlGF MoM is 0.22 MoM. Her combined screening for PE 1 in 36.

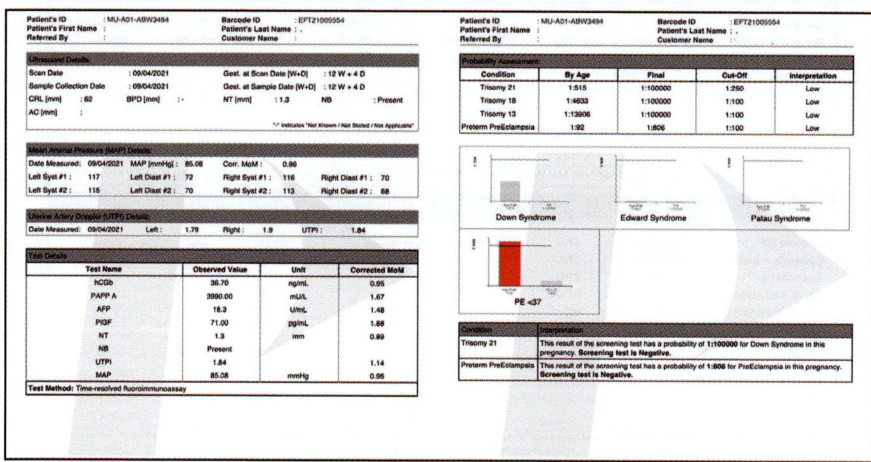

Patient's ID : MU-A01-ABW3494 Barcode ID : EFT21005554
Patient's First Name : Patient's Last Name : ,
Referred By : Customer Name :

Ultrasound Details:

Scan Date : 09/04/2021 Gest. at Scan Date [W+D] : 12 W + 4 D
Sample Collection Date : 09/04/2021 Gest. at Sample Date [W+D] : 12 W + 4 D
CRL [mm] : 62 BPD [mm] : - NT [mm] : 1.3 NB : Present
AC [mm] :

"-" indicates "Not Known / Not Stated / Not Applicable"

Mean Arterial Pressure (MAP) Details:

Date Measured: 09/04/2021 MAP [mmHg] : 85.08 Corr. MoM : 0.96
Left Syst #1 : 117 Left Diast #1 : 72 Right Syst #1 : 116 Right Diast #1 : 70
Left Syst #2 : 115 Left Diast #2 : 70 Right Syst #2 : 113 Right Diast #2 : 68

Uterine Artery Doppler (UTPI) Details:

Date Measured: 09/04/2021 Left : 1.79 Right : 1.9 UTPI : 1.84

Test Details

Test Name	Observed Value	Unit	Corrected MoM
hCGb	36.70	ng/mL	0.95
PAPP A	3990.00	mU/L	1.67
AFP	18.3	U/mL	1.48
PlGF	71.00	pg/mL	1.88
NT	1.3	mm	0.89
NB	Present		
UTPI	1.84		1.14
MAP	85.08	mmHg	0.96

Test Method: Time-resolved fluoroimmunoassay

Patient's ID : MU-A01-ABW3494 Barcode ID : EFT21005554
Patient's First Name : Patient's Last Name : ,
Referred By : Customer Name :

Probability Assessment:

Condition	By Age	Final	Cut-Off	Interpretation
Trisomy 21	1:515	1:100000	1:250	Low
Trisomy 18	1:4633	1:100000	1:100	Low
Trisomy 13	1:13906	1:100000	1:100	Low
Preterm PreEclampsia	1:92	1:806	1:100	Low

Condition	Interpretation
Trisomy 21	This result of the screening test has a probability of **1:100000** for Down Syndrome in this pregnancy. **Screening test is Negative.**
Preterm PreEclampsia	This result of the screening test has a probability of **1:806** for PreEclampsia in this pregnancy. **Screening test is Negative.**

Image courtesy: Dr Seetha Ramamurthy Pal.

1. **Is the risk above high or low?**
2. **How much dose of aspirin is recommended for prevention of PE in those identified as high risk?**
3. **What time of day should aspirin be taken and why?**
4. **How effective is aspirin in reduction of risk of PE?**
5. **Till what gestation aspirin should be continued?**
6. **Recommendations are based on which famous trial?**

Ans.

1. High risk for developing preterm PE (prior to 37 weeks)
2. Tablet aspirin 150 mg bedtime
3. Aspirin should be taken at bedtime in view of diurnal effect on its response.
4. Aspirin reduces the risk of PE by 62% before 37 weeks, and 84% by 34 weeks
5. 36 weeks
6. Aspirin for Evidence-Based Preeclampsia Prevention (ASPRE) trial.

SUGGESTED READING

1. Rolnik DL, Wright D, Poon LC, O'Gorman N, Syngelaki A, de Paco Matallana C, et al. Aspirin versus placebo in pregnancies at high risk for preterm preeclampsia. N Engl J Med. 2017;377:613-22.

STATION 10. Primigravida, 32 years old with chronic hypertension. She is on Labetalol 100 mg TDS. She has been identified as high risk as per triple test for PE screening. She has been started on aspirin 150 mg daily at bedtime.

1. **What is the association of chronic hypertension with development of PE?**
2. **How effective is the aspirin prophylaxis in preventing superimposed PE?**
3. **How should these patients be counselled?**

Ans.

1. 20% cases of chronic hypertension in pregnancy develop superimposed PE.
2. Aspirin is not much effective in preventing superimposed PE as per various studies but it has an effect on reducing fetal growth restriction and hence preterm birth. So, it should be advised to patients with chronic hypertension.
3. Patients should be counselled about increased risk for PE and need to continue aspirin prophylaxis and antihypertensive medications and need for strict compliance and maternal and fetal surveillance.

SUGGESTED READING

1. Kametas NA, Nzelu D, Nicolaides KH. Chronic hypertension and superimposed preeclampsia: screening and diagnosis. Am J Obstet Gynecol. 2022;226(2S): S1182-95.

STATION 11. G2P1L1 previous uneventful normal delivery of female baby weighing 3 kg. In this pregnancy her uterine artery PI is >95th centile. Her combined risk for PE as her risk was 1 in 40 at 13 weeks. She was started on aspirin 150 mg OD at bedtime.

1. **Which is the most important factor in determining the effectiveness?**
2. **How should these patients be followed up?**
3. **If her uterine artery PI is found to be normal at follow-up scan at 20 weeks, should aspirin be stopped?**

Ans.

1. Compliance to aspirin should be ensured. With compliance ≥90% the reduction in risk is nearly 75%.
2. Serial growth scans starting 28 weeks onwards to identify fetal growth restriction. At every visit blood pressure and proteinuria should be determined.
3. Aspirin prophylaxis should be continued till 36 weeks.

SUGGESTED READING

1. Stepan H, Galindo A, Hund M, Schlembach D, Sillman J, Surbek D. Clinical utility of sFlt-1 and PlGF in screening, prediction, diagnosis and monitoring of pre-eclampsia and fetal growth restriction. Ultrasound Obstet Gynecol. 2023;61: 168-80.

STATION 12. **A primigravida had missed her first trimester risk assessment for PE. She has presented at 20 weeks for an anomaly scan. Her uterine artery PI is >95th centile.**

1. **How is uterine artery PI measured in second and third trimester?**
2. **Can aspirin prophylaxis be offered after second trimester high risk for PE or if raised uterine artery Doppler PI is detected?**

Ans.

1. Uterine artery is measured at the crossover with external iliac artery.
2. Aspirin intervention seems ineffective when it started after 20 weeks. Although it is too late to prevent the development of PE after second-trimester prediction, the knowledge can still be useful in guiding follow-up and management of a pregnancy at risk.

STATION 13. **A 35-year-old second gravida, there is history of PE in her last pregnancy at 32 weeks. In this pregnancy, she was identified as high risk for PE with her combined first trimester screening. She was started on aspirin prophylaxis 150 mg OD. Currently, she is at 30 weeks with occasional blood pressure readings of 140/90.**

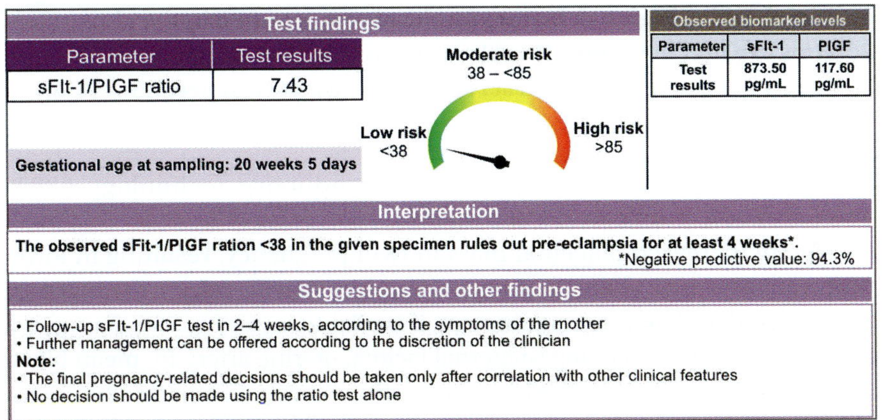

Test findings

Parameter	Test results
sFlt-1/PIGF ratio	7.43

Gestational age at sampling: 20 weeks 5 days

Observed biomarker levels

Parameter	sFlt-1	PIGF
Test results	873.50 pg/mL	117.60 pg/mL

Interpretation

The observed sFit-1/PIGF ration <38 in the given specimen rules out pre-eclampsia for at least 4 weeks*.
*Negative predictive value: 94.3%

Suggestions and other findings

- Follow-up sFlt-1/PIGF test in 2–4 weeks, according to the symptoms of the mother
- Further management can be offered according to the discretion of the clinician

Note:

- The final pregnancy-related decisions should be taken only after correlation with other clinical features
- No decision should be made using the ratio test alone

1. **How can we predict further her risk for development of PE in current pregnancy?**
2. **What is the cut off used for the tool in Question 1 above?**
3. **At what gestation can this be used?**
4. **Why cannot this tool be used in first trimester screening for PE?**

Ans.

1. Soluble fms-like tyrosine kinase-1 (sFlt-1)/PlGF ratio can be assessed.
2. In the PROGNOSIS study, a single sFlt-1/PlGF ratio cut-off (<38) was validated to rule out reliably PE within 1 week (negative predictive value >96%) and rule in PE (≥38) within 4 weeks (positive predictive value >25%).
3. Between 20 and 37 weeks
4. Flt-1 is not useful for screening for PE during the first trimester, as levels of sFlt-1 only begin to increase at 21–24 weeks of gestation in women who go on to develop PE.

SUGGESTED READING

1. Stepan H, Galindo A, Hund M, Schlembach D, Sillman J, Surbek D. Clinical utility of sFlt-1 and PlGF in screening, prediction, diagnosis and monitoring of pre-eclampsia and fetal growth restriction. Ultrasound Obstet Gynecol. 2023;61:168-80.

STATION 14. Primigravida, 39 years old, in vitro fertilization (IVF) conception, diamniotic dichorionic twin pregnancy, presented at 12 weeks for first trimester scan and screening for aneuploidy and PE.

1. **Identify four high risk factors for development of PE in the above case.**
2. **How are uterine artery Dopplers affected in twin pregnancy?**
3. **How effective is combined screening in case of twin pregnancy?**

Ans.

1. Advanced maternal age, assisted reproductive technology (ART) conception, primigravida, and multifetal gestation.
2. Due to increased placental mass in twin pregnancy, resulting in lower mean resistance in the uterine arteries, twin-specific reference ranges are preferred for Doppler examination, if available.
3. The combined screening (maternal factors, uterine artery PI, mean blood pressure, and PlGF) algorithm for singletons can also be used in twins and can identify >95% of women with twin pregnancy who will develop PE. However, the examiner should be aware that this is achieved at the cost of a 75% screen-positive rate.

SUGGESTED READING

1. Sotiriadis A, Hernandez-Andrade E, da Silva Costa F, Ghi T, Glanc P, Khalil A, et al. ISUOG Practice Guidelines: role of ultrasound in screening for and follow-up of pre-eclampsia. Ultrasound Obstet Gynecol. 2018;53:7-22.

STATION 15.

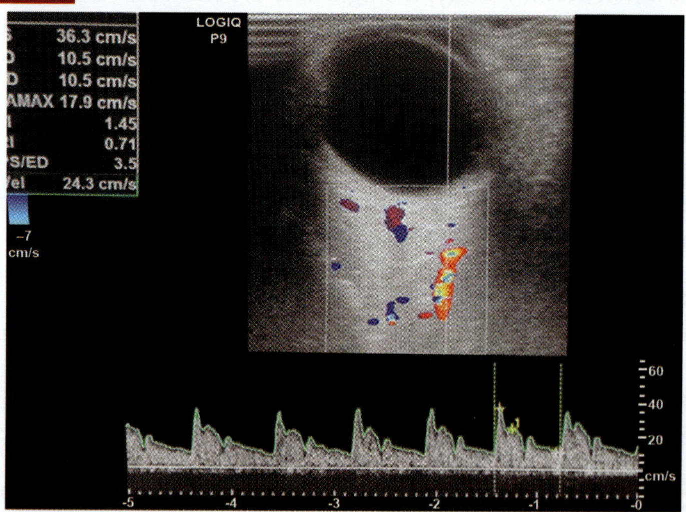

Image courtesy: Dr Jaya Chawla.

1. **Identify the vessel whose Doppler is shown in the image above.**
2. **Which is the most useful index of this Doppler for the prediction of pre-eclampsia?**
3. **What is the detection rate for preterm and term PE using this modality?**

Ans.

1. Ophthalmic artery Doppler
2. The most useful Doppler index of the ophthalmic artery is the ratio of the second to the first systolic peak velocity.
3. When screening at 32 weeks, about 60% of term PE is detected, and at 36 weeks about 70% of term PE is detected.

SUGGESTED READING

1. Nicolaides KH, Sarno M, Wright A. Ophthalmic artery Doppler in the prediction of preeclampsia. Am J Obstet Gynecol. 2022;226(2S):S1098-S1101.
2. Sarno M, Wright A, Vieira N, Sapantzoglou I, Charakida M, Nicolaides KH. Ophthalmic artery Doppler in prediction of pre-eclampsia at 35–37 weeks' gestation. Ultrasound Obstet Gynecol. 2020;56:717-24.

First Trimester Scan with Combined First Trimester Screening

Chandra Kant Garg, Megha Sharma, Saumya Srivastava

STATION 1.

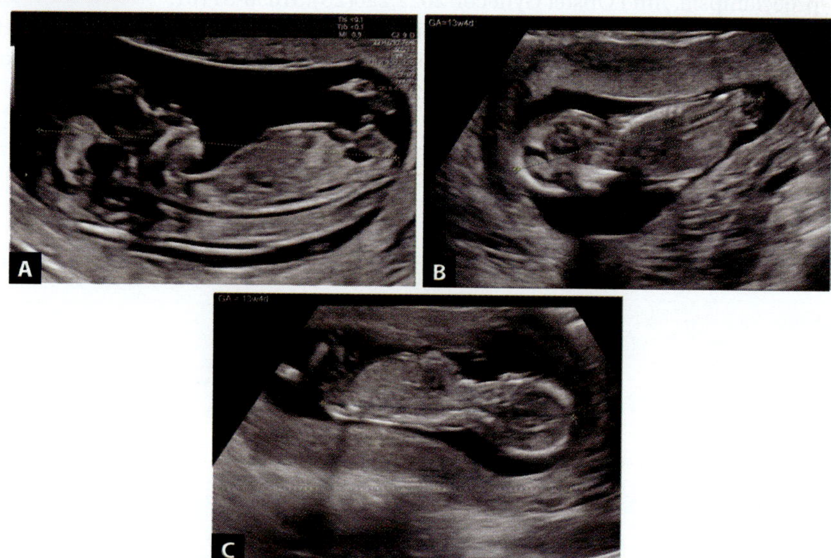

1. **What has been measured in the above images A to C and which one is the most accurate image?**
2. **How does an accurate measurement of the above parameter facilitate clinical management?**
3. **What are the criteria for a good crown-rump length (CRL) image?**
4. **What is the cutoff length for this parameter while performing the first trimester nuchal translucency (NT) scan?**

Ans.

1. Crown-rump length and image A
2. The CRL is the most accurate measurement for determining the gestational age of the baby in the first trimester. It helps us establish an estimated due date (EDD) that is more reliable than using the last menstrual period (LMP), especially if the menstrual cycles are irregular.
3. A midsagittal, magnified section of the fetus-oriented horizontally with a neutral position of head (not hyperflexed or hyperextended).

The image includes the entire length of the fetus from the top of the head (crown) to the bottom of the rump (excluding the limbs).

4. 45–84 mm.

SUGGESTED READING

1. International Society of Ultrasound in Obstetrics and Gynecology; Bilardo CM, Chaoui R, Hyett JA, Kagan KO, Karim JN, et al. ISUOG Practice Guidelines (updated): performance of 11-14-week ultrasound scan. Ultrasound Obstet Gynecol. 2023;61(1):127-43.

STATION 2.

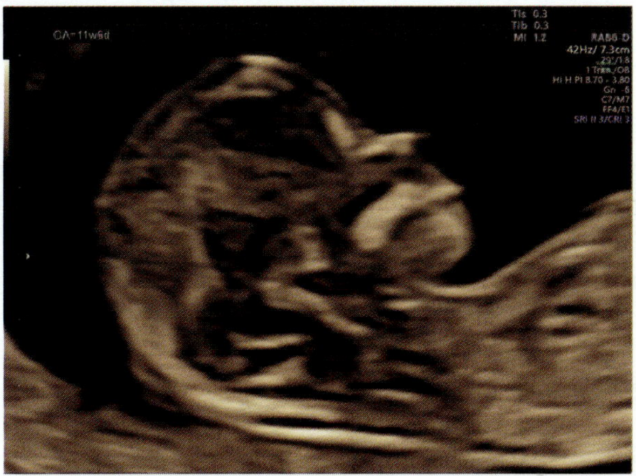

1. **Name the two most important parameters identified in this image.**
2. **What is optimal gestational age and CRL for performing this scan?**
3. **What are the criteria for an appropriate image for this scan?**
4. **How are the parameters identified in question 1 above clinically significant?**
5. **Name one parameter and one ratio that is identifiable in this scan and their clinical significance.**

Ans.

1. (1) Nuchal translucency and (2) Nasal bone (NB)
2. (1) 11+0 to 13+6 weeks of gestation and (2) CRL between 45 and 84 mm.
3. Midsagittal section with magnification so that fetal head and upper chest cover >75% of screen in neutral position of fetal head
4. To calculate the risk for common aneuploidies (i.e., trisomies 21, 13, and 18)
5. (1) Intracranial translucency (IT), (2) brainstem and brainstem-occipital bone (BS/BSOB) ratio is a measurement of the BS to BSOB distance, (3) They can be used as markers of spina bifida in fetuses.

SUGGESTED READING

1. International Society of Ultrasound in Obstetrics and Gynecology; Bilardo CM, Chaoui R, Hyett JA, Kagan KO, Karim JN, et al. ISUOG Practice Guidelines (updated): performance of 11-14-week ultrasound scan. Ultrasound Obstet Gynecol. 2023;61(1):127-43.

STATION 3.

1. **What is combined screening in first trimester?**
2. **Which hormones are measured in a dual marker test?**
3. **What is the sensitivity of dual marker test for the detection of aneuploidy when combined with maternal age?**
4. **What is the detection rate (DR) and false-positive rate (FPR) of combined screening?**

Ans.

1. It is a screening strategy which combines maternal historic factors, centiles of Nuchal transluscency along with 2 biochemical markers to calculate risk for aneuplodies
2. Beta-human chorionic gonadotropin (β-hCG) and pregnancy-associated plasma protein-A (PAPP-A)
3. 60–65%
4. DR 90–92 %; FPR 5%

SUGGESTED READING

1. Wright D, Syngelaki A, Bradbury I, Akolekar R, Nicolaides KH. First-trimester screening for trisomies 21, 18 and 13 by ultrasound and biochemical testing. Fetal Diagn Ther. 2014;35(2):118-26.

STATION 4.

Analyte	Value	Unit	
PAPP-A Free β hCG	0.7 69.9	mIU/mL ng/mL	

Ultrasound data		
Ultrasound date		**Nuchal translucency**
CRL	44 mm	**NT MoM's**
Gestational age by CRL	11 + 0	**Nasal bone**
Gestation age on the day of serum taking	11 + 3	**Measured by**

Risk

1:10

1. **What information should be provided in the test requisition form before the combined first trimester screen is done?**
2. **If first trimester combined screening is high risk, what next?**
3. **Is there any error in the report in the figure above that we can point out?**

Ans.

1. Before interpreting any combined first trimester screening report, the following parameters need to be checked:
   - Crown-rump length is between 45 mm and the maximum 84 mm.
   - *Maternal age:* The risk for trisomies increases with maternal age. The risk for Turner syndrome and triploidy does not change with maternal age.
   - *Previous affected pregnancy:* In women who had a previous pregnancy with trisomy 21, the risk of recurrence in the subsequent pregnancy is 0.75% higher than the maternal and gestational age-related risk for trisomy 21 at the time of testing.
   - In vitro fertilization (IVF)/multiple pregnancy—whether donor or self-gametes
   - Received exogenous hCG—it may interfere with the serum values of free β-hCG.
   - Maternal weight, smoking, diabetes mellitus, and ethnicity
   - Presence or absence of other markers on NT NB scan
2. Further testing to confirm fetal karyotype, i.e., chorionic villus sampling (CVS) up to 14 weeks/amniocentesis after 16 weeks with early anomaly scan
3. The CRL at which NT is measured in this report is 44 mm. The ideal CRL at which NT scan should be performed is 45–84 mm.

SUGGESTED READING

1. FMF. (2004). The 11-13+6 weeks scan. [online] Available from https://fetalmedicine.org/education/11-13-weeks-scan [Last accessed April, 2025].
2. Wright D, Syngelaki A, Bradbury I, Akolekar R, Nicolaides KH. First-trimester screening for trisomies 21, 18 and 13 by ultrasound and biochemical testing. Fetal Diagn Ther. 2014;35(2):118-26.

STATION 5.

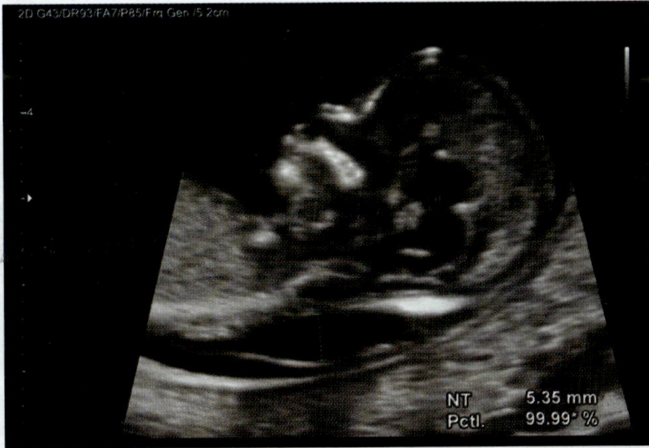

1. **What is this condition in a 12 weeks 5 days fetus?**
2. **What conditions are associated with this abnormality?**
3. **Which is the single best investigation to offer in this case?**
4. **What are the implications of 99th percentile in the presence of a normal karyotype and chromosomal microarray (CMA?)**
5. **What follow-up should be offered if the abnormality resolves in the second trimester?**

Ans.

1. Increased NT
2. Chromosomal/genetic abnormalities (i.e., Down syndrome, Turner syndrome, etc.), structural anomalies, including cardiac defects, diaphragmatic hernias, exomphalos, body stalk anomalies, and skeletal defects; certain genetic syndromes, such as congenital adrenal hyperplasia, fetal akinesia, or Noonan syndrome; hereditary hematological conditions such as Diamond–Blackfan anemia, α-thalassemia, and Fanconi's anemia
3. Chorionic villus sampling should be done for fluorescence in situ hybridization (FISH) which if normal followed by high-resolution fetal CMA study.
4. Rule out structural defects including cardiac abnormalities
5. Rule out evolving cardiac disorders and single gene disorders

SUGGESTED READING

1. Mula R, Goncé A, Bennásar M, Arigita M, Meler E, Nadal A, et al. Increased nuchal translucency and normal karyotype: perinatal and pediatric outcomes at 2 years of age. Ultrasound Obstet Gynecol. 2012;39(1):34-41.
2. Socolov D, Socolov R, Gorduza VE, Butureanu T, Stanculescu R, Carauleanu A, et al. Increased nuchal translucency in fetuses with a normal karyotype-diagnosis and management: An observational study. Medicine (Baltimore). 2017;96(29):e7521.

STATION 6. **A 27-year-old woman attends her first trimester anomaly scan at 13 weeks of gestation. The ultrasound reveals an abnormal fetal head appearance.**

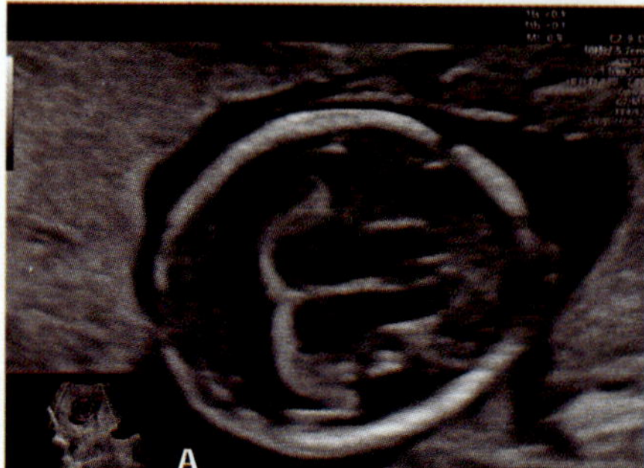

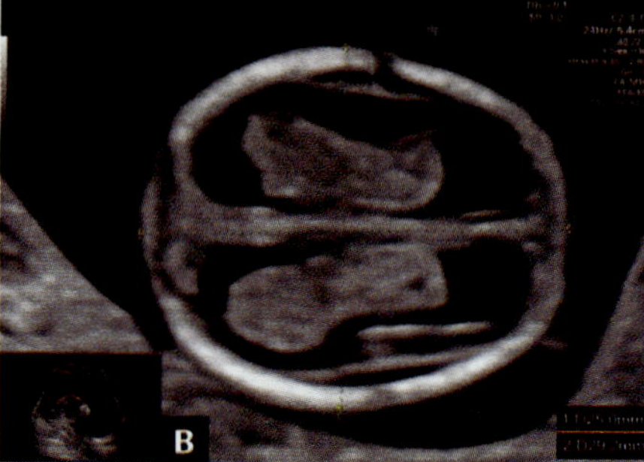

1. **Identify the first trimester anomaly.**
2. **What are the various types? Can all of these be diagnosed in the first trimester anomaly scan?**
3. **What could be other associated findings on ultrasound in such cases?**
4. **What are the most commonly associated chromosomal abnormalities?**
5. **Write the further management of this case including relevant investigations.**
6. **What is the prognosis of the case shown above?**
7. **What would be the risk of recurrence in subsequent pregnancies?**

Ans.

1. The image A and B show a common ventricle with fused thalamus suggestive of alobar holoprosencephaly.
2. The various types of holoprosencephaly are as follows:
   - *Alobar*—single ventricle with noncleavage of cerebral hemispheres
   - *Semilobar*—cerebral hemispheres and ventricles are fused anteriorly but separated posteriorly
   - *Lobar*—cerebral hemispheres are separated both anteriorly and posteriorly, but there is partial fusion of the frontal horns of the lateral ventricles, absence of septum pellucidum and abnormalities of the corpus callosum, cavum septum pellucidum, and olfactory tract.
   - *Middle interhemispheric variant* is rare type, affecting only a small part of the brain.

   Alobar holoprosencephaly is the most severe type and can be diagnosed in the first trimester. Semilobar can also be diagnosed early but the diagnosis of lobar holoprosencephaly is usually made at 18 weeks gestation and beyond.
3. Alobar and lobar holoprosencephaly are associated with microcephaly and midfacial defects in 80% of cases. Cyclopia and proboscis are commonly found in alobar holoprosencephaly. Extracerebral defects are particularly common in fetuses with trisomies 13 and 18 and those with genetic syndromes.
4. Chromosomal defects, mainly trisomy 13 or 18, are found in >50% of cases at 12 weeks' gestation. Genetic syndromes are found in 20% of cases.
5. Detailed ultrasound examination including neurosonogram, invasive testing for karyotyping, and array is advised. Fetal MRI may be useful for confirmation of diagnosis in cases of suspected lobar holoprosencephaly. If pregnancy continues, follow-up should be standard.
6. *Prognosis:* Alobar and semilobar—usually lethal within the first year of life. In lobar type, life expectancy may be normal but usually with severe developmental delay and visual impairment.
7. Recurrence in isolated cases: 6%. Part of trisomies: 1%. Part of genetic syndromes: 25–50%.

SUGGESTED READING

1. Society for Maternal-Fetal Medicine (SMFM); Monteagudo A. Holoprosencephaly. Am J Obstet Gynecol. 2020;223(6):B13-B16.

STATION 7. A 25-year-old woman attends her first trimester scan at 13 weeks of gestation. The scan reveals an abnormal appearance of the fetal skull.

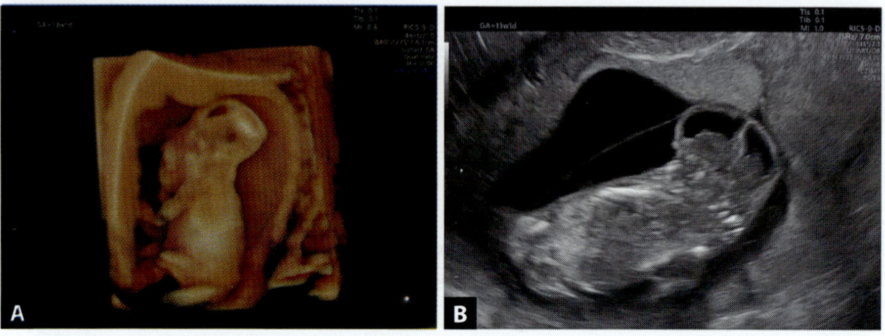

1. **Identify the abnormality in provided ultrasound images A and B. What is the incidence?**
2. **What is the prognosis of this condition?**
3. **What are the pregnancy complications associated with this condition?**
4. **What is the risk of recurrence in subsequent pregnancies and how can this risk be modified?**

Ans.

1. There is absence of cranial vault and cerebral hemispheres with exposure of intracranial content suggestive of acrania. Incidence of acrania/anencephaly is about 1 in 1,000 at 12 weeks gestation.
2. Acrania is a severe condition and is not compatible with life. Over time, the exposed brain tissue deteriorates, progressing to a condition called anencephaly.
3. There is risk of polyhydramnios in later gestation due to reduced fetal swallowing and development of fetal malpresentation and prolonged labor.
4. Acrania is the most severe form of open neural tube defect, and hence, risk of recurrence is similar with one previously affected sibling: 5% and two previously affected siblings: 10%. Supplementation of the maternal diet with folate (5 mg/day) for 3 months before and 2 months after conception reduces this risk of recurrence by about 75%.

SUGGESTED READING

1. Grosse SD, Collins JS. Folic acid supplementation and neural tube defect recurrence prevention. Birth Defects Res A Clin Mol Teratol. 2007;79:737-42.

STATION 8. A 30-year-old woman attends her routine first trimester scan at 12 weeks 6 days of gestation. During the scan, you observe an abnormal finding.

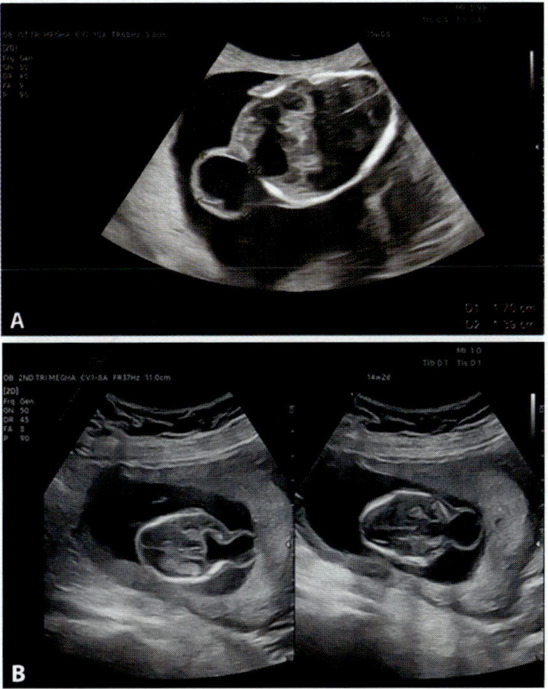

1. **Identify and explain above ultrasound images A and B.**
2. **What are the other associated abnormalities that one should look for in such a case?**
3. **How will you counsel regarding further investigations and prognosis?**
4. **What should be borne in mind while deciding the place of delivery? Are these defects amenable to surgical correction?**

Ans.

1. There is large defect in the occipital region with abnormal protrusion of brain structures through it known as occipital encephalocele. Encephaloceles are mostly occipital but can be parietal and rarely frontal. The underlying mechanism is defective closure of the anterior neural tube.
2. Chromosomal defects, mainly trisomies 13 or 18, are found in about 10% of cases. Cerebral and noncerebral defects and genetic syndromes are found in >60% of cases. The most common genetic syndrome is Meckel–Gruber syndrome which is autosomal recessive and has polydactyly, has multicystic dysplastic kidneys along with occipital encephalocele. Thus, we should look for the number of digits and the kidneys in a case of occipital encephalocele.

Other syndromes with encephalocele are Walker–Warburg syndrome (autosomal recessive; type II lissencephaly, agenesis of corpus callosum, cerebellar malformations, and cataract) and amniotic band syndrome (sporadic; single or multiple abnormalities of the extremities, craniofacial region and trunk due to the presence of amniotic bands).

3. The patient should be offered invasive testing for karyotyping and microarray. If the encephalocele is bulky, with severe microcephaly or other lethal anomalies, termination of pregnancy may be the choice due to the severe morbidity and mortality. Postpartum surgical treatment is appropriate for cases with relatively small encephalocele and without other associated lethal anomalies. Mortality for posterior encephalocele is >50% and for posterior meningocele and anterior encephalocele is about 20%. Neurological handicap remains in >50% of survivors.
   The risk of recurrence in isolated cases is 3–5%. While in autosomal recessive conditions, the risk is 25%.
4. Delivery should be planned in a tertiary care center with neonatal intensive care unit (NICU) and pediatric neurosurgery facilities. Pediatric neurosurgery is appropriate for cases with relatively small isolated encephaloceles. The procedure basically consists of removing the overlying sac and closing the defect including the dural defect. Prognosis depends on the size, content and location of the encephalocele.

SUGGESTED READING

1. Liao SL, Tsai PY, Cheng YC, Chang CH, Ko HC, Chang FM. Prenatal Diagnosis of Fetal Encephalocele Using Three-dimensional Ultrasound. J Med Ultrasound. 2012;20:(3):150-54.
2. Ong AGJ, Rolnik DL, Menezes M, Meagher S. Early Diagnosis and Differences in Progression of Fetal Encephalocele. J Ultrasound Med. 2020;39:1435-40.

STATION 9. A 22-year-old woman attends your antenatal clinic for a routine NT scan at 14 weeks of gestation. During the scan, you identify an abnormal appearance.

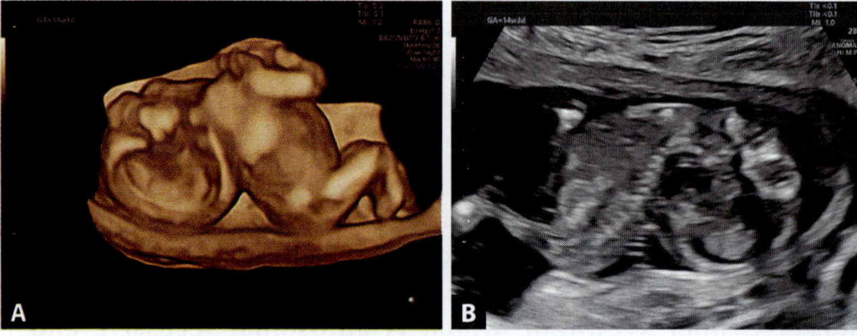

1. **Review the provided ultrasound image A and B and describe the findings.**
2. **Name the condition.**

3. **Describe the prognosis of this condition.**
4. **How to counsel?**

Ans.

1. There is fixed retroflexion of the head with abnormal cervical spine
2. Iniencephaly is a rare and lethal neural tube defect.
3. Very poor, it is not compatible with life outside the womb.
4. Empathetic counseling and discuss options of continuation versus termination of pregnancy

SUGGESTED READING

1. Holmes LB, Toufaily MH, Westgate MN. Iniencephaly. Birth Defects Res. 2018;110(2):128-33.

STATION 10. **A 28-year-old woman presents for her first trimester scan around 12 weeks of gestation. The ultrasound findings are as follows:**

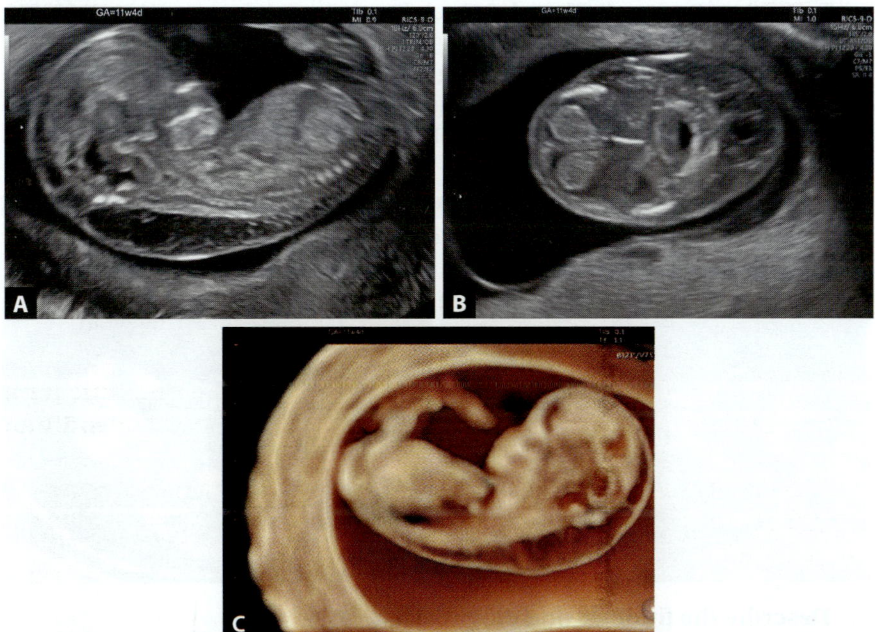

1. **Describe the ultrasound findings in the above images A to C. What is this condition called?**
2. **What is the most common abnormality associated with this presentation?**
3. **What would be the investigations indicated in the management of this case?**
4. **What is the prognosis of this condition?**

Ans.

1. NT increased with multilocular cystic structure and septation is identified in the posterior aspect of the fetal neck known as cystic hygroma. It is caused by the improper development of the lymphatic system.
2. Cystic hygroma is often associated with chromosomal abnormalities such as Turner syndrome, Down syndrome, or other trisomies.
3. Invasive testing (CVS or amniocentesis) for chromosomal analysis, follow-up ultrasound in the second trimester to assess for resolution or additional anomalies. Also, fetal echocardiography to check for heart defects (later in the pregnancy)
4. If associated with chromosomal or structural issues, the prognosis may be poor. However, in some cases, cystic hygroma can resolve spontaneously without complications.

SUGGESTED READING

1. Malone, Ciara M et al. Euploid First-Trimester Cystic Hygroma: A More Benign Entity than Previously Thought? Fetal diagnosis and therapy vol. 48,9 (2021): 667-671. doi:10.1159/000519056
2. Zheng J, Wang T, Sun H, Guan Y, Yang F, Wu J, et al. Genetic correlation between fetal nuchal translucency thickening and cystic hygroma and exploration of pregnancy outcome. Sci Rep. 2024;14(1):27191. doi: 10.1038/s41598-024-76628-y.

STATION 11. A 29-year-old woman attends her first trimester scan at 12 weeks of gestation. During the scan, you observe a midline anterior abdominal wall defect.

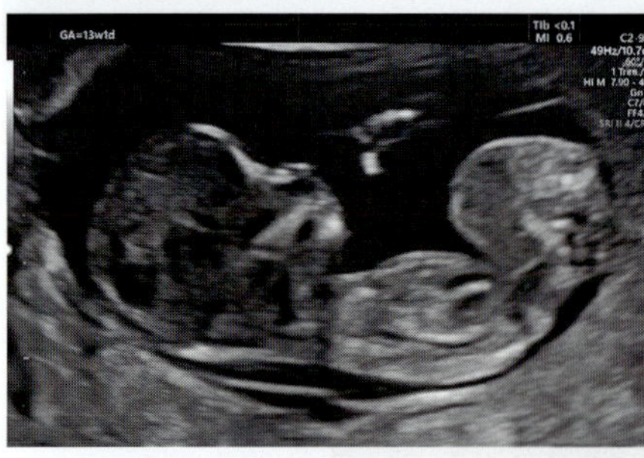

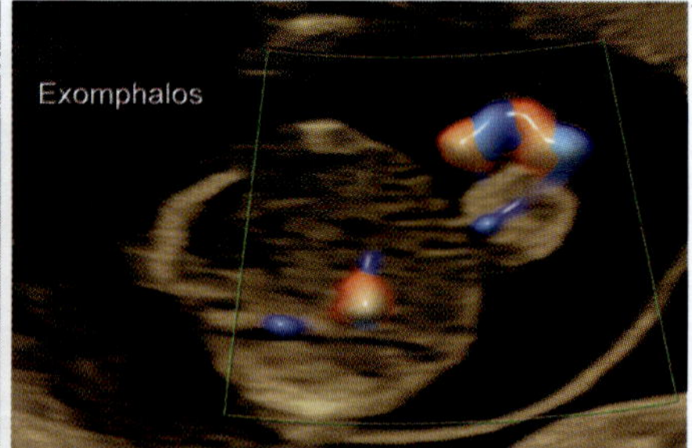

1. **Describe the findings and diagnosis.**
2. **What is the differential diagnosis?**
3. **What is the risk of association with genetic abnormalities?**
4. **How would you like to further investigate this case?**
5. **Which factors determine the fetal prognosis?**

Ans.

1. *Exomphalos:* An anterior abdominal wall defect—herniation of abdominal contents (bowel, possibly liver) into a membranous sac at the base

of the umbilical cord. The membrane covers the herniated contents. Differentiates from normal physiological gut herniation (which resolves by 11–12 weeks of gestation).

2. Gastroschisis, cloacal exstrophy, and pentalogy of Cantrell
3. Exomphalos is often associated with chromosomal abnormalities (28–30%) such as trisomy 18, trisomy 13, or other genetic syndromes like Beckwith–Wiedemann syndrome (10%). There may also be associated structural anomalies, especially involving the heart or other organs.
4. Invasive testing (CVS or amniocentesis) to evaluate for chromosomal abnormalities. Follow-up ultrasound in the second trimester for detailed anomaly scanning. Fetal echocardiography to assess for congenital heart defects.
5. The outcome depends on whether this is an isolated condition or associated with other abnormalities. Isolated exomphalos may have a better prognosis and can often be repaired surgically after birth. Presence of liver in sac and ratio of mean omphalocele diameter to transverse abdominal diameter >0.8 are associated with poor prognosis.

SUGGESTED READING

1. Shi X, Tang H, Lu J, Yang X, Ding H, Wu J. Prenatal genetic diagnosis of omphalocele by karyotyping, chromosomal microarray analysis and exome sequencing. Ann Med. 2021;53(1):1285-91.
2. Tassin M, Descriaud C, Elie C, Houfflin Debarge V, Dumez Y, Perrotin F, et al. Omphalocele in the first trimester: prediction of perinatal outcome. Prenat Diagn. 2013;33(5):497-501.
3. Țarcă E, Al Namat D, Luca AC, Lupu VV, Al Namat R, Lupu A, et al. Omphalocele and Cardiac Abnormalities-The Importance of the Association. Diagnostics (Basel). 2023;13(8):1413.

STATION 12.

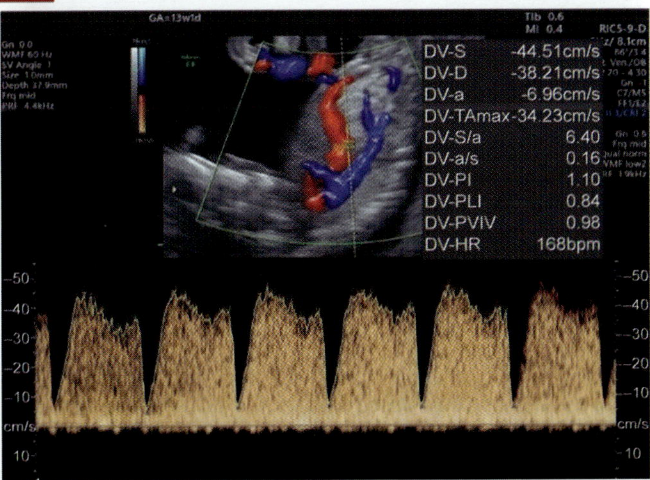

1. **Identify above Doppler wave form.**
2. **Describe the anatomy of the vessel form which the above wave form originates.**
3. **What is the function of this vessel in the fetal circulation?**
4. **What are the technical prerequisites to interrogate this vessel?**

Ans.

1. Ductus venosus (DV)
2. Small vascular connection between umbilical vein (UV) and inferior vena cava (IVC)
3. To create a jet of highly oxygenated blood to direct it on left side of heart
4. The UV, DV, and the heart should be seen together in the same frame, PD gate size 0.5–1.0 mm, low pulse-repetition frequency (PRF), insonation angle <30°, filter should be set at low frequency (50–70 Hz) and high sweep speed (2–3 cm/s)

SUGGESTED READING

1. Bhide A, Acharya G, Baschat A, Bilardo CM, Brezinka C, Cafici D, et al. ISUOG Practice Guidelines (updated): use of Doppler velocimetry in obstetrics. Ultrasound Obstet Gynecol. 2021;58(2):331-9.

STATION 13. **A 32-year-old woman attends her first trimester scan at 13 weeks of gestation. During the scan, you identify an abnormally enlarged cyst in the fetal abdomen.**

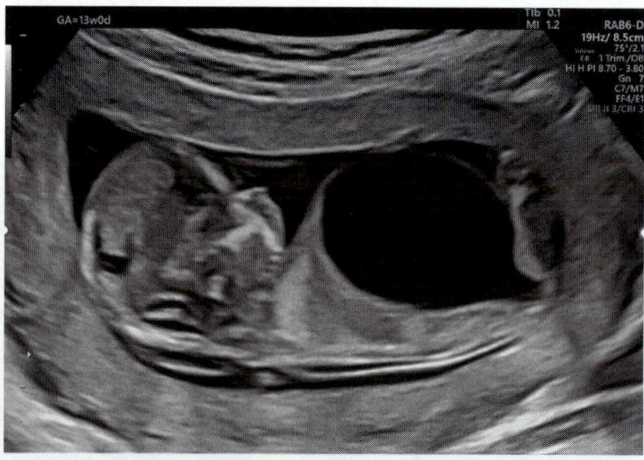

1. **Describe the ultrasound findings. What is the potential cause of this condition?**
2. **What is the differential diagnosis of cystic structure in the fetal abdomen?**
3. **What are the most common conditions associated with this condition?**

4. **What further investigations would be required and how will you follow-up?**
5. **How will you counsel the prospective parents regarding prognosis of the case?**
6. **What is the treatment or possible interventions?**

Ans.

1. Enlarged fetal bladder [longitudinal bladder diameter (LBD) > 7 mm at 10–14 weeks), no evidence of bladder emptying during the scan. This condition is called megacystis. It can result from a blockage in the urinary tract, such as posterior urethral valves, or other structural problems.
2. Cystic structures in the fetal abdomen may arise commonly from bowel (bowel atresia), bladder, gonads (ovarian cysts), or the mesentery (mesenteric cyst or intestinal duplication cysts). Rarely, they may be associated with other abdominal structures such as kidneys (renal cysts), adrenal (cysts/tumors), spleen, and liver (hepatic cysts and choledochal cysts). The most common cysts arising from the pelvis comprises megacystis and gonadal cysts, and rarely cysts due to gross bowel dilatation.
3. Megacystis occurs in 1/1,600 to 1/3,000 pregnancies. The cause may be obstructive in 60% of cases (posterior urethral valves, urethral atresia or urethral stenosis, and cloacal anomalies), nonobstructive in 30% of cases, mainly syndromic disease (megacystis-microcolon-intestinal hypoperistalsis syndrome and prune belly syndrome), and finally idiopathic or transient (10% of cases). It may also be associated with abnormalities in other systems, most commonly with structural cardiac defects (35%). When LBD is 7–15 mm, the incidence of chromosomal defects, mainly trisomies 13 and 18, is about 20%. In contrast in megacystis with LBD >15 mm, the incidence of chromosomal defects is about 10%.
4. Invasive testing (CVS or amniocentesis) to check for chromosomal abnormalities. Follow-up ultrasound at 16–18 weeks to assess bladder size and function, amniotic fluid levels. Also to check development of associated anomalies (e.g., renal or lung hypoplasia).
5. With LBD 7–14 mm, in the chromosomally normal group, there is spontaneous resolution of the megacystis in about 90% of cases. If the megacystis resolves early and is not associated with other abnormalities, the prognosis may be good. If it persists and leads to other complications, the prognosis may depend on the severity of kidney and lung involvement. In LBD >15 mm, in chromosomally normal group, the condition is invariably associated with progressive obstructive uropathy leading to hydronephrosis and dysplastic kidneys.
6. In certain cases, procedures such as vesicoamniotic shunting may be considered later in pregnancy to relieve the obstruction.

SUGGESTED READING

1. Fontanella F, Duin L, Adama van Scheltema PN, Cohen-Overbeek TE, Pajkrt E, Bekker M, et al. Antenatal Workup of Early Megacystis and Selection of Candidates for Fetal Therapy. Fetal Diagn Ther. 2019;45(3):155-61.
2. Lesieur E, Barrois M, Bourdon M, Blanc J, Loeuillet L, Delteil C, et al. Megacystis in the first trimester of pregnancy: Prognostic factors and perinatal outcomes. PLoS One. 2021;16(9):e0255890.

STATION 14. A 30-year-old woman came for her first trimester screening at 12 weeks of gestation. She has past history of preeclampsia. Her mean pulsatility index (PI) is 2.45.

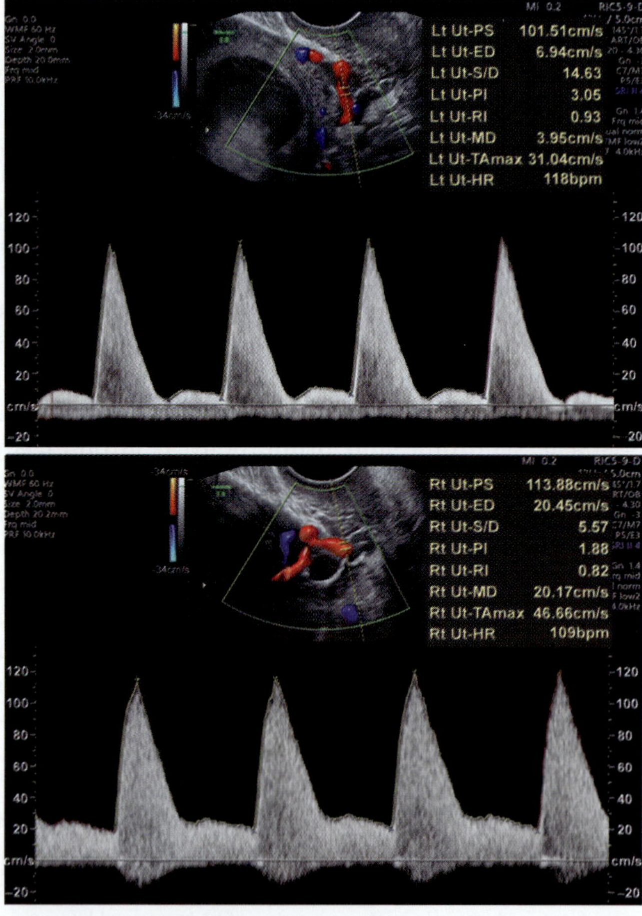

1. **How to conduct a uterine artery Doppler?**
2. **What is the purpose of uterine artery Doppler?**
3. **Describe the management of increased risk of preecplampsia.**
4. **Describe follow-up and monitoring.**

Ans.

1. Put color Doppler to identify the uterine artery near the internal os. Place the sample gate 1 cm distal to the crossover of the uterine artery with the external iliac artery. Record at least three consecutive waveforms with good quality on each side. Calculate the mean PI by averaging both sides.
2. This test measures blood flow in the uterine arteries, which supply blood to the placenta. If the blood flow is normal, the risk of preeclampsia is low, and no additional measures are needed. If we find increased resistance in the uterine arteries, it may indicate a higher risk of preeclampsia or related complications.
3. Low-dose aspirin (150 mg) at bedtime from now until 36 weeks to improve placental function and reduce the risk of preeclampsia.
4. Pregnancy needs to be monitored with additional scans to check fetal growth and amniotic fluid levels.

SUGGESTED READING

1. Sotiriadis A, Hernandez-Andrade E, da Silva Costa F, Ghi T, Glanc P, Khalil A, et al. ISUOG Practice Guidelines: role of ultrasound in screening for and follow-up of pre-eclampsia. Ultrasound Obstet Gynecol. 2019;53(1):7-22.

STATION 15. A 32-year-old woman attends a high-risk clinic at 20 weeks of gestation. She has a history of chronic hypertension and is concerned about preeclampsia. You are asked to perform an ophthalmic artery Doppler and explain its significance.

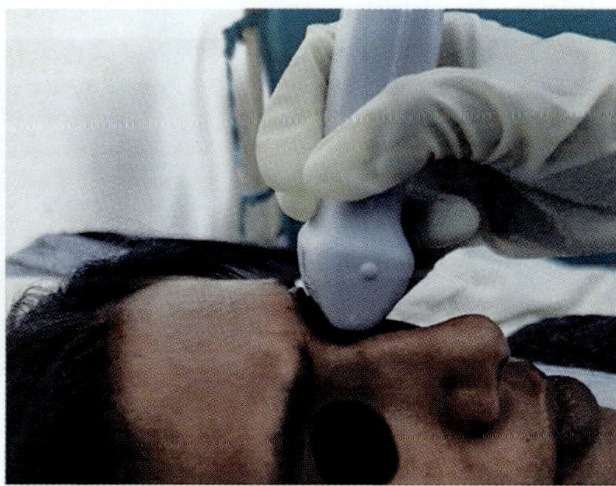

1. **How to perform the ophthalmic artery Doppler?**
2. **What is the purpose of this test?**
3. **How should the results be interpreted?**
4. **Describe further follow-up and management.**

Ans.

1. Use a high-frequency linear probe for the ultrasound. Identify the ophthalmic artery as it crosses the optic nerve within the orbit using color Doppler. Place the sample gate over the vessel to obtain a spectral waveform. Record three consistent waveforms to assess the peak systolic velocity (PSV) and PI.
2. The ophthalmic artery Doppler is a noninvasive way to assess vascular changes that occur during pregnancy. It helps us detect early signs of systemic vascular resistance, which is linked to the risk of developing preeclampsia.
3. Normal resistance in the ophthalmic artery, indicating low risk of preeclampsia. Increased PI or RI, suggesting higher risk of preeclampsia due to systemic vascular dysfunction.
4. If the results are normal, no additional interventions are required. If the Doppler indicates increased risk, we will recommend starting low-dose aspirin (150 mg at bedtime) to reduce the risk of preeclampsia.

SUGGESTED READING

1. Kusuma RA, Nurdiati DS, Al Fattah AN, Danukusumo D, Abdullah S, Sini I. Ophthalmic artery Doppler for pre-eclampsia prediction at the first trimester: a Bayesian survival-time model. J Ultrasound. 2023;26(1):155-62.

STATION 16. **A 29-year-old woman came for first-trimester ultrasound at 12 weeks of gestation. She is undergoing a combined screening for chromosomal abnormalities. You are tasked with performing tricuspid Doppler and explaining its significance.**

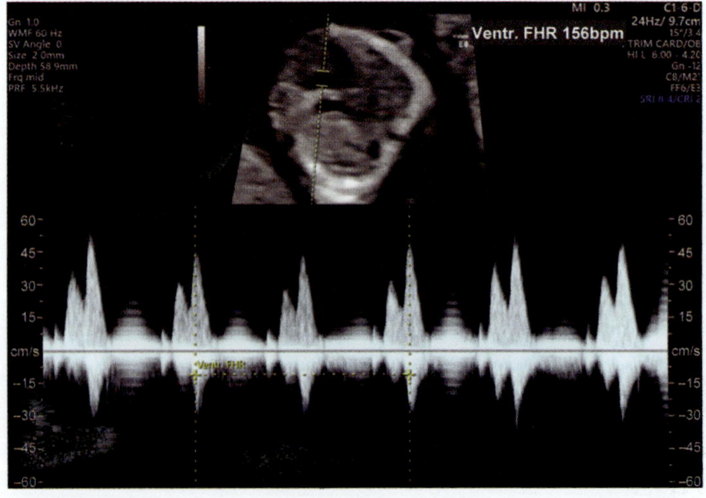

1. **How to acquire a tricuspid Doppler waveform?**
2. **What does this waveform interrogate?**

3. **What is a normal finding?**
4. **What is an abnormal finding?**

Ans.

1. Uses an apical view of the fetal thorax to visualize the four-chamber heart. Focuses on the right atrium and right ventricle. Activates color Doppler to identify the tricuspid valve inflow and regurgitation jets. Places the pulsed Doppler sample gate at the level of the tricuspid valve to obtain waveforms. Records at least three consecutive waveforms to assess for regurgitation.
2. The tricuspid Doppler test assesses blood flow through the tricuspid valve of fetus
3. Normal blood flow through the tricuspid valve without evidence of regurgitation suggests a lower risk for abnormalities
4. Abnormal finding shows tricuspid regurgitation (TR) as blood flowing back into the right atrium during systole with a velocity exceeding 60 cm/second for >50% of systole.

SUGGESTED READING

1. Falcon O, Auer M, Gerovassili A, Spencer K, Nicolaides KH. Screening for trisomy 21 by fetal tricuspid regurgitation, nuchal translucency and maternal serum free β-hCG and PAPP-A at 11 + 0 to 13 + 6 weeks. Ultrasound Obstet Gynecol. 2006;27:151-5.

STATION 17.

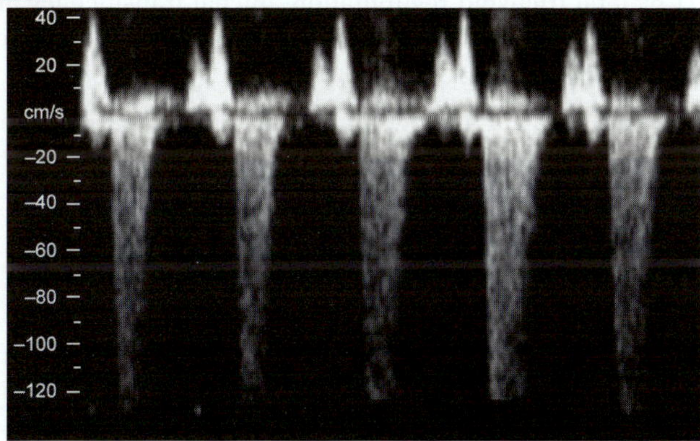

1. **Identify the first trimester ultrasound marker shown in image above.**
2. **What is the ideal way to obtain a tricuspid waveform?**
3. **How can we say that the waveform shows TR?**
4. **What conditions are associated with TR?**
5. **How will you follow a fetus with TR?**

Ans.

1. Tricuspid regurgitation
2. PD sample gate must be 2–3 mm, place across tricuspid valves (medial, central, and lateral), set PRF to visualize waves of up to 100 cm/sec velocity with sweep speed 2–3 cm/sec
3. Tricuspid regurgitation is diagnosed if the regurgitant jet has a velocity of >60 cm/sec and lasts for more than half of the systole, since aortic or pulmonary arterial blood flow at this gestation can produce a maximum velocity of 50 cm/sec.
4. Tricuspid regurgitation at 11–13 weeks' gestation is a common finding in fetuses with trisomies 21, 18, and 13 and in those with major cardiac defects. Tricuspid regurgitation is found in about 1% of euploid fetuses, in 55% of fetuses with trisomy 21 and in one-third of fetuses with trisomy 18 and trisomy 13.
5. If there is TR, we should include it in the algorithm for combined first trimester risk calculation to refine the a priori risk for fetal aneuploidy. Based on the revised risk, we may recommend further testing, such as noninvasive prenatal testing (NIPT) or CVS, to evaluate for chromosomal abnormalities. Additionally, a detailed fetal echocardiogram is recommended to check for structural heart issues besides the second trimester anomaly scan.

SUGGESTED READING

1. Falcon O, Auer M, Gerovassili A, Spencer K, Nicolaides KH. Screening for trisomy 21 by fetal tricuspid regurgitation, nuchal translucency and maternal serum free β-hCG and PAPP-A at 11 + 0 to 13 + 6 weeks. Ultrasound Obstet Gynecol. 2006;27:151-5.

STATION 18.

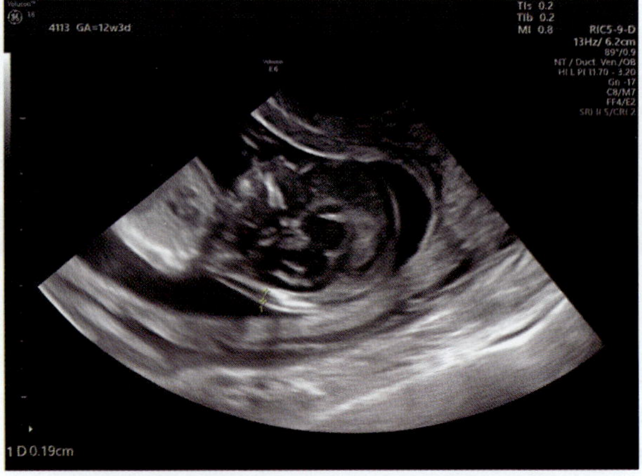

Image courtesy: Dr Seetha Ramamurthy Pal.

History
Ethnic origin: South Asian (Indian, Pakistani, Bangladeshi).
Parity: 1.
Maternal weight: 67.2 kg.
Smoking in this pregnancy: no; Diabetes Mellitus: no.
Conception: spontaneous;
last period: 23 January 2021 EDD by dates: 30 October 2021

First Trimester Ultrasound
Gestational age: **11 weeks + 6 days** from CRL EDD by scan: 30 October 2021

Crown-rump length (CRL) 51.7 mm
Nuchal translucency (NT) 1.85 mm
Chromosomal markers:
Nasal bone: present.

Maternal Serum Biochemistry
Sample **2119002184**, taken on: 16 April 2021, analysed on: 17 April 2021. Equipment: Roche.

Free ß-hCG 22.35 IU/l equivalent to 0.707 MoM
PAPP-A 0.916 IU/l equivalent to 0.401 MoM

FMF Operator: saumya srivastav, FMF Id: 142489

Condition	*Background risk*	*Adjusted risk*
Trisomy 21	1: 106	1: 703
Trisomy 18	1: 1250	1: 13281
Trisomy 13	1: 2943	1: 4328

The background risk for aneuploidies is based on maternal age (40 years). The adjusted risk is the risk at term, calculated on the basis of the background risk, ultrasound factors (fetal nuchal translucency thickness, nasal bone) and maternal serum biochemistry (PAPP-A, free beta-hCG).
All biochemical markers are corrected as necessary according to several maternal characteristics including racial origin, weight, height, smoking, method of conception and parity.

Mrs X, a 40-year-old lady G2P1L1, came at 12 weeks for routine first trimester aneuploidy screening. She has pregestational diabetes and is on insulin. Her ultrasound image and combined double marker report are given above.

1. **What is the final risk of trisomy 21 mentioned in this combined double marker report?**
2. **Point out two errors in the report.**
3. **On reassessment with correct parameters, the trisomy 21 risk came as 1:13. What should be the next investigation advised to her?**
4. **What are the other pregnancy risks associated with this type of combined double marker report?**

Ans.

1. The adjusted risk of trisomy 21 mentioned in the report is 1:703.
2. There are two errors seen in the report—the maternal diabetes status is not considered and absent NB is taken as present for risk assessment.
3. 1:13 is high risk for trisomy 21, hence, invasive diagnostic testing for fetal chromosomal study should be offered.
4. Beside increased risk of trisomy 21, there is also increased risk of fetal growth restriction (FGR), preeclampsia, gestational hypertension, placental abruption, and prematurity associated with low PAPP-A values (≤0.4 MoM).

SUGGESTED READING

1. Bardi F, Kagan KO, Bilardo CM. First-trimester screening strategies: A balance between costs, efficiency and diagnostic yield. Prenat Diagn. 2023;43(7):865-72.

2. Papamichail M, Fasoulakis Z, Daskalakis G, Theodora M, Rodolakis A, Antsaklis P. Importance of Low Pregnancy Associated Plasma Protein-A (PAPP-A) Levels During the First Trimester as a Predicting Factor for Adverse Pregnancy Outcomes: A Prospective Cohort Study of 2636 Pregnant Women. Cureus. 2022;14(11):e31256.

STATION 19.

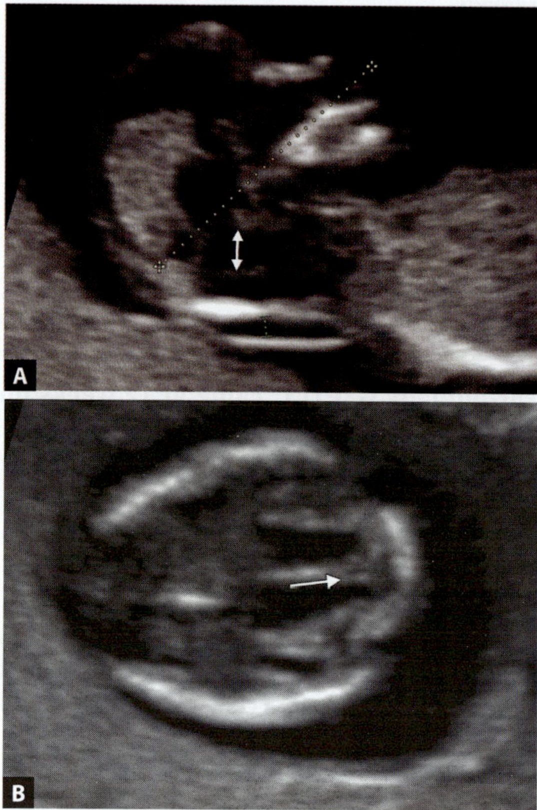

1. **What is the posterior fossa abnormality seen in image A of this fetus?**
2. **Which is the sonographic sign seen in image B?**
3. **Which fetal structure should be evaluated properly with these sonographic signs?**

Ans.

1. There is increased BS thickness with reduced BS: BS:BSOB and IT is not well demarcated in image A. There is also posterior and downward displacement of the junction of the midbrain and BS below the maxillo-occipital line.
2. *"Crash sign":* Posterior displacement of the mesencephalon and deformation against the occipital bone in the axial view of fetal head

caused by cerebrospinal fluid (CSF) leak and reduced arachnoid space in fetuses with open spina bifida.

3. Fetal spine should be evaluated in all three planes (axial, sagittal, and coronal) for any evidence of open neural tube defect, when above sonographic signs are present.

SUGGESTED READING

1. Lachmann R, Chaoui R, Moratalla J, Picciarelli G, Nicolaides KH. Posterior brain in fetuses with open spina bifida at 11 to 13 weeks. Prenat Diagn. 2011;31(1):103-6.
2. Ramkrishna J, Araujo Júnior E, Peixoto AB, Da Silva Costa F, Meagher S. Maxillo-occipital line: a sonographic marker for screening of open spina bifida in the first trimester of pregnancy. J Matern Fetal Neonatal Med. 2019;32(24):4073-9.
3. Ushakov F, Sacco A, Andreeva E, Tudorache S, Everett T, David AL, et al. Crash sign: new first-trimester sonographic marker of spina bifida. Ultrasound Obstet Gynecol. 2019;54(6):740-5.

STATION 20.

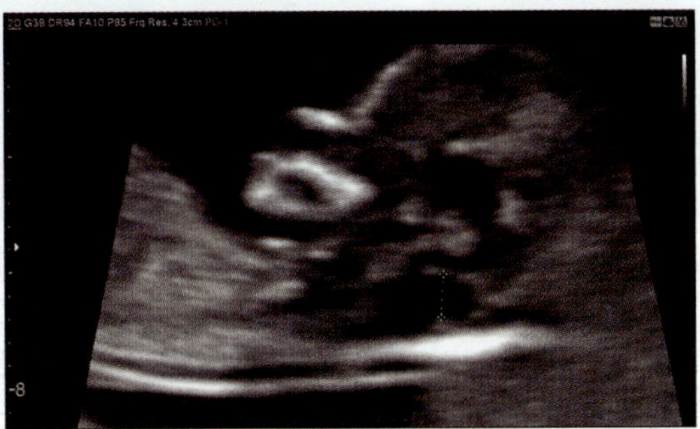

1. **What are the four lines and three spaces in the fetal brain?**
2. **Identify the abnormality shown in above image.**
3. **What are the possible associations with this condition?**
4. **What should be the follow-up protocol for this fetus?**

Ans.

1. Three spaces are: IT, cisterna magna, and NT. Four lines are the posterior surface of midbrain, posterior border of BS, anterior border of the choroid plexus of fourth ventricle, and occipital bone.
2. There is increased IT with posterior displacement of choroid plexus of fourth ventricle giving a posterior fossa cystic appearance.
3. There is increased risk of posterior fossa abnormality in these fetuses and follow-up is needed in mid trimester to look for Blake's pouch cyst, Dandy–Walker malformation, and abnormal development of cerebellum and vermis.
4. Patients should be called back at 16–18 weeks gestational age for early evaluation of fetal brain and again at 20–22 weeks for evaluation of cerebellum and vermis as part of a neurosonogram.

SUGGESTED READING

1. Martinez-Ten P, Illescas T, Adiego B, Estevez M, Bermejo C, Wong AE, et al. Non-visualization of choroid plexus of fourth ventricle as first-trimester predictor of posterior fossa anomalies and chromosomal defects. Ultrasound Obstet Gynecol. 2018;51(2):199-207.
2. Volpe P, De Robertis V, Volpe G, Boito S, Fanelli T, Olivieri C, et al. Position of the choroid plexus of the fourth ventricle in first- and second-trimester fetuses: a novel approach to early diagnosis of cystic posterior fossa anomalies. Ultrasound Obstet Gynecol. 2021;58:568-75.

STATION 21.

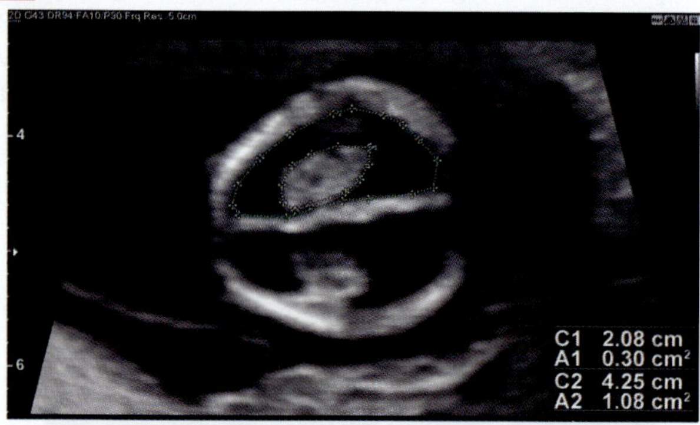

1. **Explain the sonographic finding in a 13 weeks fetus, shown in above image.**
2. **What are the first sonographic criteria for this above condition?**
3. **What is the standard management in these cases?**
4. **What sign is this called?**

Ans.

1. The choroid plexus area to lateral ventricle area is 0.28, which is suggestive of first trimester ventriculomegaly.
2. The first trimester criteria for ventriculomegaly are ratio of choroid plexus area to lateral ventricle area <0.5 and choroid plexus length to lateral ventricle length <0.7 when measured in axial plane.
3. Second trimester ultrasound is suggested at 16 weeks for intracranial evaluation and an early anomaly scan for any other structural abnormality. Based on sonographic findings, invasive diagnostic testing is indicated for any genetic association. Intrauterine infections (particularly cytomegalovirus and toxoplasmosis) should be screened for in mother and diagnostic testing offered by amniocentesis beyond 20 weeks gestation if infections are suspected on maternal serology. Detailed neurosonography should be offered at 20–22 weeks gestational age and fetal brain MRI can be done after 24 weeks gestational age.
4. Dry brain sign.

SUGGESTED READING

1. Giorgione V, Haratz KK, Constantini S, Birnbaum R, Malinger G. Fetal cerebral ventriculomegaly: What do we tell the prospective parents? Prenat Diagn. 2022;42(13):1674-81.
2. Prasad S, Di Fabrizio C, Eltaweel N, Kalafat E, Khalil A. First-trimester choroid-plexus-to-lateral-ventricle disproportion and prediction of subsequent ventriculomegaly. Ultrasound Obstet Gynecol. 2023;62(2):234-40.

STATION 22.

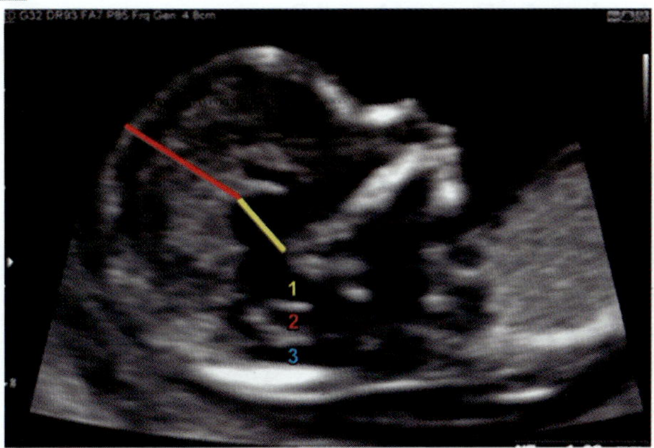

1. **What are the anechoic spaces marked 1, 2, and 3 in the midsagittal view of a 13 weeks fetus shown in above image?**
2. **What are the boundaries of the space marked as 2?**
3. **What is the clinical importance of space marked 2?**
4. **What measurements do the yellow line and red line signify?**
5. **What is the clinical importance of measurement of structures marked by yellow and red lines?**

Ans.

1. The anechoic space marked above are: (1) BS, (2) IT or fourth ventricle, and (3) cisterna magna.
2. Intracranial translucency or the fourth ventricle is bounded anteriorly by the posterior margin of BS and posteriorly by the choroid plexus of the fourth ventricle.
3. A diminished size of IT (<1.5 mm) is suggestive of an open neural tube defect and an increased size (>2.5 mm) is suggestive of an evolving posterior cranial fossa abnormality.
4. The structure marked in the yellow line is the midbrain diameter and the red line is the falx diameter.
5. An increase in the ratio of midbrain diameter to falx diameter (>1) gives an early clue to the potential first trimester diagnosis of agenesis of corpus callosum.

SUGGESTED READING

1. Lachmann R, Sodre D, Barmpas M, Akolekar R, Nicolaides KH. Midbrain and falx in fetuses with absent corpus callosum at 11-13 weeks. Fetal Diagn Ther. 2013;33(1):41-6.
2. Volpe N, Dall'Asta A, Di Pasquo E, Frusca T, Ghi T. First-trimester fetal neurosonography: technique and diagnostic potential. Ultrasound Obstet Gynecol. 2021;57(2):204-14.

STATION 23. G3P1011 was referred for anterior abdominal wall defect at 12 weeks. Look at the images A and B.

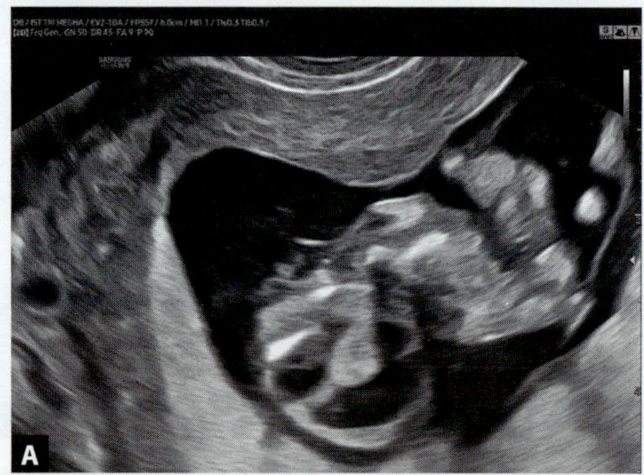

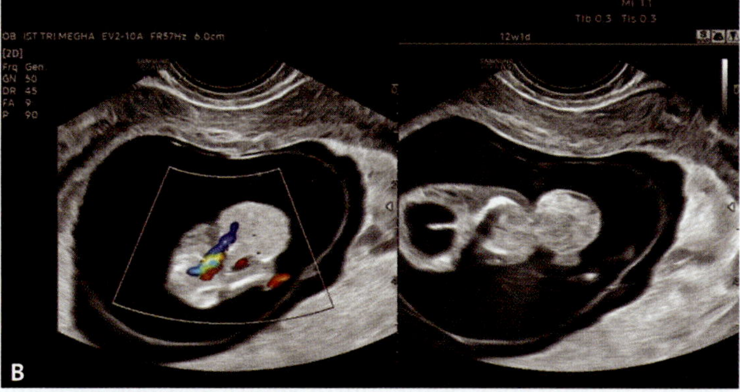

1. **What is the provisional diagnosis?**
2. **What are the associated features of the condition?**
3. **What is the etiology for this condition?**
4. **The patient is anxious about the recurrence in the next pregnancy and wants further testing. What will you advise her?**

Ans.

1. The images A and B depict a fetus with multiple congenital abnormalities—irregular tissue mass, exencephaly, spinal deformity, omphalocele, and short cord suggestive of limb-body wall complex (LBWC) or body stalk anomaly.

2. Limb-body wall complex refers to a combination of multiple malformations involving the craniofacial structures, thoracoabdominal wall, extremities, and spine. The classic clinical triad of LBWC includes a craniofacial defect (characteristically *exencephaly* or *encephalocele* with facial cleft), *limb deformity*, and body wall malformation with *evisceration*.
3. Theories regarding the etiology of LBWC include early amnion rupture causing mechanical injury, defective development in the germinal disk, and vascular disruption during embryogenesis.
4. The anomaly, though lethal, is not generally associated with chromosomal abnormalities or genetic syndromes. The risk of recurrence is usually negligible and hence no genetic testing is required.

SUGGESTED READING

1. Jain JA, Fuchs KM. Limb-Body Wall Complex. In: Copel JA, D'Alton ME, Feltovich H, Gratacós E, Krakow D, Odibo AQ (Eds), et al. Obstetric Imaging: Fetal Diagnosis and Care, 2nd edition. Philadelphia, PA: Elsevier; 2018.

STATION 24.

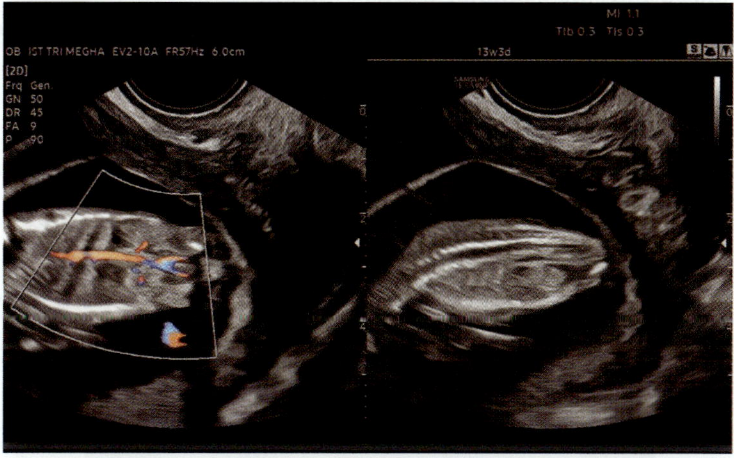

1. **Identify the anatomical structures shown in the above image.**
2. **What conditions can be associated with absence of these anatomical structures?**
3. **What is the prognosis for the case in question 2 above and how will you counsel such patients?**
4. **What is the risk of recurrence if the structure in question 1 is absent bilaterally?**

Ans.

1. The image shows bilateral (B/L) kidneys appearing on either side of the spine with both the renal arteries arising from the aorta.

2. Renal agenesis is nonvisualization of one or both the kidneys.
   a. Unilateral renal agenesis—nonvisualization of one kidney with normal bladder and amniotic fluid. Color Doppler demonstrates a single renal artery. There may be compensatory hypertrophy of the contralateral kidney.
   b. Bilateral renal agenesis—nonvisualization of the kidneys and bladder in combination with anhydramnios >17 weeks gestation. Renal arteries are not visualized on color Doppler. Adrenal glands assume discoid shape and move laterally and inferiorly—lying down adrenals. It leads to Potter's sequence (pulmonary hypoplasia, flat facies, and talipes)
3. In the majority of cases, renal agenesis is a sporadic and isolated abnormality. Chromosomal defects, mainly trisomy 18, are found in 1–2% of cases. Associated syndromes are found in 10% of cases. The most common are: Fraser syndrome (autosomal recessive condition characterized by renal agenesis, laryngeal atresia, cryptophthalmos, and syndactyly) and VACTERL association [vertebral and ventricular septal defects, anal atresia, tracheoesophageal fistula, renal anomalies, radial dysplasia and single umbilical artery (SUA)].
   Bilateral is lethal, usually in the neonatal period due to pulmonary hypoplasia. Unilateral has a normal prognosis. In some patients, there may be vesicoureteric reflux.
4. *Recurrence:* Nonsyndromic—3%. In 15% of cases, one of the parents has unilateral renal agenesis and in these families the risk of recurrence is increased.

SUGGESTED READING

1. Society for Maternal-Fetal Medicine (SMFM); Jelin A. Renal agenesis. Am J Obstet Gynecol. 2021;225(5):B28-B30.

STATION 25.

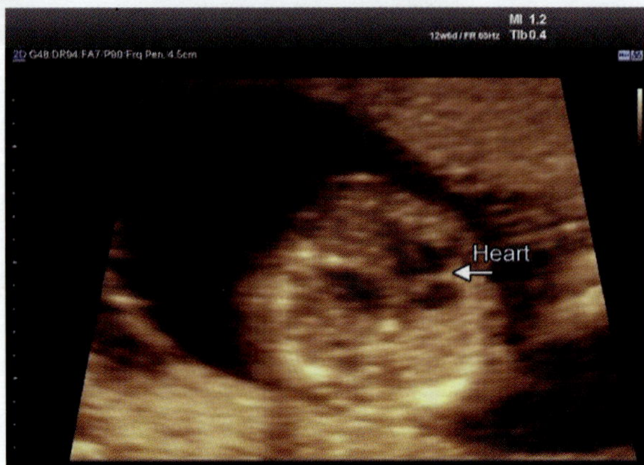

1. **The image is a cross section of the fetal chest at 12 weeks. What is your provisional diagnosis?**
2. **What are the associated syndromes and conditions?**
3. **What are the prognostic factors of the condition?**
4. **Is there any prenatal treatment available?**

Ans.

1. The image shows a cystic structure in the fetal chest pushing the heart toward the other side, likely congenital diaphragmatic hernia (CDH).
2. Chromosomal defects, mainly trisomies 18 or 13 and occasionally tetrasomy 12p or Pallister–Killian syndrome, are found in 20% of cases. Genetic syndromes are found in 10% of cases. The most common is Fryns syndrome (autosomal recessive; anophthalmia, facial cleft, micrognathia, ventriculomegaly, and diaphragmatic hernia). Defects in other systems, mainly craniofacial and cardiac, are found in 20% of cases.
3. Reported survival rate is approximately 85% for cases of isolated CDH. The prognosis is associated with several risk factors that can be assessed prenatally, including liver herniation, stomach herniation, low fetal lung volume, and low lung area-to-head circumference ratio (LHR) on prenatal ultrasound, as well as the presence of chromosomal abnormalities, concurrent anomalies, and hydrops fetalis. Liver herniation is usually found to be associated with a poorer prognosis than other hernias.
   Assessment of severity is by measurement of contralateral lung area in a transverse section of the chest to head circumference ratio (LHR). An observed to expected LHR of ≤25% is considered severe, moderate if 26–45%, and mild if >45%.
4. The prenatal management of CDH involves the endoscopic insertion of an inflatable balloon into the trachea with consequent retention of fluid produced by the lungs which may stimulate lung growth, a procedure known as fetoscopic endoluminal tracheal occlusion (FETO). The balloon is inserted at 26 weeks' gestation and removed endoscopically at 34 weeks. If this is not possible, delivery is ideally by cesarean section and ex utero intrapartum treatment (EXIT). An EXIT procedure is performed as an adjunct to cesarean section and involves the fetal head and neck being removed from the uterus through a standard lower segment incision, and the airway then is able to be established while the baby remains connected to the placenta.

SUGGESTED READING

1. Grivell RM, Andersen C, Dodd JM. Prenatal interventions for congenital diaphragmatic hernia for improving outcomes. Cochrane Database Syst Rev. 2015;2015(11):CD008925.

2. Sperling JD, Sparks TN, Berger VK, Farrell JA, Gosnell K, Keller RL, et al. Prenatal Diagnosis of Congenital Diaphragmatic Hernia: Does Laterality Predict Perinatal Outcomes? Am J Perinatol. 2018;35(10):919-24.

STATION 26. **A 29-year-old G2P1L1 patient visits her obstetrician with the findings of an open neural tube defect and other findings as shown below images A and B:**

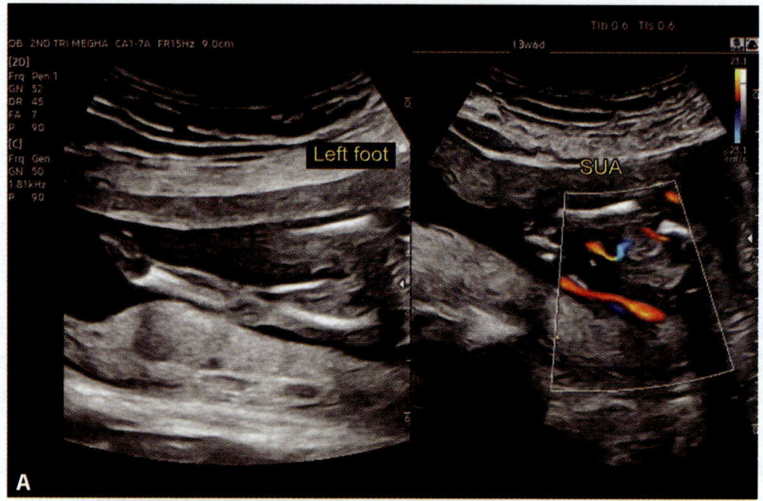

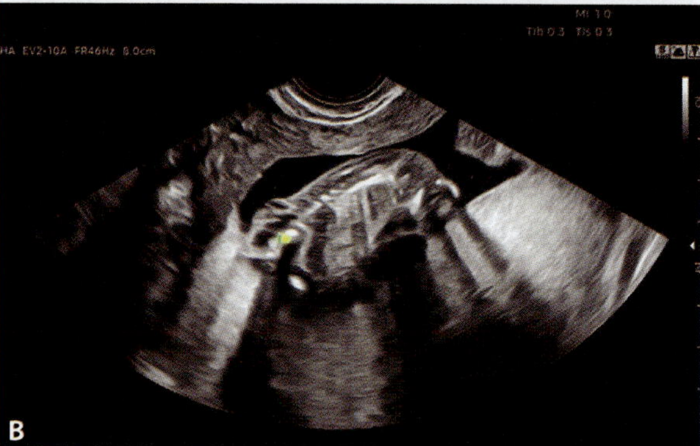

1. **What are the findings that can be seen in the above images A and B?**
2. **What other system abnormalities can be associated with the above images A and B?**

3. **What prenatal counseling will you offer this woman?**
4. **How would you follow-up this patient in the absence of skeletal and neural tube defect?**

Ans.

1. Single umbilical artery and unilateral club foot.
2. The incidence of SUA is around 1%. Chromosomal abnormalities, mainly trisomies 18, 13, and triploidy, are found in 5% of cases. Abnormalities affecting cardiovascular, skeletal, gastrointestinal, genitourinary, and central nervous systems are found in 20% of cases.
3. SUA is associated with a sevenfold increase in risk of trisomy 18. A high proportion of trisomy 18 fetuses have other major defects that are easily detectable at the 11–14-week scan and many other abnormalities that are detectable at 16–20 weeks. However, in the above case the findings of club feet, SUA, and spina bifida warrant further invasive testing for karyotyping or array to rule out chromosomal aneuploidies especially Edwards syndrome.
4. Isolated SUA may be associated with fetal growth restriction (<5th percentile) in 10% of cases. Stillbirth, usually in association with growth restriction, is twice as common as in the general population. So, in isolated cases of SUA, combined first trimester screening can be done to ascertain the risk of common aneuploidies. If low risk, the pregnancy can be followed up with serial growth monitoring starting 32 weeks. Option of NIPT can be given to the patients. Prenatal invasive testing is not warranted in cases of isolated SUA.

SUGGESTED READING

1. Indications for Outpatient Antenatal Fetal Surveillance: ACOG Committee Opinion, Number 828. Obstet Gynecol. 2021;137(6):e177-e197.
2. Rembouskos G, Cicero S, Longo D, Sacchini C, Nicolaides KH. Single umbilical artery at 11-14 weeks' gestation: relation to chromosomal defects. Ultrasound Obstet Gynecol. 2003;22(6):567-70.

STATION 27. **A 21-year-old primigravida presents at 13 weeks gestation with the following scan images A and B and a heart rate of 80 beats/min.**

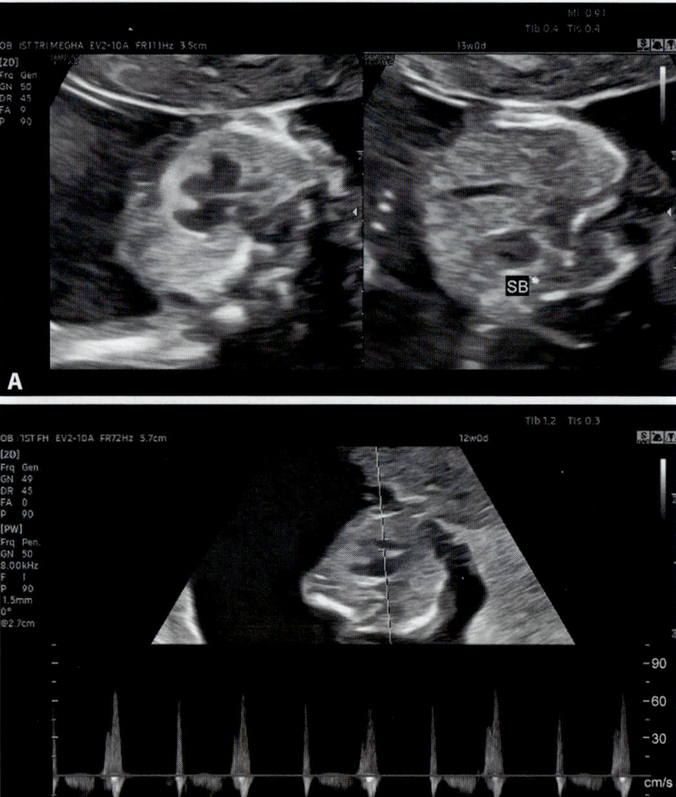

1. **Describe the findings and identify the cardiac abnormality.**
2. **Can all cardiac abnormalities be diagnosed in the early anomaly scan? Name three fetal malformations that can be picked up with 100% certainty at the time of the first trimester early anomaly scan.**
3. **What is the prognosis in this case?**
4. **Name the syndrome associated with this presentation.**

Ans.

1. Stomach and apex of the heart lie on the opposite side indicating a situs abnormality, situs inversus, or heterotaxy. The heart also looks abnormal with nonvisualization of the crux and bradycardia.
2. All cardiac abnormalities cannot be diagnosed at the 12–13 weeks scan.

   During the first trimester anomaly scan, some abnormalities are always detectable, some are potentially detectable while others are not detectable.

Abnormalities always detectable in the nuchal scans are as follows:	*Abnormalities sometimes detectable on nuchal scans:*
• Acrania • Encephalocele • Alobar holoprosencephaly • Iniencephaly • Exomphalos • Gastroschisis • Megacystis • Body stalk anomaly • Limb reduction • Cystic hygroma	• Diaphragmatic hernia • Bilateral renal agenesis • Lethal CardiacHDs • Lethal skeletal dysplasias • Isolated bone shortening • Polydactyly • Facial clefts • Open spina bifida • Talipes

3. The prognosis in situs abnormalities depends on the associated cardiac abnormalities and other systemic associations. Since here it is associated with complete atrioventricular septal defect (AVSD) and heart block likely left isomerism, the prognosis is usually poor with high morbidity and mortality as heart block may lead to hydrops and intrauterine deaths.
4. Situs inversus may be associated with ciliary dyskinesia or Kartagener syndrome.

SUGGESTED READING

1. Grande M, Arigita M, Borobio V, Jimenez JM, Fernandez S, Borrell A. First-trimester detection of structural abnormalities and the role of aneuploidy markers. Ultrasound Obstet Gynecol. 2012;39(2):157-63.
2. Lambert TE, Kuller J, Small M, Rhee E, Barker P. Abnormalities of Fetal Situs: An Overview and Literature Review. Obstet Gynecol Surv. 2016;71(1):33-8.

CHAPTER 4

Non-invasive Prenatal Screening

Sumitra Bachani, Sakshi Yadav

STATION 1. A 28-year-old pregnant lady with singleton pregnancy comes for advice on prenatal screening at 12 weeks gestation. She is keen to get noninvasive prenatal screen (NIPS).

1. **What information would you need to gather before ordering the test?**
2. **What is the origin of fetal cells in maternal plasma?**
3. **How does fetal fraction (FF) increase with gestational age after 20 weeks?**

Ans.

1. - Maternal age and gestational age
   - Type of conception
   - Any ultrasound findings/nuchal translucency (NT) scan report
   - History of any chromosomal disorders in previous pregnancies
2. Apoptosis of syncytiotrophoblasts of placenta
3. It increases 1.0% per week after 20 weeks until term

SUGGESTED READING

1. American College of Obstetricians and Gynecologists' Committee on Practice Bulletins—Obstetrics; Committee on Genetics; Society for Maternal-Fetal Medicine. Screening for Fetal Chromosomal Abnormalities: ACOG Practice Bulletin, Number 226. Obstet Gynecol. 2020;136(4):e48-e69.
2. Wang E, Batey A, Struble C, Musci T, Song K, Oliphant A. Gestational age and maternal weight effects on fetal cell-free DNA in maternal plasma. Prenat Diagn. 2013;33(7):662-6.

STATION 2.

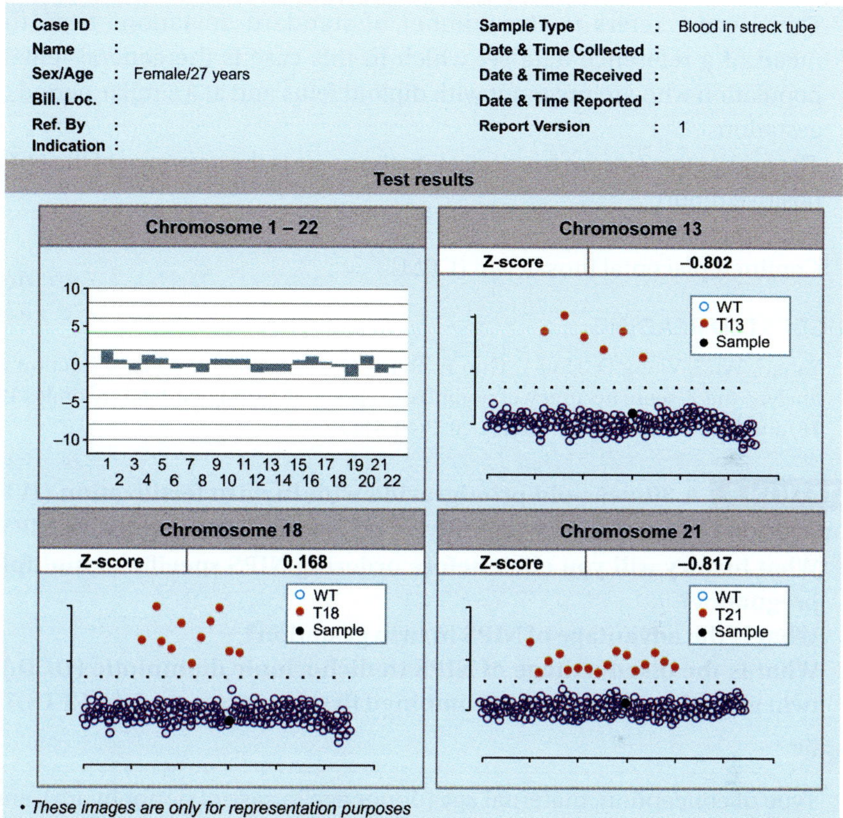

Case ID :		**Sample Type** :	Blood in streck tube
Name :		**Date & Time Collected** :	
Sex/Age :	Female/27 years	**Date & Time Received** :	
Bill. Loc. :		**Date & Time Reported** :	
Ref. By :		**Report Version** :	1
Indication :			

Test results

• *These images are only for representation purposes*

Refer to the above image which is a part of a report of noninvasive prenatal screen.

1. **What do Z-scores denote about the test?**
2. **What is the significance of Z-score in interpreting the report?**
3. **What other parameter should be seen while interpreting the Z scores?**
4. **If in a NIPS report the FF is 30% but the Z-score is only plus 4 points higher than baseline, what is the possible condition?**

Ans.

1. The Z-score refers to the number of standard deviations from the mean of a reference data set which in this case is the general female population who are pregnant with diploid fetus and at a similar period of gestation.
2. The higher the Z-score from baseline the more is the accuracy of the NIPS positive report.
3. Fetal fraction
4. Confined placental mosaicism (CPM)

SUGGESTED READING

1. Yang J, Wu J, Wang D, Hou Y, Guo F, Zhang Q, et al. Combined fetal fraction to analyze the Z-score accuracy of noninvasive prenatal testing for fetal trisomies 13, 18, and 21. J Assist Reprod Genet. 2023;40(4):803-10.

STATION 3. A 30-year-old primigravida with in vitro fertilization (IVF) conception twin gestation wants advice on prenatal screening with NIPS.

1. **What history will you elicit before ordering NIPS specific to multiple pregnancy?**
2. **What is the advantage of NIPS in twin gestation?**
3. **What is the disadvantage of NIPS in dichorionic diamniotic (DCDA) twin gestation compared to combined first trimester screen (CFTS)?**

Ans.

1. Type of conception, maternal age (donor age in case of donor ovum), and gestational age
2. Cell-free DNA (cfDNA) yields the highest detection rates (DRs) and the lowest false-positive rates (FPRs) than other screening tests.
3. Individual twin risk cannot be detected by NIPS in DCDA twin which can be reported in CFTS.

SUGGESTED READING

1. American College of Obstetricians and Gynecologists' Committee on Practice Bulletins-Obstetrics; Committee on Genetics; Society for Maternal-Fetal Medicine. Screening for fetal chromosomal abnormalities: ACOG Practice Bulletin, No. 226. Obstet Gynecol. 2020;136(4):e48-e69.

STATION 4. A 29-year-old primigravida patient was referred to fetal medicine outpatient department (OPD) for consultation at 26 weeks of pregnancy for prenatal genetic counseling. Her NT/nasal bone (NB) was within normal limits and level 2 ultrasound reported no abnormalities.

Her a priori risk was 1:950. She opted for NIPS and the following report was released.

Noninvasive prenatal testing–(NIPT)

NIPT screens a maternal blood sample for chromosomal aneuploidy in fetal DNA using the following methodology:
- Extraction of fetal cell-free DNA from the maternal blood sample
- High throughput sequencing of the extracted fetal cell-free DNA
- Calculation of molecular mass of fetal DNA in all chromosomes

Based on the scope, NIPT can screen the following conditions:
- Whole Genome - 23 pairs of human chromosomes
- Common chromosomal abnormality:
  Trisomy 13 (Patau's syndrome)
  Trisomy 18 (Edward's syndrome)
  Trisomy 21 (Down's syndrome)

NIPT is capable of genome-wide aneuploidy detection of the whole fetal genome (23 pairs of chromosomes). Test results with the inerpretation of risk for Trisomy 13, Trisomy 18, Trisomy 21 and sex chromosome aneuploidies will be provided. This test confers an accuracy of up to 99% on the detection of fetal chromosomal aneuploidy.

Test results summary

Autosomal aneuploidies	Risk	Test results	Aneuploidy risk
Chromosome 13	●	Low risk group	<1/10000
Chromosome 18	●	Low risk group	<1/10000
Chromosome 21	●	Low risk group	<1/10000
Sex chromosome	●	High risk group	<1/20
Other chromosomes	●	Low risk group	–

1. **She asks if NIPS is confirmatory for sex chromosome aneuploidy (SCA), how will you counsel her?**
2. **What should be done to confirm the diagnosis?**
3. **What is the detection rate for trisomy 21 with NIPS since this was a case of high risk for trisomy 21?**

Ans.

1. Positive predictive value (PPV) of NIPS for fetal SCAs is 32%. The PPV of different SCA abnormalities such as 45,X, 47,XXX, 47,XXY, 47,XXY, and 45,Y is 17.5%, 60.0%, 56.5%, 100%, and 0%, respectively.
2. Invasive testing (amniocentesis) for fetal karyotype for confirmation
3. Detection rate for trisomy 21 is >99% with a FPR of 1%.

SUGGESTED READING

1. Lyu Z, Huang C. Systematic analysis of the causes of NIPS sex chromosome aneuploidy false-positive results. Mol Genet Genomic Med. 2022;10(7):e1963.

STATION 5. **A 29-year-old primigravida patient was referred to fetal medicine OPD for consultation at 26 weeks of pregnancy for prenatal genetic counseling. Her level 2 ultrasound showed the following image. Her a priori risk is 1:950.**

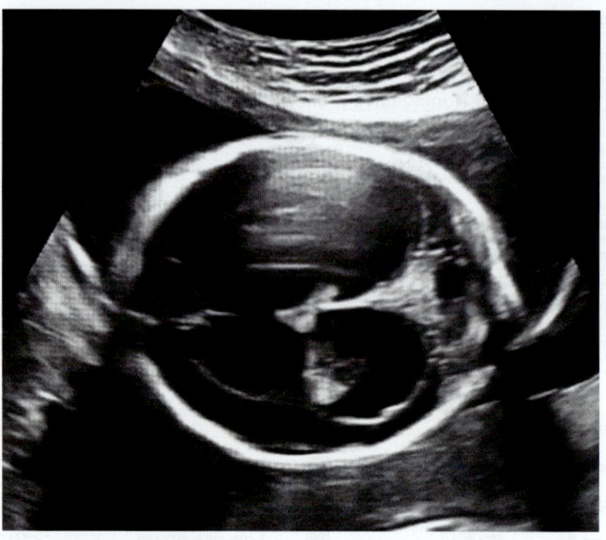

1. **Would you offer her NIPS?**
2. **She got her NIPS done despite counseling which is low risk. Would you offer her invasive testing?**
3. **What are the chromosomal abnormalities that can be detected by NIPS?**

Ans.

1. No, NIPS should not be offered in fetuses with structural abnormalities.
2. Yes, if a fetal structural abnormality is identified, invasive diagnostic testing is indicated after counseling, regardless of a negative NIPS screen result.
3. Aneuploidies of 13, 18, and 21; rare autosomal trisomies (RATs); sex chromosome aneuploidies; microdeletion/microduplication syndromes; and triploidy.

SUGGESTED READING

1. Gregg AR, Skotko BG, Benkendorf JL, Monaghan KG, Bajaj K, Best RG, et al. Noninvasive prenatal screening for fetal aneuploidy, 2016 update: a position statement of the American College of Medical Genetics and Genomics. Genet Med. 2016;18(10):1056-65.

STATION 6. **A 28-year-old primigravida singleton pregnancy at 14 weeks was referred to fetal medicine specialist in view of NIPT report—*no call.***

Case ID	:		Sample Type	: Blood in streck tube
Name	:		Date & Time collected	:
Sex/Age	:	Female/27 years	Date & Time received	:
Bill. Loc.	:		Date & Time reported	:
Ref. By	:		Report version	: 1
Indication	:			

Noninvasive prenatal testing – (NIPT)

Comment	:	The provided blood sample was processed for test but due to low fetal fraction no result can be obtained.
Advise	:	Repeat sample

--------- End of Report ---------

1. **What are the various methods of NIPS?**
2. **What is the failure rate as per the methodology used?**
3. **What are the various causes of "no call" result?**

Ans.

1. • Massive parallel shotgun sequencing (MPSS)
   • Chromosome-selective/targeted sequencing
   • Single nucleotide polymorphism (SNP)-based approach
2. • Massive parallel shotgun sequencing (lowest failure rates of 1.58%)
   • Chromosome-selective/targeted sequencing (3.56% failure rate)
   • SNP-based approach (highest failure rate of 6.39%)
3. Low FF (<4%), obesity (inverse relationship with free fraction), increasing maternal age, maternal chromosomal abnormalities, large chromosomal segments with homozygosity, anticoagulation with low molecular weight heparin (LMWH), twin gestations, IVF, and aneuploidy (any 4).

SUGGESTED READING

1. Gregg AR, Skotko BG, Benkendorf JL, Monaghan KG, Bajaj K, Best RG, et al. Noninvasive prenatal screening for fetal aneuploidy, 2016 update: a position statement of the American College of Medical Genetics and Genomics. Genet Med. 2016;18(10):1056-65.
2. Yaron Y. The implications of noninvasive prenatal testing failures: a review of an under discussed phenomenon. Prenat Diagn. 2016;36(5):391-6.

STATION 7. **For the above patient reason for no call result is mentioned as FF of 3.2%.**

1. **What can be the causes of low FF in NIPS?**
2. **What is the further management for this patient after primary failed NIPS testing?**
3. **As per the American College of Medical Genetics and Genomics (ACMG), why is repeat blood draw not recommended?**

Ans.

1. Advanced maternal age, chromosomal abnormality, obesity, twin gestation, fetal growth restriction, and assisted reproductive technology (any 4)
2. - Offer invasive diagnostic testing without repeating the cfDNA test, as test failure due to low FF itself increases risk of fetal aneuploidy (up to 5%)
   - Detailed level 2 ultrasound
3. Repeat blood draw is not recommended given the marginal rate of increase in cfDNA before 20 weeks' gestation (0.1% per week). There is 40–50% test failure rate from resampling.

SUGGESTED READING

1. Gregg AR, Skotko BG, Benkendorf JL, Monaghan KG, Bajaj K, Best RG, et al. Noninvasive prenatal screening for fetal aneuploidy, 2016 update: a position statement of the American College of Medical Genetics and Genomics. Genet Med. 2016;18(10):1056-65.

STATION 8. A 26-year-old pregnant women with low-risk pregnancy with NIPS suggestive of high risk for Down syndrome.

1. **What is the false-positive rate by NIPT?**
2. **What is the most widely accepted cause of false-positive NIPT?**
3. **Which regulator has issued a warning regarding false-positive result with NIPT?**
4. **What invasive testing will you offer her?**
5. **What are maternal origins of false-positive noninvasive prenatal testing results?**

Ans.

1. 0.13%
2. Confined placental mosaicism
3. The United States Food and Drug Administration (USFDA)
4. Chorionic villus sampling (CVS) and amniocentesis can be offered but amniocentesis would be preferred in view of placental origin for both cfDNA and CVS; hence risk of CPM would be still present with CVS.
5. Maternal mosaicism, leiomyomas, malignancy, organ transplantation, and blood transfusion

SUGGESTED READING

1. Raymond Y, Fernando S, Menezes M, Mol BW, McLennan A, da Silva Costa F, et al. Placental, maternal, fetal, and technical origins of false-positive cell-free DNA screening results. Am J Obstet Gynecol. 2024;230(4):381-9.

STATION 9. **A woman at 13 weeks spontaneous connection undergoes NIPS which is reported as high risk for trisomy 21.**

1. **What is the likelihood that a positive NIPS is true positive?**
2. **If she opts to undergo invasive testing and the report confirms no aneuploidy, then what is the residual risk of chromosomal abnormality?**
3. **What is the likelihood of there being a confined placental mosaicism (CPM) on CVS?**
4. **What should be done in a case of CPM?**

Ans.

1. 90%
2. 2%
3. 1–2%
4. Amniocentesis and karyotyping of fetal DNA

SUGGESTED READING

1. Gil MM, Accurti V, Santacruz B, Plana MN, Nicolaides KH. Analysis of cell-free DNA in maternal blood in screening for aneuploidies: updated meta-analysis. Ultrasound Obstet Gynecol. 2017;50(3):302-14. Update in: Ultrasound Obstet Gynecol. 2019;53(6):734-42.

STATION 10. **The a priori risk for aneuploidy in a woman with singleton pregnancy at 15 weeks gestation is 1 in 100 for trisomy 21. She opts to undergo the targeted imaging for fetal anomalies (TIFFA) scan at 17 weeks. Later at 20 weeks gestation, she also opts for NIPS.**

1. **What will be the final posterior risk for trisomy 21 after a normal anomaly scan?**
2. **How will the final posterior risk for aneuploidy be calculated?**
3. **How much is the risk reduction in trisomy 21, 18, and 13 if no other markers for aneuploidy are present and NIPS is low risk?**
4. **What will be the final posterior risk if after the serum screen risk was 1 in 3 for trisomy 18 and ultrasound was normal?**

Ans.

1. 1 in 33,300
2. The posterior risk of aneuploidy for a given patient can be obtained by multiplying the prior risk with the negative likelihood ratios on ultrasonography.
3. The risks for trisomies 21, 18, and 13 are reduced by a factor of 333, 47, and 100, respectively.
4. 1 in 141

SUGGESTED READING

1. Gil MM, Accurti V, Santacruz B, Plana MN, Nicolaides KH. Analysis of cell-free DNA in maternal blood in screening for aneuploidies: updated meta-analysis. Ultrasound Obstet Gynecol. 2017;50(3):302-14. Update in: Ultrasound Obstet Gynecol. 2019;53(6):734-42.

STATION 11. **Mrs XY, a 28-year-old lady, G2P1L1A0, conceived by IVF. She visited hospital at 12 weeks. NT/NB scan was done and reported normal. She opted for noninvasive prenatal screening. But after 10 days, this was the report.**

Fetal fraction 2%		
Chromosomal abnormality	*Risk*	*Z-score*
Trisomy 21	N/A	–
Trisomy 13	N/A	–
Trisomy 18	N/A	–
Sex chromosomal abnormality	N/A	–
Test failure		

1. **What could be the reason for test failure in this case?**
2. **What is the criterion for low FF?**
3. **Mention three causes for low FF in IVF conception?**
4. **If she opts for redrawing, what is the rate of increase in FF per day in first trimester and second trimester?**

Ans.

1. Due to low FF
2. <4%
3. Theories suggest:
   a. Small placental mass in IVF pregnancies
   b. Increased maternal cfDNA due to increased inflammation and cellular damage
   c. Increase BMI in women conceiving with IVF
4. From 10 to 12.5 weeks of gestation, FF increased by 0.44% per week; from 12.5 and 20 weeks of gestation, it increased at a rate of 0.083% per week; and after approximately 20 weeks, FF increased steadily at a rate of 0.821%.

SUGGESTED READING

1. Deng C, Liu S. Factors Affecting the Fetal Fraction in Noninvasive Prenatal Screening: A Review. Front Pediatr. 2022;10:812781.
2. Kamath V, Chacko MP, Kamath MS. Non-invasive Prenatal Testing in Pregnancies Following Assisted Reproduction. Curr Genomics. 2022;23(5):326-36.

STATION 12. **Mrs AB, a 39-year-old lady, G1P0A0, conceived by IVF with donor ova. She had normal NT/NB scan at 12 weeks and had intermediate risk for trisomy 21 (1:450) and low risk for trisomies 13/18. The dual report showed maternal age of 39 years. She was counseled and opted to undergo noninvasive prenatal screening. Her NIPS is low risk for trisomy 13/18/21 and sex chromosomes.**

1. **Whose age is to be mentioned in dual report in case of IVF pregnancy with donor ova?**
2. **In case of donor ova, which NIPS technique should be used (MPSS or SNP-based)?**
3. **Mention two other parameters to be looked in the NIPS report along with aneuploidy risk?**
4. **What is the relation of Z-score with aneuploidy risk?**

Ans.

1. Age of donor
2. In case of donor ovum pregnancies, MPSS should be used. SNP-based technique is not routinely used.
3. Fetal fraction and Z-scores for aneuploidies should also be seen.
4. Higher Z-score in case of high risk for any aneuploidy has more PPV.

SUGGESTED READING

1. Lee TJ, Rolnik DL, Menezes MA, McLennan AC, da Silva Costa F. Cell-free fetal DNA testing in singleton IVF conceptions. Hum Reprod. 2018;33(4):572-8.

STATION 13. **A 39-year-old patient, G2A1, comes with IVF conception (self-egg) at 13 weeks for NT/NB scan which showed twin gestation with one live fetus with crown-rump length (CRL) corresponding to 13 weeks with normal NT/NB scan and other fetus with CRL corresponding to 9 weeks with no cardiac activity.**

1. **What is this phenomenon known as?**
2. **Can we offer combined screening to this patient?**
3. **On what basis, the risk is calculated in first trimester?**
4. **Her early anomaly scan at 17 weeks was normal and other sac showed vanishing twin with fetal pole. Will you now offer screening test or invasive diagnostic test in view of advanced maternal age?**

Ans.

1. Vanishing twin pregnancy
2. No. In case of vanishing twin with fetal pole, biochemical screening can be false positive due the possibility of aneuploidy in the vanished twin.
3. The risk is calculated on the basis of first trimester scan markers like NT/NB/DV/TV flow.

4. In view of advanced maternal age, the option of amniocentesis should be discussed. As her anomaly scan is normal and fetal pole is still present, again biochemical screening/NIPS cannot be done.

SUGGESTED READING

1. D'Antonio F, Khalil A. Screening and diagnosis of chromosomal abnormalities in twin pregnancy. Best Pract Res Clin Obstet Gynaecol. 2022;84:229-39.

STATION 14. A 23-year-old patient, G1P0, visited at 7 weeks for early pregnancy scan. Her scan showed two gestational sacs with one showing live fetus with CRL of 7 weeks and other sac showed a tiny fetal pole with no cardiac activity. She was again called at 13 weeks for NT/NB scan. The scan showed a live fetus with CRL corresponding to 13 weeks 3 days with normal NT of 1.8 mm and NB seen and other sac with a small fetal pole.

1. **Which screening test should be advised for her at present gestation?**
2. **What happens to biochemical markers [pregnancy-associated plasma protein A (PAPA-A) and β-human chorionic gonadotropin (β-hCG)] in first trimester in presence of vanishing twin?**
3. **For how long approximately the fetal DNA is present after fetal demise?**

Ans.

1. At present, only NT/NB-based screening can be offered to her.
2. There is not so much change in β-hCG, however, levels of PAPP-A may significantly increase.
3. Cell-free fetal DNA mostly seen up to 8 weeks, however, it may be present as long as 15 weeks.

SUGGESTED READING

1. Lee DR, Lee S, Lee SJ. The effect of a vanishing twin on first- and second-trimester maternal serum markers and ultrasound screening for aneuploidy. Obstet Gynecol Sci. 2023;66(6):477-83.
2. Spencer K, Staboulidou I, Nicolaides KH. First trimester aneuploidy screening in the presence of a vanishing twin: implications for maternal serum markers. Prenat Diagn. 2010;30(3):235-40.

STATION 15. A 28-year-old pregnant patient with twin gestation with NT/NB showing fetus A with CRL corresponding to 13 weeks, NT 1.6 mm and NB seen and fetus B with CRL corresponding to 13 weeks 2 days, NT 1.2 mm and NB seen.

1. **What two options of aneuploidy screening will you discuss with her at this gestation?**
2. **She opted for NIPS, and it showed high risk for trisomy 21 in fetus A and low risk for fetus B. Will you do amniocentesis for confirmation only for fetus A or both the fetuses? And why?**

Ans.

1. Combined screening and NIPS.
2. We will test both the fetuses A as well as B, as NIPS cannot differentiate between the twins.

SUGGESTED READING

1. Palomaki GE, Chiu RWK, Pertile MD, Sistermans EA, Yaron Y, Vermeesch JR, et al. International Society for Prenatal Diagnosis Position Statement: cell free (cf) DNA screening for Down syndrome in multiple pregnancies. Prenat Diagn. 2021;41(10):1222-32.

STATION 16. A 38-year-old pregnant patient, spontaneous conception, with monochorionic diamniotic (MCDA) twins with fetus A with CRL of 12 weeks and fetus B with CRL of 12 weeks 2 days, with normal NT/NB for both fetuses.

1. **Can NIPS be done for MCDA twin gestation?**
2. **What is the failure rate of NIPS in case of twin gestation?**
3. **She went ahead with NIPS, however, there was no call for this test. What could be the reason for this?**

Ans.

1. Yes, NIPS can be done for both DCDA/MCDA types of twins.
2. Failure rate in case of twins is higher as compared to singleton, up to 2–13%, mean of 3.4%.
3. Low FF in case of twins. Although the FF is higher as compared to singleton pregnancy; however, the increase in FF is not just double and per fetus fraction is sometimes less compared to singleton.

SUGGESTED READING

1. Palomaki GE, Chiu RWK, Pertile MD, Sistermans EA, Yaron Y, Vermeesch JR, et al. International Society for Prenatal Diagnosis Position Statement: cell free (cf)DNA screening for Down syndrome in multiple pregnancies. Prenat Diagn. 2021;41(10):1222-32.

STATION 17.

Fetal fraction		*12.9%*	
Result details: aneuploidies (Basic)			
Chromosome tested	*Aneuploidy*	*LLR score (Trisomy)*	*High risk LLR cut-off (Trisomy)*
Chromosome 21	Low risk	–31.06	≥2.5
Chromosome 18	Low risk	–49.1	≥3
Chromosome 13	Low risk	–41.23	≥3
Sex chromosomal aneuploidies	High risk for XXX		

A young 24-year-old primigravida gravies with normal NT/NB scan opted for NIPS. Her NIPS result showed low risk for T21/13/18 and high risk for sex chromosomal aneuploidy.

1. **Write three sex chromosomal abnormalities which can be detected by NIPS.**
2. **What is the detection rate and PPV for sex chromosomal aneuploidies?**
3. **Reasons for low PPV for monosomy X?**

Ans.

1. Turner (monosomy X), Klinefelter syndrome (XXY), XXX, and XYY syndrome.
2. Overall detection rate for any SCA is around 99.6%. The PPVs for NIPS is around 29.5% for 45,X, 54% for XXX, 74% for XXY, and 74.5% for XYY.
3. PPV for 45,X may be lower due to:
    a. Higher rates of placental mosaicism for monosomy X
    b. Maternal mosaicism for 45,X

SUGGESTED READING

1. Dungan JS, Klugman S, Darilek S, Malinowski J, Akkari YMN, Monaghan KG, et al. Noninvasive prenatal screening (NIPS) for fetal chromosome abnormalities in a general-risk population: An evidence-based clinical guideline of the American College of Medical Genetics and Genomics (ACMG). Genet Med. 2023;25(2):100336. Erratum in: Genet Med. 2023;25(8):100874.

STATION 18. Regarding various technologies in NIPS.

1. **Name three different types of technologies used in NIPS?**
2. **Name three conditions where SNP-based technology cannot be used?**

Ans.

1. Different technologies include:
    a. Whole genome sequencing by MPSS
    b. Targeted sequencing by:
        i. SNP-based
        ii. Rolling circle amplification NIPT technology
        iii. Target capture sequences (TACS) using long DNA probes
2. Cannot be used in (1) egg donation, (2) surrogate pregnancies, and (3) consanguinity.

SUGGESTED READING

1. Kypri E, Ioannides M, Achilleos A, Koumbaris G, Patsalis P, Stumm M. Non-invasive prenatal screening tests – update 2022. J Lab Med. 2022;46(4):311-20.

STATION 19. **A 35-year-old primigravida visits at 11 weeks 3 days. Her NT/NB scan was normal. She did not do any combined screening. She did her NIPS and the result shows trisomy 16.**

1. **What is the probable cause for trisomy 16?**
2. **Will you do CVS or amnio to confirm the diagnosis?**
3. **Which microdeletions have been recently recommended by ACMG to be screened by NIPS?**

Ans.

1. Mostly due to CPM
2. Amnio will be done to confirm the diagnosis in fetus.
3. ACMG has recently advocated the screening for 22q11del syndrome by NIPS as it is quite common and variable phenotypes.

SUGGESTED READING

1. Dungan JS, Klugman S, Darilek S, Malinowski J, Akkari YMN, Monaghan KG, et al. Noninvasive prenatal screening (NIPS) for fetal chromosome abnormalities in a general-risk population: An evidence-based clinical guideline of the American College of Medical Genetics and Genomics (ACMG). Genet Med. 2023;25(2):100336. Erratum in: Genet Med. 2023;25(8):100874.

STATION 20.

Fetal fraction		*11.3%*	
Result details: aneuploidies (Basic)			
Chromosome tested	*Aneuploidy*	*LLR score (Trisomy)*	*High risk LLR cut-off (Trisomy)*
Chromosome 21	Low risk	–19.27	≥2.5
Chromosome 18	High risk for trisomy 18	340	≥3
Chromosome 13	Low risk	–24.14	≥3
Sex chromosomal aneuploidies	Low risk		

A 37-year-old primigravida patient visited at 13 weeks with normal NT/NB scan. Her NIPS was done which revealed high risk for trisomy 18. Her early scan revealed structurally normal fetus and thick globular placenta.

1. **What could be the two reasons for high risk for trisomy 18?**
2. **In structurally normal fetus, what is the probability that the fetus is actually affected with trisomy 18?**

3. Amniotic fluid analysis showed normal chromosomes, however fetus developed early-onset fetal growth restriction (FGR) at 24 weeks. How would you confirm the CPM?

Ans.

1. Reasons for high-risk trisomy 18:
    - Confined placental mosaicism
    - Fetus with trisomy 18
2. In structurally normal fetus, very low probability of trisomy 18 in fetus.
3. Confined placental mosaicism can be confirmed by placental biopsy followed by fluorescence in situ hybridization (FISH) to confirm trisomy 18 mosaicism.

SUGGESTED READING

1. Cao P, Bui HV, Tran LPG, Nguyen OT, Giang H, Tran N. May a positive non-invasive prenatal testing alarm a confined placental mosaicism in FGR pregnancies?. Ultrasound Obstet Gynecol. 2020;56:183-3.
2. Raymond Y, Fernando S, Menezes M, Mol BW, McLennan A, da Silva Costa F, et al. Placental, maternal, fetal, and technical origins of false-positive cell-free DNA screening results. Am J Obstet Gynecol. 2024;230(4):381-9.

CHAPTER 5

Screening in Multifetal Gestations

Seetha Ramamurthy Pal

STATION 1.

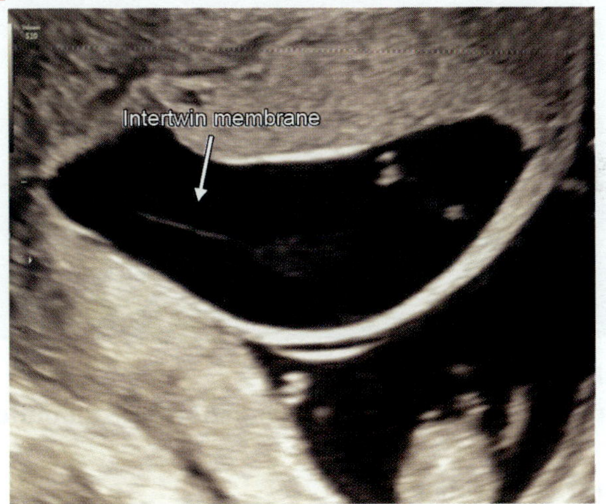

1. **Identify the type of triplets.**
2. **Can a combined first trimester screening be offered?**
3. **What is the best method of screening?**

Ans.

1. Dichorionic triamniotic triplets
2. No. Though the risk of aneuploidy in a trizygotic triplet is higher than in singleton or dizygotic pregnancies, serum screening is not validated in both trichorionic triamniotic triplets and dichorionic triamniotic triplets.
3. Nuchal translucency (NT)-based screening with maternal age is the best option.

SUGGESTED READING

1. Gibson JL, Castleman JS, Meher S, Kilby MD. Updated guidance for the management of twin and triplet pregnancies from the National Institute

for Health and Care Excellence guidance, UK: What's new that may improve perinatal outcomes? Acta Obstet Gynecol Scand. 2020;99(2):147-52.
2. Kim M, Oh J, Kim H, Lee S, Park C, Park J, et al. Performance of Down's syndrome screening in triplet pregnancy with combination of maternal age and nuchal translucency. Ultrasound Obstet Gynaecol. 2016;48(S1):107.

STATION 2.

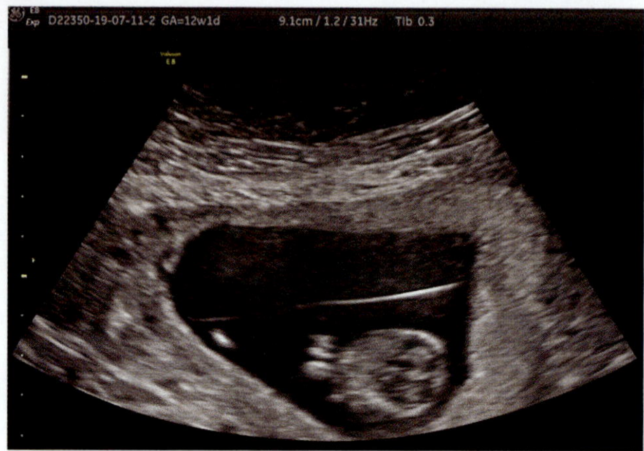

1. **What is the type of placentation?**
2. **What is the risk of T21 in each monochorionic diamniotic (MCDA) twins?**
3. **How is the risk calculated?**
4. **What is the sensitivity of combined first trimester screening (FTS) in MCDA twins?**

Ans.

1. MCDA twins
2. The risk of trisomy 21 is calculated per pregnancy because the twins share the same karyotype.
3. Risk is calculated by taking the average of NT of both the fetuses and average of the calculated risk.
4. 87% for a false positive rate (FPR) of 5%

SUGGESTED READING

1. Khalil A, Sotiriadis A, Baschat A, Bhide A, Gratacós E, Hecher K, et al. ISUOG Practice Guidelines (updated): role of ultrasound in twin pregnancy. Ultrasound Obstet Gynecol. 2025;65(2):253-76.

STATION 3.

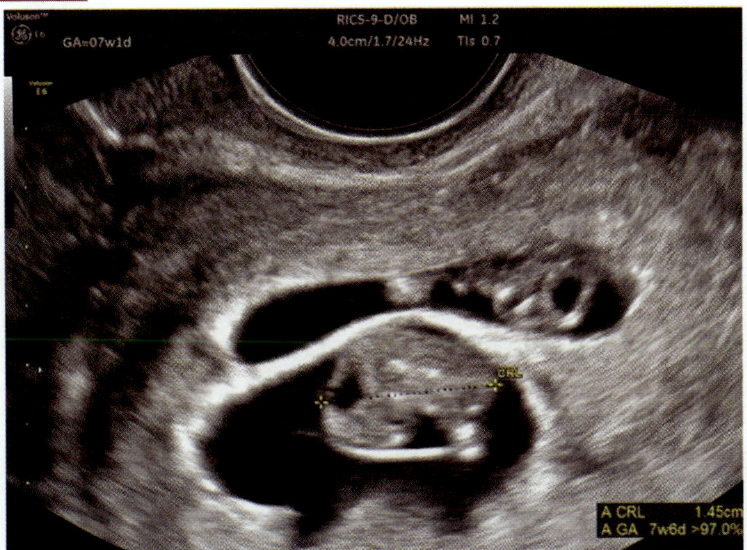

1. **Identify the type of placentation.**
2. **Sensitivity of combined first trimester screening (CFTS) in such twins.**
3. **What is the aneuploidy risk in each of the twins?**
4. **How is the risk calculated?**

Ans.

1. Dichorionic diamniotic (DCDA) placentation
2. 86% for FPR of 5%
3. In dizygotic twins the maternal age-related risk for chromosomal abnormalities for each fetus is the same as in singleton pregnancies. Therefore, in a woman with dichorionic twins the chance that at least one fetus is affected by a chromosomal defect is twice as high as in singleton pregnancies.
4. The risk is calculated per fetus as 90% of them are dizygotic, so have different karyotypes.

SUGGESTED READING

1. Khalil A, Sotiriadis A, Baschat A, Bhide A, Gratacós E, Hecher K, et al. ISUOG Practice Guidelines (updated): role of ultrasound in twin pregnancy. Ultrasound Obstet Gynecol. 2025;65(2):253-76.
2. The Fetal Medicine Foundation, the 11–13 weeks scan/education.

STATION 4.

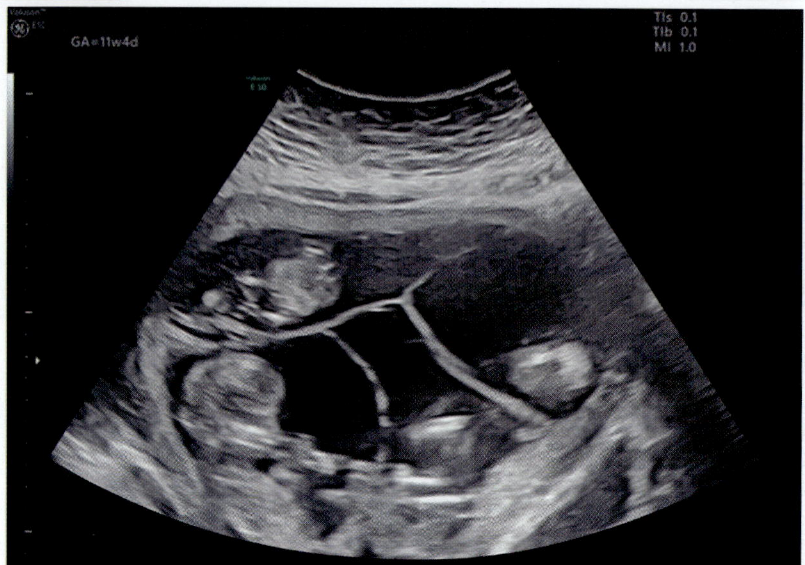

1. **How is labelling of fetuses done in multiple pregnancies?**
2. **Can CFTS be offered in higher order multiples?**
3. **Can noninvasive prenatal screening (NIPS) be offered in higher order multiples?**
4. **What type of screening can be offered in higher order multiples?**

Ans.

1. Labelling of fetuses is done in an anticlockwise fashion with the fetus near the os as twin A. Labelling should be a descriptive one, based on lateral or vertical orientation of the gestational sac, placental site (if relevant) and cord insertions of each fetus.
2. CFTS cannot be offered in higher order multiples as there is no study validating the role of serum screening in higher order multiples.
3. No, NIPS is also not validated for higher order multiple pregnancies.
4. Screening in higher order multiples is usually by maternal age combined with ultrasound markers such as NT.

SUGGESTED READING

1. Odibo AO, Lawrence-Cleary K, Macones GA. Screening for aneuploidy in twins and higher-order multiples: is first-trimester nuchal translucency the solution? Obstet Gynecol Surv. 2003;58(9):609-14.

STATION 5. A 28-year-old primigravida, conceived with IVF with DCDA twins, comes for CFTS. The scan shows discordant NT with NT >95th centile in one twin.

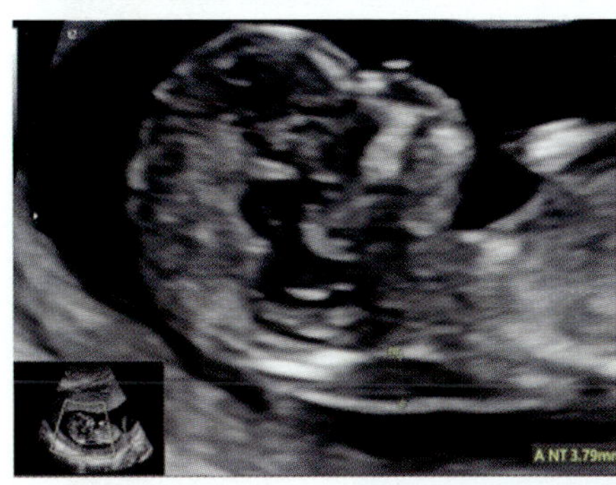
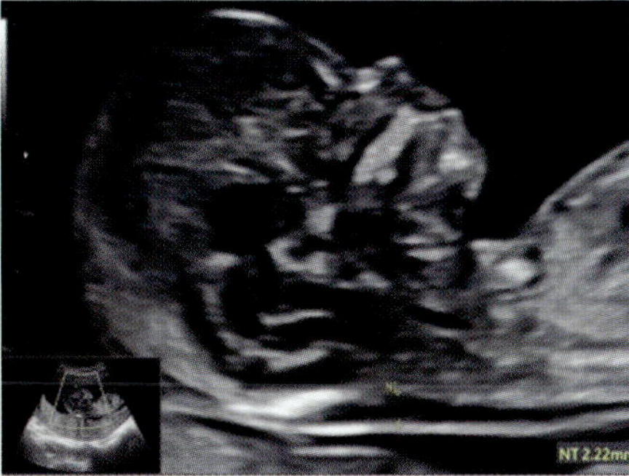

1. **How is NT discordance defined as?**
2. **What are the implications of discordant NT in DCDA twins?**
3. **What are the implications of discordant NT in MCDA twins?**
4. **What is the sensitivity of discordant NT in predicting twin-to-twin transfusion syndrome (TTTS) in MCDA twins?**
5. **Can non-invasive prenatal testing (NIPT) be offered?**

Ans.

1. Nuchal translucency discordance is commonly defined as a discrepancy in NT of at 20% between the two fetuses.
2. In DC twin pregnancies with no major fetal abnormalities, the incidence of NT ≥95th percentile in one or both fetuses is associated with increased risk of aneuploidy in that particular fetus.
3. The finding in one or both fetuses of NT ≥95th percentile, and more so NT >99th percentile, is associated with a 10% increased risk of fetal loss or need for endoscopic laser surgery at <20 weeks' gestation.
4. Discordance in NT of ≥20% is found in around 25% of monochorionic twins and has <50% sensitivity for predicting TTTS.
5. NIPT should not be offered in the presence of increased NT. Ideally invasive testing of both fetuses is recommended to rule out aneuploidy or genetic syndromes.

SUGGESTED READING

1. Cimpoca B, Syngelaki A, Litwinska E, Muzaferovic A, Nicolaides KH. Increased nuchal translucency at 11-13 weeks' gestation and outcome in twin pregnancy. Ultrasound Obstet Gynecol. 2020;55(3):318-25.

STATION 6. **Shown below is the NIPS report of a primigravida with DCDA twins.**

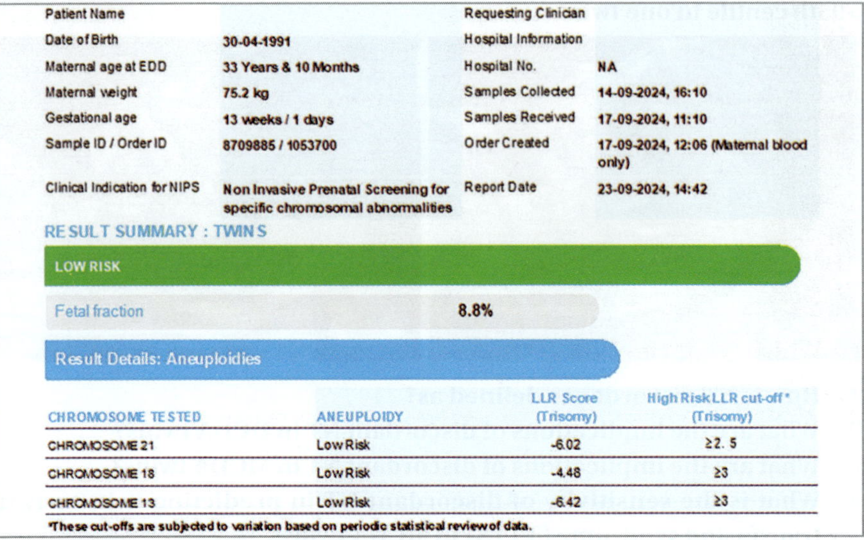

Patient Name		Requesting Clinician	
Date of Birth	30-04-1991	Hospital Information	
Maternal age at EDD	33 Years & 10 Months	Hospital No.	NA
Maternal weight	75.2 kg	Samples Collected	14-09-2024, 16:10
Gestational age	13 weeks / 1 days	Samples Received	17-09-2024, 11:10
Sample ID / Order ID	8709885 / 1053700	Order Created	17-09-2024, 12:06 (Maternal blood only)
Clinical Indication for NIPS	Non Invasive Prenatal Screening for specific chromosomal abnormalities	Report Date	23-09-2024, 14:42

RESULT SUMMARY : TWINS

LOW RISK

Fetal fraction 8.8%

Result Details: Aneuploidies

CHROMOSOME TESTED	ANEUPLOIDY	LLR Score (Trisomy)	High Risk LLR cut-off* (Trisomy)
CHROMOSOME 21	Low Risk	-6.02	≥2. 5
CHROMOSOME 18	Low Risk	-4.48	≥3
CHROMOSOME 13	Low Risk	-6.42	≥3

*These cut-offs are subjected to variation based on periodic statistical review of data.

1. **What is the sensitivity of NIPT in twins?**
2. **Can we use NIPT in twins discordant for fetal anomaly or NT?**
3. **What is the limitation of NIPT in twins?**

Ans.

1. Overall sensitivity of NIPS in twins is 95%.
2. No. As a general rule, NIPS should never be done in the presence of a fetal structural anomaly or NT >95th centile.
3. Screen positive needs invasive testing from both the fetuses as NIPS does not identify which fetus is at risk.

SUGGESTED READING

1. Gil MM, Galeva S, Jani J, Konstantinidou L, Akolekar R, Plana MN et al. Screening for trisomies by cfDNA testing of maternal blood in twin pregnancy: update of The Fetal Medicine Foundation results and meta-analysis. Ultrasound Obstet Gynecol. 2019;53:734-42.
2. Khalil A, Archer R, Hutchinson V, Mousa HA, Johnstone ED, Cameron MJ, et al. Noninvasive prenatal screening in twin pregnancies with cell-free DNA using the IONA test: a prospective multicenter study. Am J Obstet Gynecol. 2021; 225(1).

STATION 7. **A 28-year-old DCDA twins with early embryonic demise of one twin.**

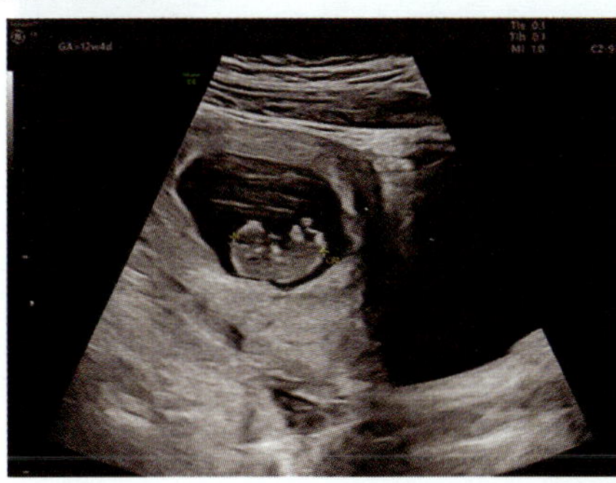
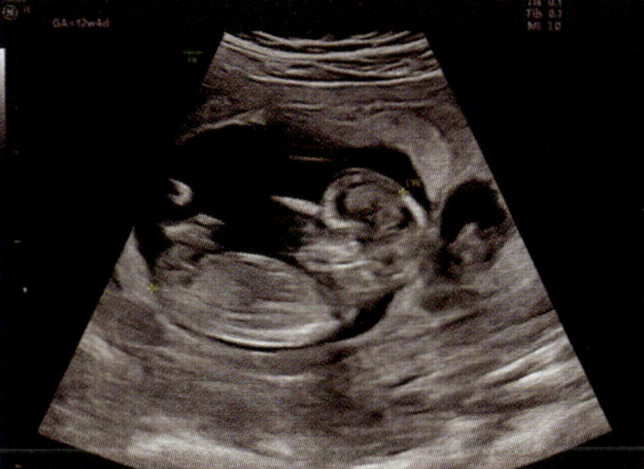

1. **Which serum marker gets affected in a vanishing twin?**
2. **What is the ideal method of screening in vanishing twin?**
3. **What is the minimum interval beyond which serum screening can be done?**
4. **Vanishing twin in cases of MCDA twins can be sign of future_________.**

Ans.

1. Pregnancy-associated plasma protein-A (PAPP-A). PAPP-A multiples of the median (MoM) are higher both in the group with an empty gestational sac and in those with a dead embryo; in the latter group, the effect of a vanishing twin on PAPP-A MoM is larger the closer the demise of the twin is to blood sampling.
2. First-trimester screening for trisomy in pregnancies with a vanishing twin should rely on a combination of maternal age, fetal nuchal translucency thickness only or with serum free beta-human chorionic gonadotropin (β-hCG), without the use of serum PAPP-A.
3. Minimum interval is 14 weeks.
4. Twin reversed arterial perfusion (TRAP) sequence

SUGGESTED READING

1. Chaveeva P, Wright A, Syngelaki A, Konstantinidou L, Wright D, Nicolaides KH. First-trimester screening for trisomies in pregnancies with vanishing twin. Ultrasound Obstet Gynecol. 2020;55(3):326-31.

STATION 8. **A 35-year-old woman, conceived on intrauterine insemination (IUI) with DCDA twins with USG findings of twin A at CFTS screening.**

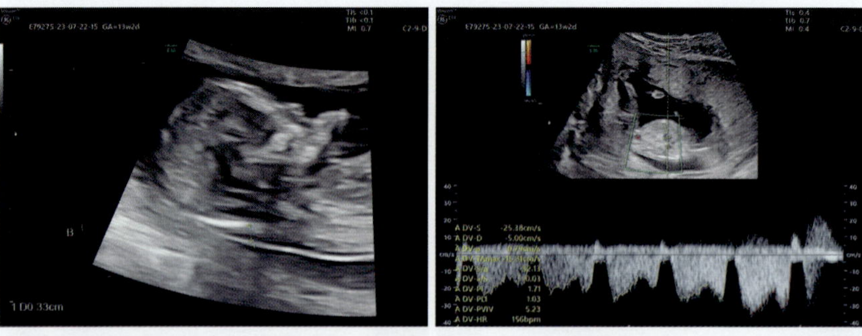

1. **Describe the ultrasound findings?**
2. **What is the next step?**
3. **Which invasive test is preferred in DCDA twins?**
4. **What is the most essential step before invasives in multiple pregnancy?**

Ans.

1. Increased NT, hypoplastic NB, and "a" wave reversal in ductus venosus in one twin.
2. Ideally invasive testing should be the next step.
3. Both chorionic villus sampling (CVS) and amniocentesis can be done; however CVS has the advantage of providing early results.
4. The most essential step before an invasive procedure is correct mapping and labelling of the fetuses using as many details as possible.

SUGGESTED READING

1. Khalil A, Sotiriadis A, Baschat A, Bhide A, Gratacós E, Hecher K, et al. ISUOG Practice Guidelines (updated): role of ultrasound in twin pregnancy. Ultrasound Obstet Gynecol. 2025;65(2):253-76.

STATION 9.

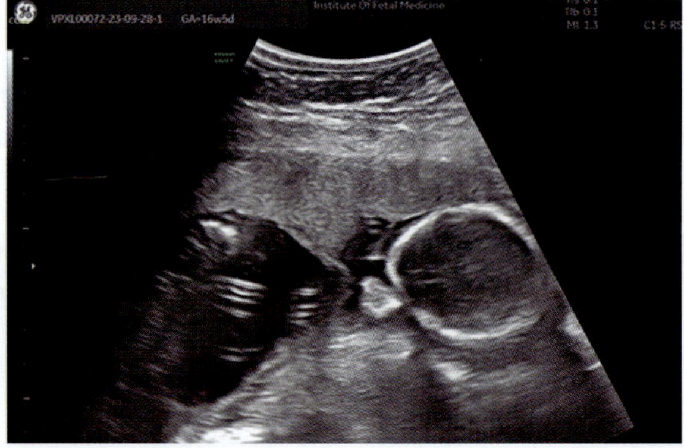

1. **What is the recommended method to perform invasives in twins?**
2. **Which is better—two puncture technique or single puncture technique?**
3. **What is the risk of fetal loss for invasives in multiple pregnancy?**

Ans.

1. Regarding invasives in multiple pregnancy, sampling of both the sacs is recommended. In MCDA twins, if fetal growth and anatomy are concordant, single sac sampling can be done.
2. Generally, two-puncture technique is preferred.
   With two-puncture technique there is a small risk of sampling same sac twice and with single-puncture technique, there is a risk of inadvertent amniotomy of the intertwin membrane. The risk of fetal loss has not been shown to be increased with the two-puncture compared with the single-puncture technique.
3. 2% risk of fetal loss. No increase in risk over baseline risk.

SUGGESTED READING

1. Di Mascio D, Khalil A, Rizzo G, Buca D, Liberati M, Martellucci CA, et al. Risk of fetal loss following amniocentesis or chorionic villus sampling in twin pregnancy: systematic review and meta-analysis. Ultrasound Obstet Gynecol. 2020;56(5):647-55.

STATION 10. **Attached is the quantitative fluorescent polymerase chain reaction (QF-PCR) report following amniocentesis of DCDA twins with NT >95th centile in one fetus.**

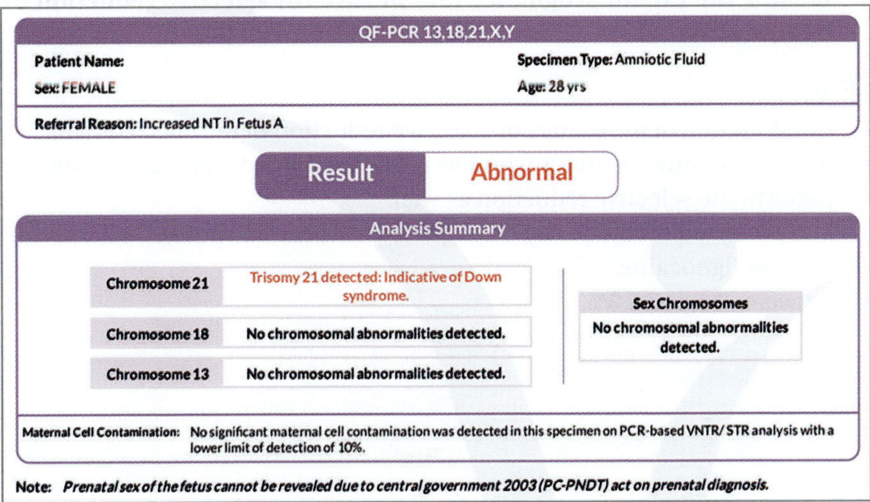

QF-PCR 13,18,21,X,Y

Patient Name:
Specimen Type: Amniotic Fluid
Sex: FEMALE
Age: 28 yrs

Referral Reason: Increased NT in Fetus A

Result Abnormal

Analysis Summary

Chromosome 21	Trisomy 21 detected: Indicative of Down syndrome.
Chromosome 18	No chromosomal abnormalities detected.
Chromosome 13	No chromosomal abnormalities detected.

Sex Chromosomes
No chromosomal abnormalities detected.

Maternal Cell Contamination: No significant maternal cell contamination was detected in this specimen on PCR-based VNTR/ STR analysis with a lower limit of detection of 10%.

Note: *Prenatal sex of the fetus cannot be revealed due to central government 2003 (PC-PNDT) act on prenatal diagnosis.*

ABOUT THIS TEST:

Prenatal Aneuploidy Test evaluates genetic information in the sample (amniotic fluid/CVS/POC) provided, to detect aneuploidy of chromosomes 13, 18, 21, X or Y. This test does not detect other chromosomal or structural anomalies. Low level mosaicism involving chromosomes 13, 18, 21 X or Y may not be detected by this procedure.

PRENATAL ANEUPLOIDY TEST REPORT			
Patient Name	Fetus of	Order ID/Sample ID	722468/8100240
Gender	NK	Sample Type	Amniotic fluid
Maternal Age	28 Years	Date and Time of Samples Receipt	15.08.2023 15:30
Mother's Sample ID	8100242	Order Booked Date and Time	16.08.2023 13:16
Referring Clinician		Date of report Generation	**21.08.2023**

CLINICAL DIAGNOSIS / SYMPTOMS / HISTORY

The subject (Fetus B) is being tested for common chromosomal abnormalities by QF-PCR analysis. The antenatal findings revealed (DCDA twins), Twin A with increased nuchal translucency (>95th centile) and absent nasal bone.

REPORT SUMMARY

No aneuploidy detected in Chromosomes 21, 18, 13 and sex chromosomes

Condition Tested	Result	Interpretation:
TRISOMY 21	No aneuploidy detected.	Results are consistent with two copies of chromosomes 21,18, 13 and two sex chromosomes. The Amniotic fluid is not contaminated with maternal cells/tissues. Note : No maternal alleles (markers) were found in the fetal genotype at 11 loci which is consistent with either egg donor or surrogate pregnancy. A detailed history and clinical correlation are recommended.
TRISOMY 18	No aneuploidy detected.	
TRISOMY 13	No aneuploidy detected.	
Sex Chromosomes	No aneuploidy detected.	

Testing method:

DNA is isolated from amniotic fluid/CVS/POC and using Devyser Compact v3 kit the markers specific to the chromosomes 13, 18, 21, X and Y are amplified. The amplified markers are then subjected to capillary electrophoresis. The data is analysed using GeneMapper TM (Thermofisher) and interpreted to determine aneuploidy of fetus for specific chromosomes.

1. **What are the further options?**
2. **What is the most essential part of selective reduction following invasive testing?**
3. **What is the preferred method of selective reduction in DCDA twins?**
4. **What is the rate of pregnancy loss in cases of selective reduction in DCDA twins?**

Ans.

1. Continuation of pregnancy or selective reduction of the affected twin.
2. Ideally the same operator who has performed the diagnostic test should perform the selective reduction as well.
3. The preferred method is by USG-guided intracardiac potassium chloride (KCl) or lignocaine.
4. Between 2.1 and 5.8%.

SUGGESTED READING

1. Beriwal S, Impey L, Ioannou C. Multifetal pregnancy reduction and selective termination. Obstet Gynaecol. 2020;22(4):284-92.

STATION 11. A 38-year-old P1 + 0, conceived spontaneously with MCDA twins with one twin with signs of acrania.

1. **What are the further options?**
2. **What is the best method of termination in MCDA twins?**
3. **Why cannot KCl be used for selective reduction in MCDA twins?**
4. **What are the complications that can happen?**

Ans.

1. Selective reduction of the affected twin. For conditions that are lethal and carry a high risk of intrauterine demise, selective reduction of the affected twin should be done to protect the healthy cotwin against the adverse effects of spontaneous demise of the other.
2. Selective fetal reduction can be done by bipolar cord coagulation, radiofrequency ablation or intrafetal laser ablation.
3. Injection of KCl in the affected twin can cause demise of the surviving twin due to the presence of vascular anastomosis between the twins.
4. In MCDA twins, fetal loss is higher when the procedure is performed before 18 weeks of gestation. The overall survival is higher with bipolar cord coagulation (BCC) [BCC 84% vs. radiofrequency ablation (RFA) 73%], but the incidence of preterm premature rupture of membranes (PPROM) is lower with RFA.

SUGGESTED READING

1. Beriwal S, Impey L, Ioannou C. Multifetal pregnancy reduction and selective termination. Obstet Gynaecol. 2020;22(4):284-92.

STATION 12. A 28-year-old primigravida, conceived by in vitro fertilization and embryo transfer (IVF-ET) and DCDA twins has come with a quadruple screening report at 17 weeks which shows high risk of T21 in one twin.

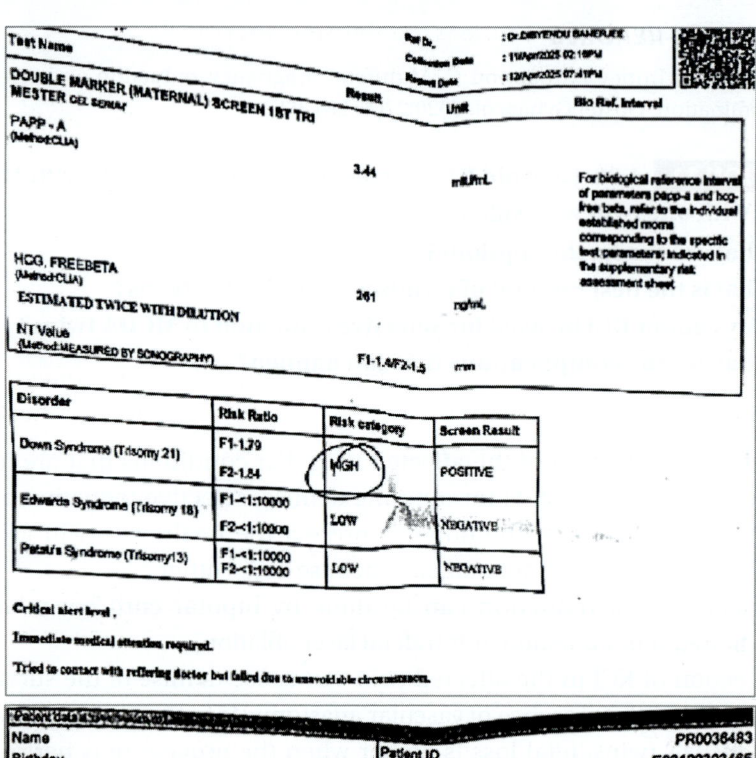

Ref Dr. : Dr. DIBYENDU BANERJEE
Collection Date : 11/Apr/2025 02:18PM
Report Date : 12/Apr/2025 07:41PM

Test Name	Result	Unit	Bio Ref. Interval
DOUBLE MARKER (MATERNAL) SCREEN 1ST TRIMESTER GEL SERUM			
PAPP - A (Method:CLIA)	3.44	mIU/mL	For biological reference interval of parameters papp-a and hcg-free beta, refer to the individual established moms corresponding to the specific test parameters; indicated in the supplementary risk assessment sheet
HCG, FREEBETA (Method:CLIA) ESTIMATED TWICE WITH DILUTION	261	ng/mL	
NT Value (Method:MEASURED BY SONOGRAPHY)	F1-1.4/F2-1.5	mm	

Disorder	Risk Ratio	Risk category	Screen Result
Down Syndrome (Trisomy 21)	F1-1.79 F2-1.84	HIGH	POSITIVE
Edwards Syndrome (Trisomy 18)	F1-<1:10000 F2-<1:10000	LOW	NEGATIVE
Patau's Syndrome (Trisomy13)	F1-<1:10000 F2-<1:10000	LOW	NEGATIVE

Critical alert level .

Immediate medical attention required.

Tried to contact with reffering doctor but failed due to unavoidable circumstances.

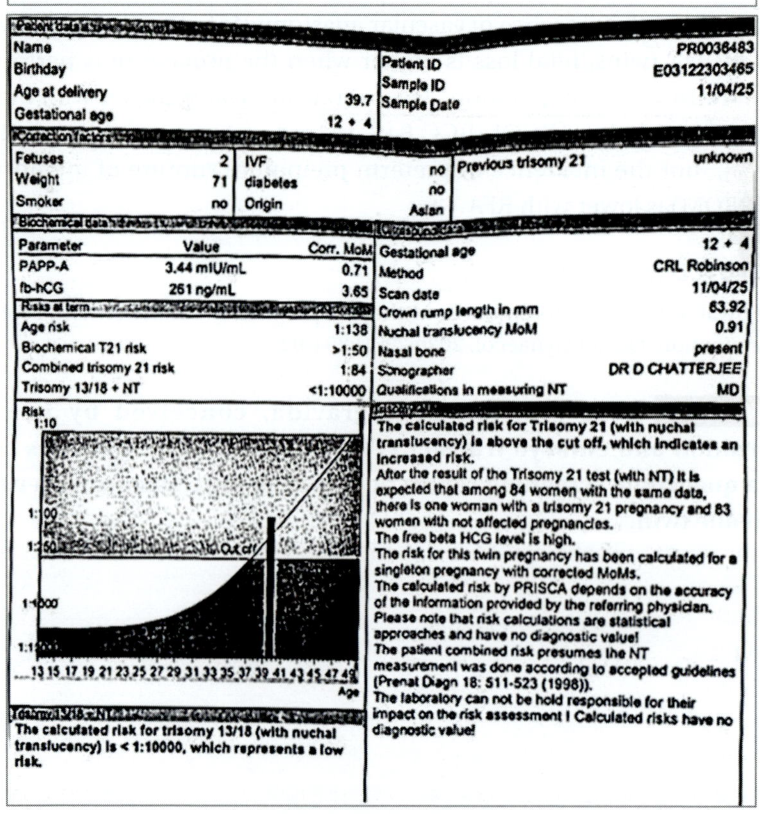

Patient data

Name		Patient ID	PR0036483
Birthday		Sample ID	E03122303465
Age at delivery	39.7	Sample Date	11/04/25
Gestational age	12 + 4		

Correction factors

Fetuses	2	IVF	no	Previous trisomy 21	unknown
Weight	71	diabetes	no		
Smoker	no	Origin	Asian		

Biochemical data

Parameter	Value	Corr. MoM
PAPP-A	3.44 mIU/mL	0.71
fb-hCG	261 ng/mL	3.65

Risks at term

Age risk	1:138
Biochemical T21 risk	>1:50
Combined trisomy 21 risk	1:84
Trisomy 13/18 + NT	<1:10000

Gestational age	12 + 4
Method	CRL Robinson
Scan date	11/04/25
Crown rump length in mm	63.92
Nuchal translucency MoM	0.91
Nasal bone	present
Sonographer	DR D CHATTERJEE
Qualifications in measuring NT	MD

The calculated risk for Trisomy 21 (with nuchal translucency) is above the cut off, which indicates an increased risk.
After the result of the Trisomy 21 test (with NT) it is expected that among 84 women with the same data, there is one woman with a trisomy 21 pregnancy and 83 women with not affected pregnancies.
The free beta HCG level is high.
The risk for this twin pregnancy has been calculated for a singleton pregnancy with corrected MoMs.
The calculated risk by PRISCA depends on the accuracy of the information provided by the referring physician.
Please note that risk calculations are statistical approaches and have no diagnostic value!
The patient combined risk presumes the NT measurement was done according to accepted guidelines (Prenat Diagn 18: 511-523 (1998)).
The laboratory can not be hold responsible for their impact on the risk assessment ! Calculated risks have no diagnostic value!

Trisomy 13/18 + NT

The calculated risk for trisomy 13/18 (with nuchal translucency) is < 1:10000, which represents a low risk.

1. **How effective is quadruple screening in twins?**
2. **What is the next most appropriate option?**
3. **Can genetic sonogram be used as a screening method for aneuploidy?**

Ans.

1. Second trimester serum screening in twins leads to a high false-positive rate (about 10%) for a detection rate of 50–70%, depending on the number of markers used and the chorionicity. This method of screening in twins should not be offered.
2. Next most appropriate option is NIPS.
3. At present, there is insufficient evidence to make any recommendation about the use of second trimester genetic sonogram (soft markers) in twins for aneuploidy screening.

SUGGESTED READING

1. Audibert F, Gagnon A; Genetics Committee of the Society of Obstetricians and Gynaecologists of Canada; Prenatal Diagnosis Committee of the Canadian College of Medical Geneticists. Prenatal screening for and diagnosis of aneuploidy in twin pregnancies. J Obstet Gynaecol Can. 2011;33(7):754-67.

STATION 13. **A 28-year-old woman with DCDA twins had an anomaly scan which revealed the following findings in twin A.**

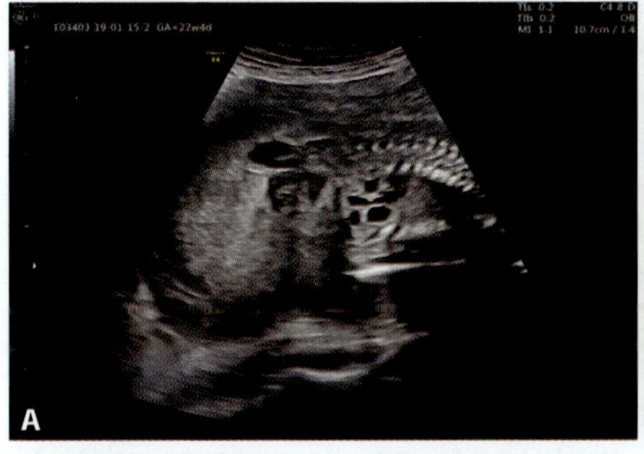
A

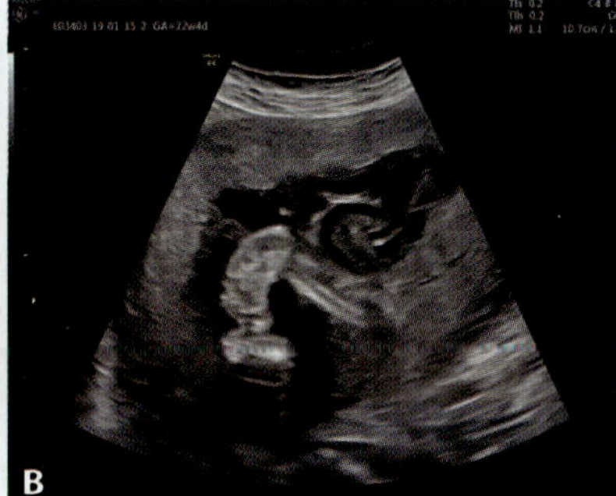
B

1. **Describe the ultrasound findings.**
2. **What is the protocol for screening structural anomalies in twins?**
3. **What are the further options?**
4. **How does it differ in MCDA twins?**

Ans.

1. The ultrasound images A and B show an open neural tube defect and talipes in one twin.
2. The risk of fetal anomaly is greater in twins compared with singleton pregnancy. The rate per fetus in dizygotic twins is probably the same as that in singletons, whereas it is two-to-three times higher in monozygotic

twins. Further MCDA twins have a higher chance of cardiac and brain abnormalities, hence fetal echocardiography should be performed in all MCDA twins.

3. Expectant management or selective termination of the affected twin by intracardiac KCl or lignocaine.
4. In MCDA twins, injection of KCl is not an option because of the risk to the healthy cotwin. Instead, cord occlusion, intrafetal laser ablation or RFA of the affected twin is necessary. The survival rate of the cotwin is approximately 80% and the risk of premature rupture of the membranes and preterm birth prior to 32 weeks is 20%.

SUGGESTED READING

1. Khalil A, Sotiriadis A, Baschat A, Bhide A, Gratacós E, Hecher K, et al. ISUOG Practice Guidelines (updated): role of ultrasound in twin pregnancy. Ultrasound Obstet Gynecol. 2025;65(2):253-76.

STATION 14.

1. **What is the risk of preterm births in multiple pregnancy?**
2. **What is the best method to screen for preterm labor in twin pregnancies?**
3. **Is prophylactic cervical cerclage indicated in low-risk asymptomatic twins?**
4. **What is the role of progesterone in prevention of preterm births in twins?**

Ans.

1. Both spontaneous and iatrogenic preterm births are more common in twins than in singleton pregnancy. More than half of twins are born before 37 weeks of gestation (60% and 12% of twin births occur before 37 and 32 weeks of gestation, respectively). The risk increases to 35% in trichorionic triamniotic (TCTA) triplets.
2. In asymptomatic women, a cervical length ≤25 mm at 20–24 weeks by transvaginal sonography (TVS), was the most accurate predictor of preterm birth before 32 and before 34 weeks.
3. No, prophylactic cerclage is not indicated in asymptomatic women with twins.
4. Vaginal progesterone does not prevent preterm birth, nor does it improve perinatal outcomes in unselected twin gestations, but it appears to reduce the risk of preterm birth occurring at early gestational ages

and of neonatal morbidity and mortality in twin gestations with a sonographic short cervix. It may be considered in twin pregnancy with cervical length ≤25 mm.

SUGGESTED READING

1. Conde-Agudelo A, Romero R, Rehal A, Brizot ML, Serra V, Da Fonseca E, et al. Vaginal progesterone for preventing preterm birth and adverse perinatal outcomes in twin gestations: a systematic review and meta-analysis. Am J Obstet Gynecol. 2023;229(6):599-616.e3.
2. Khalil A, Sotiriadis A, Baschat A, Bhide A, Gratacós E, Hecher K, et al. ISUOG Practice Guidelines (updated): role of ultrasound in twin pregnancy. Ultrasound Obstet Gynecol. 2025;65(2):253-76.

STATION 15. A 24-year-old MCDA twins at 22 weeks with growth discordance and Doppler abnormalities in twin B.

DOB,Age	24			*AB*			
Sex	Female			*Ectopic*			
				Fetus	2		
LMP	14.11.2022	*DOC*		*EDD(LMP)*	21.08.2023	*GA(LMP)*	21w3d
A GA(AUA)	21w6d	*B GA(AUA)*	19w3d				
A EDD(AUA)	18.08.2023	*B EDD(AUA)*	04.09.2023				
Perf. Phys.		*Ref. Phys.*				*Sonographer*	KOLKATA
Comment		*Indication*					

EFW (Hadlock)		*Value*	*Range*	*Age*	*Range*	*GP (Hadlock)*
A	*AC/BPD*	512g		22w3d		91.6%
B	*AC/BPD*	275g		19w0d		<1%

	2D Measurements	*AUA*	*Value*	*m1*	*m2*	*m3*	*Meth.*	*GP*	*GA*
A	*BPD (Hadlock)*	✓	5.26 cm	4.42	5.26		last	69.7%	22w0d
A	*OFD (HC)*		6.85 cm	6.06	6.85		last		
A	*HC (Hadlock)*	✓	19.51 cm	17.04	19.51		last	52.7%	21w5d
A	*HC* (Hadlock)*	☐	19.13 cm	16.56	19.13			37.8%	21w3d
A	*FL (Hadlock)*	✓	3.85 cm	3.08	3.85		last	71.6%	22w2d
A	*AC (Hadlock)*	✓	17.89 cm	14.08	13.69	17.89	last	82.9%	22w5d
A	*Cereb (Hill)*	✓	2.14 cm	2.00	2.14		last	24.6%	20w2d
A	*CM*		7.25 mm	3.59	7.25		last		
A	*Vp*		6.43 mm	5.87	6.43		last		
A	*NF*		4.06 mm	2.24	4.06		last		
B	*BPD (Hadlock)*	✓	4.44 cm	4.44			avg.	1.3%	19w3d
B	*OFD (HC)*		5.94 cm	5.94			avg.		
B	*HC (Hadlock)*	✓	16.75 cm	16.75			avg.	<1%	19w3d
B	*HC* (Hadlock)*	☐	16.39 cm	16.39				<1%	19w1d
B	*FL (Hadlock)*	✓	3.11 cm	3.11			avg.	2.9%	19w5d
B	*AC (Hadlock)*	☐	13.59 cm	13.59			avg.	1.2%	19w0d
B	*Cereb (Hill)*	✓	2.02 cm	2.02			avg.	6.9%	19w3d
B	*CM*		3.04 mm	3.04			avg.		
B	*Vp*		7.73 mm	7.73			avg.		
B	*NF*		2.37 mm	2.37			avg.		

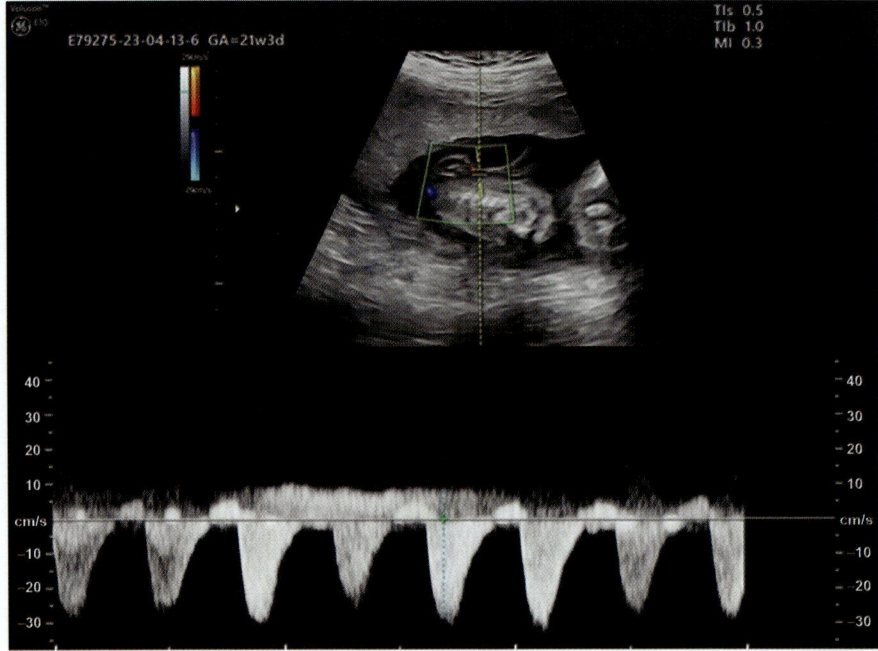

1. **How is screening for fetal growth restriction (FGR) done in multiple pregnancy?**
2. **How is growth discordance defined in twins?**
3. **How is FGR classified in MCDA twins?**
4. **How is FGR managed in twin pregnancies?**

Ans.

1. In DCDA twins, ultrasound monitoring needs to be done every 4 weeks and every 2 weeks in MCDA twins to screen for FGR.
2. Selective FGR is defined as a condition in which one fetus has estimated fetal weight (EFW) <10th centile and the intertwin EFW discordance is >25%.
3. Classification of selective fetal growth restriction (sFGR) in monochorionic twins depends on the pattern of end-diastolic velocity at umbilical artery Doppler and is divided into type I, where the umbilical artery Doppler waveform has positive end-diastolic flow. In type II, there is absent or reversed end-diastolic flow (AREDF) and in type III, there is a cyclical/intermittent pattern of AREDF.
4. In dichorionic pregnancies, sFGR should be followed as in growth-restricted singletons but there is limited evidence to guide the management of monochorionic twins affected by sFGR and is guided by the Doppler analysis.

SUGGESTED READING

1. Khalil A, Sotiriadis A, Baschat A, Bhide A, Gratacós E, Hecher K, et al. ISUOG Practice Guidelines (updated): role of ultrasound in twin pregnancy. Ultrasound Obstet Gynecol. 2025;65(2):253-76.

STATION 16.

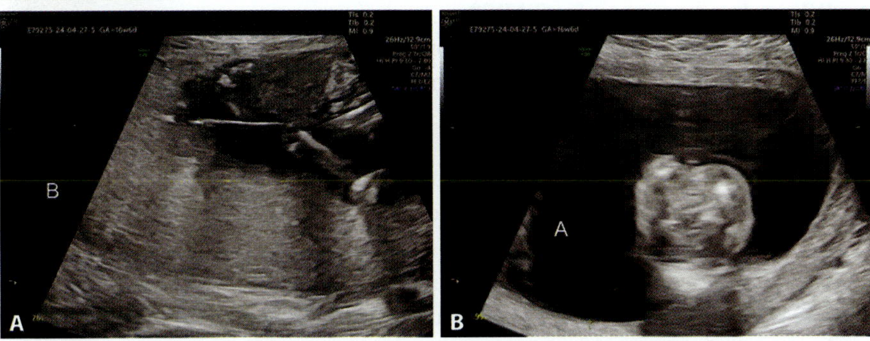

The above images A and B show an MCDA twin pregnancy with deepest vertical pocket (DVP) of 8 cm in one twin and 1.5 cm in the other twin.

1. **What is the diagnosis here?**
2. **How do we screen for this condition?**
3. **What is the best method of staging this condition?**
4. **What is the treatment of choice for the above condition?**

Ans.

1. Twin-twin transfusion syndrome.
2. In early pregnancy, discordant Crown-Rump length (CRL), NT and ductus venosus can be used to predict TTTS, however, discordant CRL has low predictive value whereas discordant DV and combination of discordant NT and DV have better predictive values with RR of 12 and 21 respectively. In second trimester, screening for TTTS should start at 16 weeks, with scans repeated every 2 weeks thereafter and if amniotic fluid discordance found, screening should be done weekly to exclude progression to TTTS.
3. Quintero staging still remains the best method of staging TTTS.
4. Laser ablation of the communicating vessels is the treatment of choice for TTTS at Quintero stages II, III, and some selective cases of stage I

SUGGESTED READING

1. Khalil A, Sotiriadis A, Baschat A, Bhide A, Gratacós E, Hecher K, et al. ISUOG Practice Guidelines (updated): role of ultrasound in twin pregnancy. Ultrasound Obstet Gynecol. 2025;65(2):253-76.

2. Stagnati V, Zanardini C, Fichera A, Pagani G, Quintero RA, Bellocco R, et al. Early prediction of twin-to-twin transfusion syndrome: systematic review and meta-analysis. Ultrasound Obstet Gynecol. 2017;49(5):573-82.

STATION 17.

1. **What is twin anemia-polycythemia sequence (TAPS)?**
2. **When do you screen for TAPS?**
3. **How is this condition screened for?**
4. **What are the treatment options for the same?**

Ans.

1. Twin anemia-polycythemia sequence is defined as the presence of anemia in the donor twin and polycythemia in the recipient twin in monochorionic twin pregnancy.
2. Screening for TAPS should be done in:
   a. All monochorionic twin pregnancies from 20 weeks' gestation
   b. Monochorionic diamniotic twins complicated by TTTS and
   c. Monochorionic diamniotic twins treated by fetoscopic laser surgery
3. Monochorionic diamniotic twins are screened for development of TAPS using ultrasound assessment of middle cerebral artery (MCA) peak systolic velocity (PSV) every 2 weeks and TAPS is diagnosed when:
   a. There is a combination of MCA-PSV ≥1.5 MoM in the anemic twin and ≤0.8 MoM in the polycythemic twin.
   b. MCA-PSV discordance ≥1 MoM
4. The management options depend on the gestational age at diagnosis, parental choice, severity of the disease, and technical feasibility of intrauterine therapy and should be individualized. The commonest options include conservative management, early delivery, laser ablation, or intrauterine blood transfusion (IUT) for the anemic twin, combined IUT for the anemic twin and partial exchange transfusion to dilute the blood of the polycythemic twin.

SUGGESTED READING

1. Khalil A, Sotiriadis A, Baschat A, Bhide A, Gratacós E, Hecher K, et al. ISUOG Practice Guidelines (updated): role of ultrasound in twin pregnancy. Ultrasound Obstet Gynecol. 2025;65(2):253-76.
2. Khalil A, Gordijn S, Ganzevoort W, Thilaganathan B, Johnson A, Baschat AA, et al. Consensus diagnostic criteria and monitoring of twin anemia-polycythemia sequence: Delphi procedure. Ultrasound Obstet Gynecol. 2020;56(3):388-94.

SECTION 2

Organ Specific Anomalies

6. **Facial and Neck Abnormalities**
   Selvaraj Ravi Lakshmy

7. **Abnormalities of Thorax**
   Chanchal, Neha Gupta, Vrunda Appannagari

8. **Congenital Abnormalities of the Heart: Structural Defects and Arrhythmias**
   Bijoy K Balakrishnan, Alok Varshney

9. **Congenital Abnormalities of the Gastrointestinal Tract and Abdominal Wall**
   Tulika Ranjan Joshi

10. **Congenital Abnormalities of the Kidney and Urinary Tract**
    Chinmayee Ratha

11. **Central and Peripheral Nervous System Abnormalities**
    Akshatha Prabhu, Anita Kaul

12. **Skeletal Dysplasia**
    Manisha Kumar, Apoorva Kulshreshtha

CHAPTER 6

Facial and Neck Abnormalities

Selvaraj Ravi Lakshmy

STATION 1.

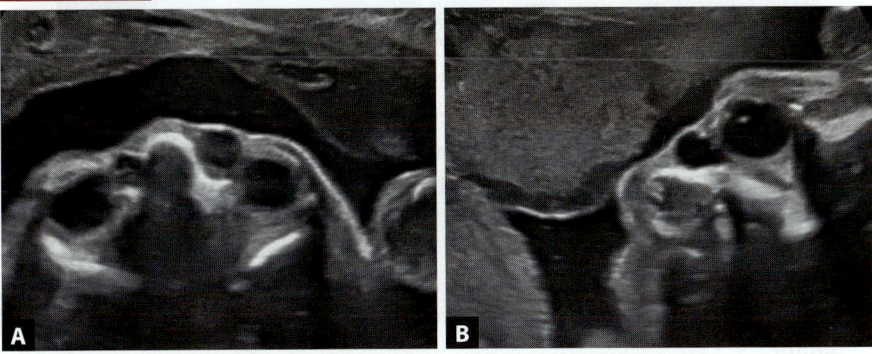

1. **Identify the condition shown in above images A and B.**
2. **Name two differential diagnoses for this condition.**
3. **What is the prognosis?**
4. **What is the recurrence risk?**

Ans.

1. Cysts seen at the medial aspect of the orbit—dacryocystocele.
2. Anterior encephalocele, lymphangioma.
3. They resolve spontaneously in the third trimester or within first 6 months of birth.
4. No increased risk of recurrence.

SUGGESTED READING

1. Kim YH, Lee YJ, Song MJ, Han BH, Lee YH, Lee KS. Dacryocystocele on prenatal ultrasonography: diagnosis and postnatal outcomes. Ultrasonography. 2015;34(1):51-7.

STATION 2.

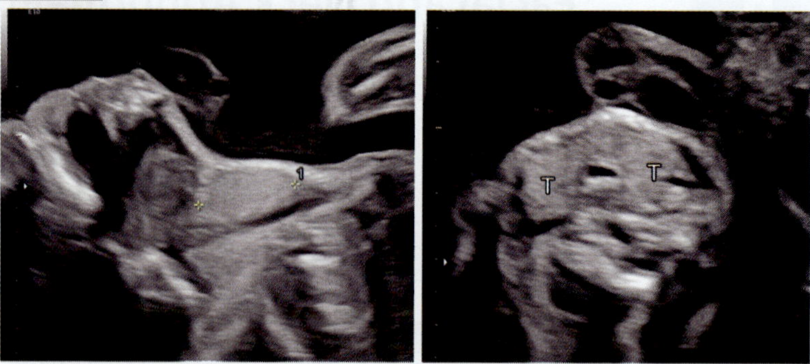

1. **Identify the condition shown above.**
2. **What is the etiology behind this condition?**
3. **What is the maternal history relevant to this condition?**
4. **What is the autosomal recessive condition associated with this finding?**

Ans.

1. Anterior cervical echogenic mass suggestive of an enlarged thyroid—fetal goiter.
2. Transplacentally transferred maternal autoantibodies, maternal antithyroid drugs, inadequate or excessive iodine availability, thyroid dyshormonogenesis.
3. Intake of antithyroid drugs.
4. Thyroid dyshormonogenesis.

SUGGESTED READING

1. Figueiredo CM, Falcão I, Vilaverde J, Freitas J, Oliveira MJ, Godinho C, et al. Prenatal diagnosis and management of a fetal goiter hypothyroidism due to dyshormonogenesis. Case Rep Endocrinol. 2018;2018(1):9564737.
2. Taff C. Prenatal diagnosis and treatment of fetal goiter. J Diagnostic Med Sonogr. 2016;32(1):40-3.

STATION 3.

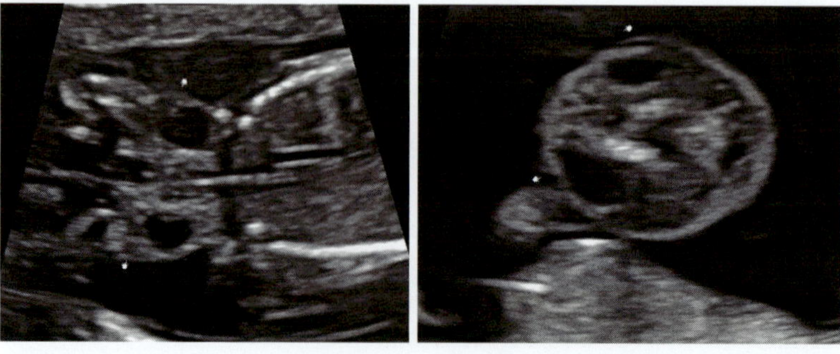

1. **Identify the condition.**
2. **What are the common associations with this condition?**
3. **What is the prognosis?**
4. **Write two differential diagnoses.**

Ans.

1. Anechoic cystic structures located on either side of the neck—dilated jugular lymph sacs.
2. Aneuploidy such as Trisomy 21 and Turner's syndrome.
3. If it is an isolated condition with no other aneuploidy markers, structural anomaly, and chromosomal abnormalities, this condition can resolve by itself.
4. Lymphangioma, hemangioma, branchial cleft cyst.

SUGGESTED READING

1. Bekker MN, Haak MC, Rekoert-Hollander M, Twisk J, Van Vugt JM. Increased nuchal translucency and distended jugular lymphatic sacs on first-trimester ultrasound. Ultrasound Obstet Gynecol. 2005;25(3):239-45.
2. De Mooij YM, Bekker MN, Spreeuwenberg MD, Van Vugt JM. Jugular lymphatic sacs in first-trimester fetuses with normal nuchal translucency. Ultrasound Obstet Gynecol. 2009;33(4):394-8.

STATION 4.

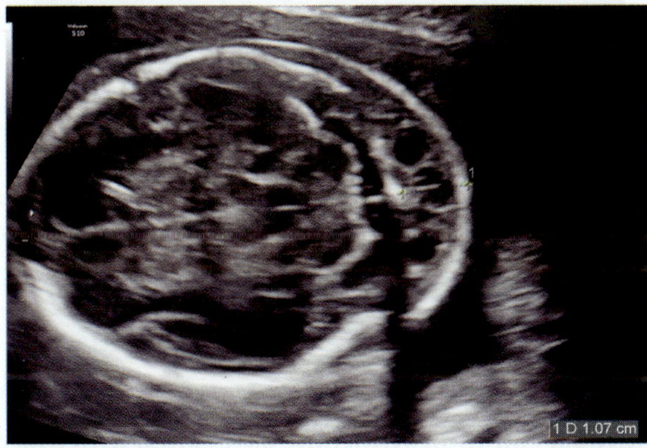

1. **Identify this condition.**
2. **What is the most common association with this condition?**
3. **Name a few genetic disorders in which this finding can be present.**
4. **What is the most common aneuploidy associated with this condition?**

Ans.

1. Nuchal fold thickness in transcerebellar plane is greater than 6 mm—thickened nuchal fold with septations.
2. Cystic hygroma, nonimmune hydrops.

3. Aneuploidy, arthrogryposis, single gene disorders such as Noonan's syndrome, etc.
4. Trisomy 21 and Turner's syndrome.

SUGGESTED READING

1. Cho JY, Kim KW, Lee YH, Toi A. Measurement of nuchal skin fold thickness in the second trimester: influence of imaging angle and fetal presentation. Ultrasound Obstet Gynecol. 2005;25(3):253-7.
2. Li L, Fu F, Li R, Liu Z, Liao C. Prenatal diagnosis and pregnancy outcome analysis of thickened nuchal fold in the second trimester. Medicine. 2018;97(46): e13334.

STATION 5.

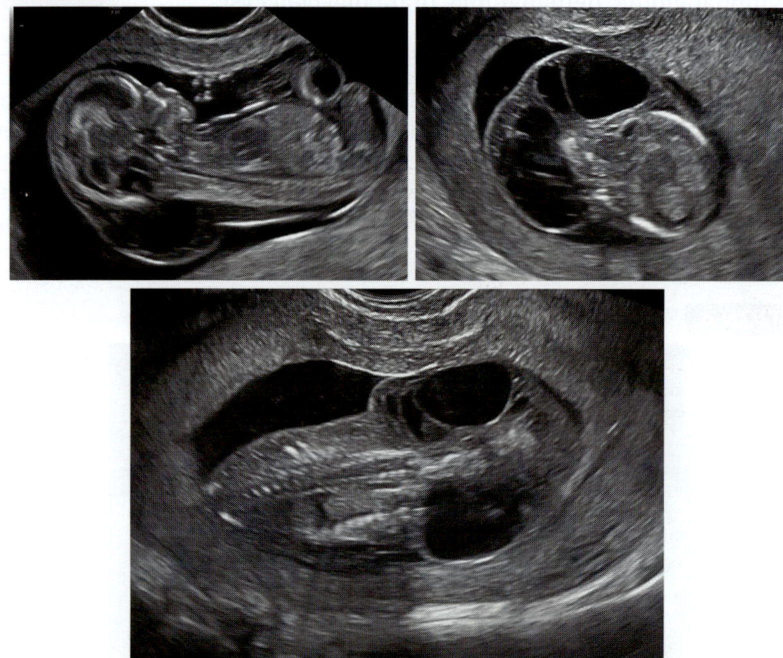

1. **Identify the condition.**
2. **What is the most common syndrome associated with this condition?**
3. **What are the other common associations with this condition? Name three.**
4. **What is the importance of ultrasonography (USG) phenotype in this condition.**

Ans.

1. Multiple septated cystic structures located in the occipito-cervical region of the fetal neck—cystic hygroma seen at 11–14 weeks scan.

2. Trisomy 21 and Turner syndrome.
3. Noonan syndrome, lethal multiple pterygium syndrome, Neu-Laxova syndrome, Fryns syndrome, nonimmune hydrops.
4. The presence of other structural anomalies in cystic hygroma namely hypoplastic left heart, presence of contractures and pterygium, associated central nervous system (CNS) anomalies can point toward a particular syndromic association.

SUGGESTED READING

1. Graesslin O, Derniaux E, Alanio E, Gaillard D, Vitry F, Quéreux C, et al. Characteristics and outcome of fetal cystic hygroma diagnosed in the first trimester. Acta obstetricia et gynecologica Scandinavica. 2007;86(12):1442-6.

STATION 6.

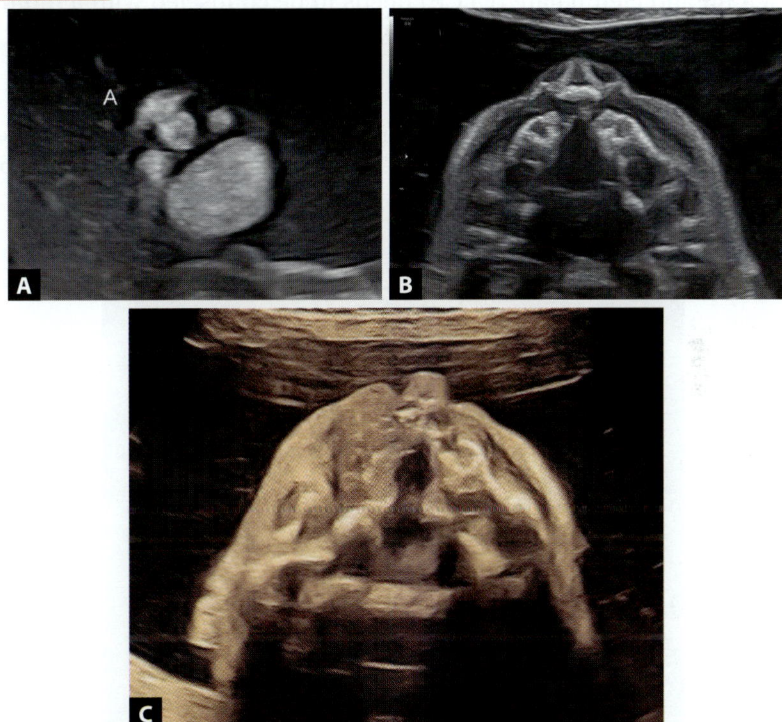

1. **Identify the diagnosis.**
2. **Enumerate the findings that lead to the diagnosis.**
3. **What are the other common associations with this condition?**
4. **How will you counsel the patient?**

Ans.

1. Complete bilateral cleft lip and palate.

2. The findings that lead to a diagnosis of complete bilateral cleft lip and palate are as follows:
   a. Nose chin view demonstrating bilateral paramedian cleft of the upper lip.
   b. Axial view of the palate showing detached premaxilla, and bilateral paramedian cleft in alveolar ridge.
   c. Axial view demonstrating midline disruption in the bony posterior edge of the secondary palate.
3. Trisomy 13, Trisomy 18, holoprosencephaly spectrum, posterior fossa anomalies, velo-cardio facial syndrome.
4. The presence of other structural anomalies and known genetic syndromes have to be ruled out in this condition. Offer invasive testing. In the event of a normal chromosomal microarray, isolated bilateral cleft lip and cleft palate (CLCP) needs to be counseled with a multidisciplinary team along with the maxilla-facial surgeon.

SUGGESTED READING

1. Selvaraj LR, Ziyaullah T. Syndromes and Associations. First and Mid Trimester Ultrasound Diagnosis of Orofacial Clefts: An Atlas and Guide. Singapore: Springer; 2021.

STATION 7.

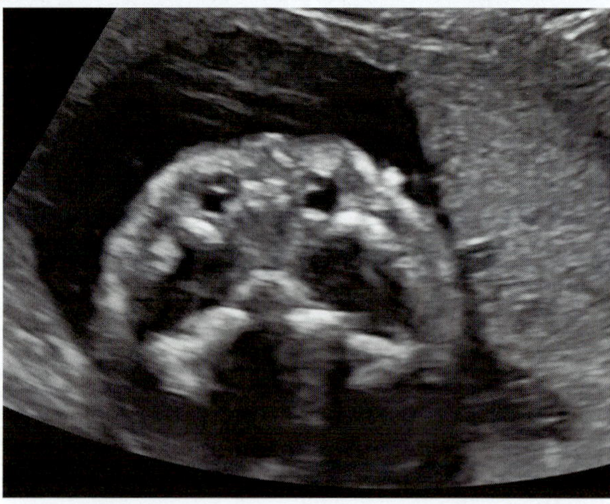

1. **Identify the condition.**
2. **What is the most common association in brain with this finding?**
3. **What is the common genetic syndrome associated with this condition?**
4. **What is the first line of investigation to evaluate for the common genetic syndrome?**

Ans.

1. Axial view of fetal face shows bilateral microphthalmia (small-sized orbits) with hypotelorism (decreased interorbital distance).
2. Holoprosencephaly
3. Trisomy 13
4. Fetal karyotype

SUGGESTED READING

1. Murthy BR. Imaging of Fetal Brain and Spine: An Atlas and Guide. Singapore: Springer; 2019.

STATION 8.

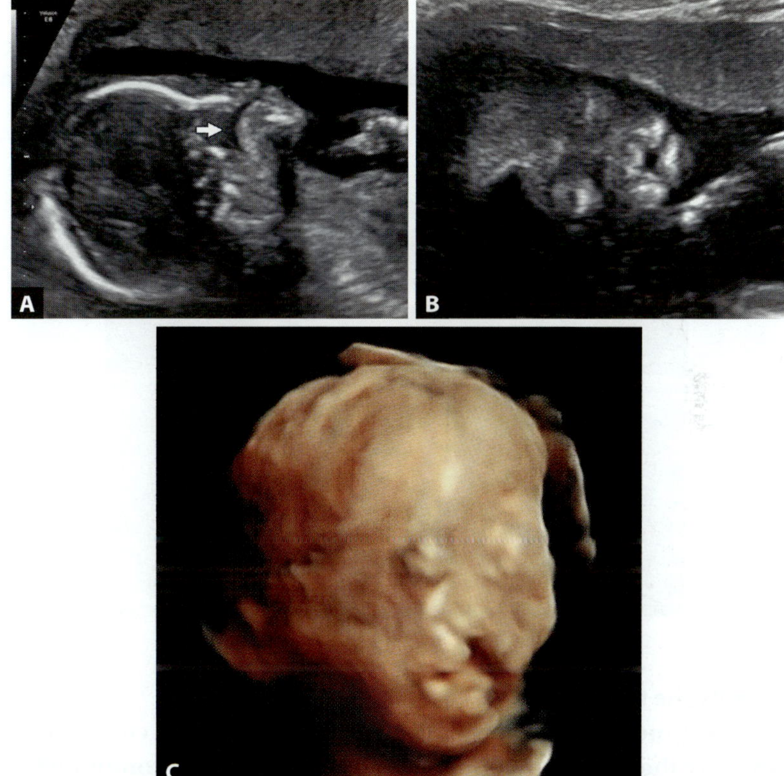

1. **Name the findings in each of the above images A to C.**
2. **What is the diagnosis?**
3. **What is the most common chromosomal abnormality associated with this condition?**
4. **How do you differentiate them from bilateral cleft lip and palate?**

Ans.

1. a. Absence of maxillary line (arrow) in sagittal section.
   b. Absence of median process in nose chin view.
   c. Absent nose, nasal septum, and nostrils.
2. Arrhinia with median cleft lip and palate.
3. Trisomy 13
4. In bilateral cleft lip and palate, there is a presence of premaxillary protrusion in midsagittal profile of face. Nose chin view shows bilateral paramedian clefts with the presence of median process. In median cleft lip and palate, there is absence of premaxilla with the absence of median process in nose chin view.

SUGGESTED READING

1. Selvaraj LR, Ziyaullah T. Syndromes and Associations. First and Mid Trimester Ultrasound Diagnosis of Orofacial Clefts: An Atlas and Guide. Singapore: Springer; 2021. pp. 155-67.

STATION 9.

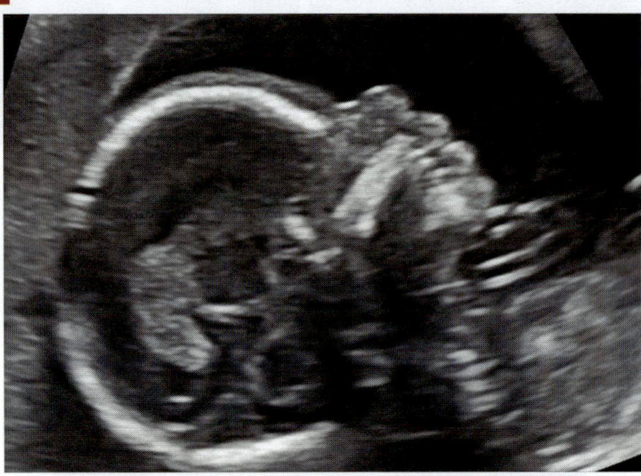

Image courtesy: Selvaraj Ravi Lakshmy

1. **Identify the finding.**
2. **Name the most common genetic association with this condition.**
3. **What are the other soft markers associated with this condition?**
4. **List the soft markers in the order of increasing significance in the perspective of isolated likelihood ratio.**

Ans.

1. Unossified nasal bone
2. Trisomy 21

3. Thickened nuchal fold, aberrant right subclavian artery, pyelectasis, ventriculomegaly, echogenic intracardiac foci, short femur, short humerus, echogenic bowel
4. Short femur, short humerus, intracardiac echogenic focus, mild hydronephrosis, echogenic bowel, increased nuchal fold, ventriculomegaly, aberrant right subclavian artery (ARSA), absent or hypoplastic nasal bone.

SUGGESTED READING

1. Agathokleous M, Chaveeva P, Poon LC, Kosinski P, Nicolaides KH. Meta-analysis of second-trimester markers for trisomy 21. Ultrasound Obstet Gynecol. 2013;41(3):247-61.

STATION 10.

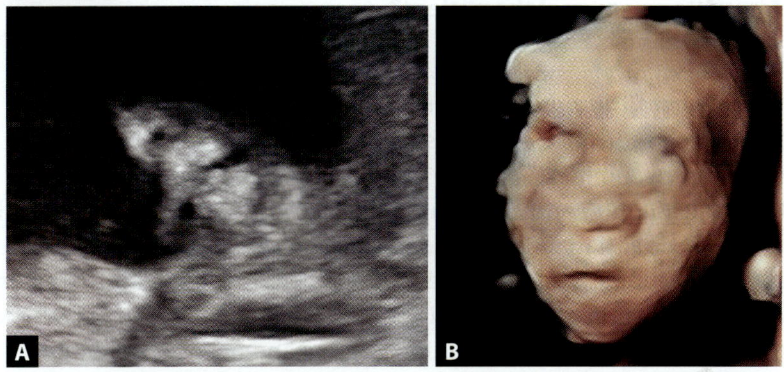

1. **Identify the finding in the nose chin view in image A.**
2. **Name the closest differential diagnosis of this condition.**
3. **Name the most common structural and syndromal association with this condition.**
4. **Name any nonchromosomal syndrome associated with this condition.**

Ans.

1. Single nostril seen in nose chin view suggestive of cebocephaly.
2. Ethmocephaly
3. Holoprosencephaly—Trisomy 13
4. Smith-Lemli-Opitz syndrome

SUGGESTED READING

1. Schinzel A, Savoldelli G, Briner J, Schmid W. Prenatal ultrasonographic diagnosis of holoprosencephaly two Stations of cebocephaly and two of cyclopia. Arch Gynecol. 1984;236(1):47-53.

STATION 11.

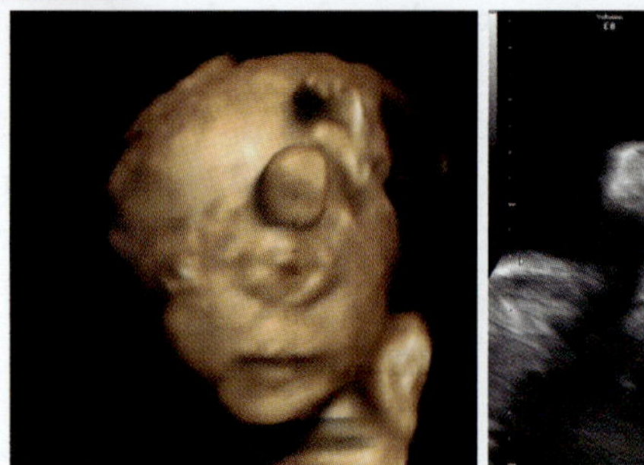

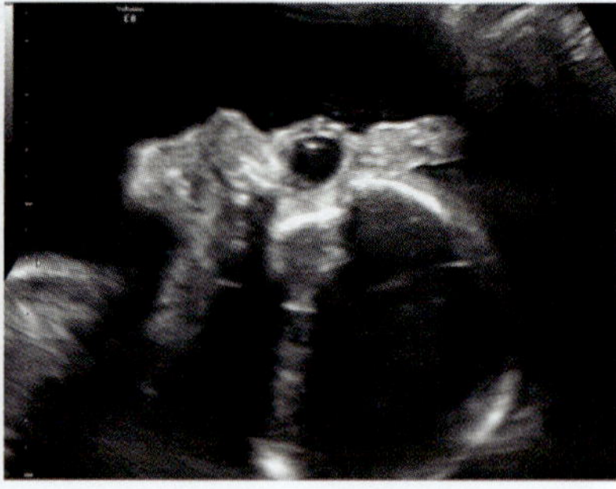

1. **Identify the findings.**
2. **What is the most common association with this finding?**
3. **What are the four types of this association?**
4. **How will you counsel the patient?**

Ans.

1. A single midline orbit with presence of a tubular process above the orbit which is the proboscis, absence of nose—cyclopia.
2. Holoprosencephaly
3. Types of holoprosencephaly are alobar, semilobar, lobar, and middle hemispheric variant.
4. Invasive testing has to be offered for fetal karyotyping with DNA storage to evaluate for aneuploidy like Trisomy 13. Cyclopia is seen in alobar and semilobar types and this condition is lethal and needs termination.

SUGGESTED READING

1. Murthy BR. Imaging of Fetal Brain and Spine: An Atlas and Guide. Singapore: Springer; 2019.

STATION 12.

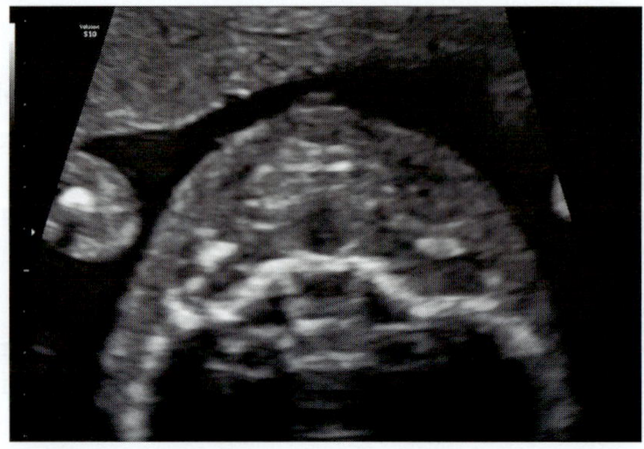

1. **What is the anatomical landmark shown in this picture?**
2. **What is the significance of the anatomical landmark?**
3. **Will this landmark rule out cleft of the secondary palate?**
4. **What are the other signs to evaluate secondary palate in mid-trimester?**

Ans.

1. Posterior palatal line seen between the two pterygoid processes marks the edge of the bony secondary palate.
2. Intact posterior palatal line signifies that the bony secondary palate is intact.
3. This anatomical landmark evaluates only for cleft of the bony secondary palate and does not rule out an isolated cleft of the soft palate.
4. Equal sign—demonstrating the uvula is another marker to evaluate the secondary palate in mid-trimester.

SUGGESTED READING

1. Selvaraj LR, Ziyaullah T. Syndromes and Associations. First and Mid Trimester Ultrasound Diagnosis of Orofacial Clefts: An Atlas and Guide. Singapore: Springer; 2021.
2. Wilhelm L, Borgers H. The 'equals sign': a novel marker in the diagnosis of fetal isolated cleft palate. Ultrasound Obstet Gynecol. 2010;36(4):439-44.

STATION 13.

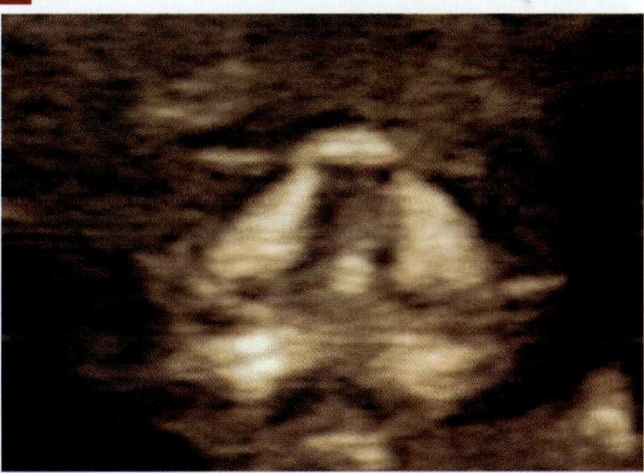

1. **Name the triangle shown in this image.**
2. **Label the anatomical landmarks of this triangle.**
3. **Identify the abnormality shown in this image in the retronasal triangle (RNT).**
4. **What is the clinical significance of the finding?**

Ans.

1. Retronasal triangle
2. The apex of the triangle is formed by the nasal bones, base formed by the palate, and the side walls formed by the frontal process of maxilla.
3. Defect in the base of the triangle.
4. Complete absence of the base of the triangle can be seen in bilateral cleft lip and palate and median cleft lip and palate.

SUGGESTED READING

1. Sepulveda W, Wong AE, Martinez-Ten P, Perez-Pedregosa J. Retronasal triangle: a sonographic landmark for the screening of cleft palate in the first trimester. Ultrasound Obstet Gynecol. 2010;35(1):7-13.

STATION 14.

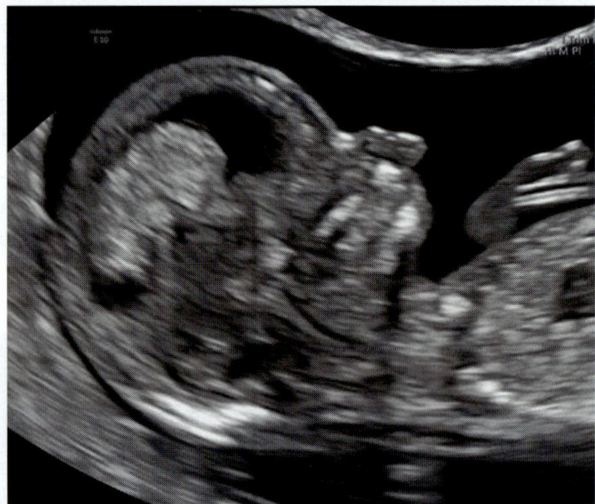

1. **Describe the findings in the midsagittal view of the face.**
2. **What is the diagnosis?**
3. **What are the additional views which help to confirm the diagnosis?**
4. **What forms the posterior aspect of the maxillary line in this image?**

Ans.

1. The midsagittal profile view of the face shows—presence of maxillary gap sign, absence of superimposed line sign, and presence of premaxillary protrusion.

2. Features suggestive of complete bilateral cleft lip and palate.
3. Additional views are namely the RNT view and axial view of palate. The RNT view will show absence of base of the triangle. Axial view of the palate will show bilateral paramedian defects with protrusion of premaxilla.
4. Vomer is seen in the posterior aspect of the maxillary line.

SUGGESTED READING

1. Selvaraj LR, Ziyaullah T. Syndromes and Associations. First and Mid Trimester Ultrasound Diagnosis of Orofacial Clefts: An Atlas and Guide. Singapore: Springer; 2021. pp. 155-67.

STATION 15.

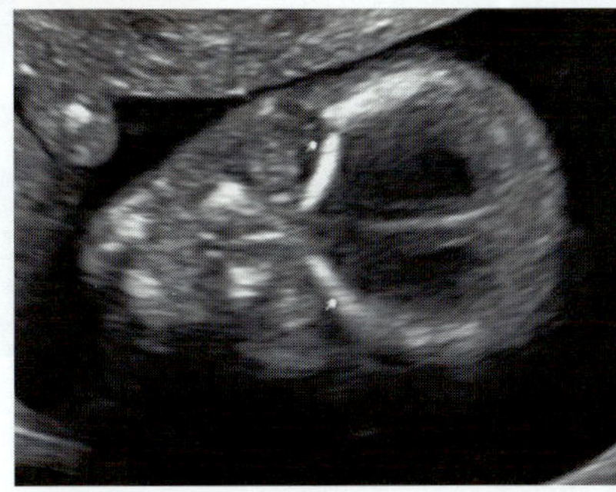
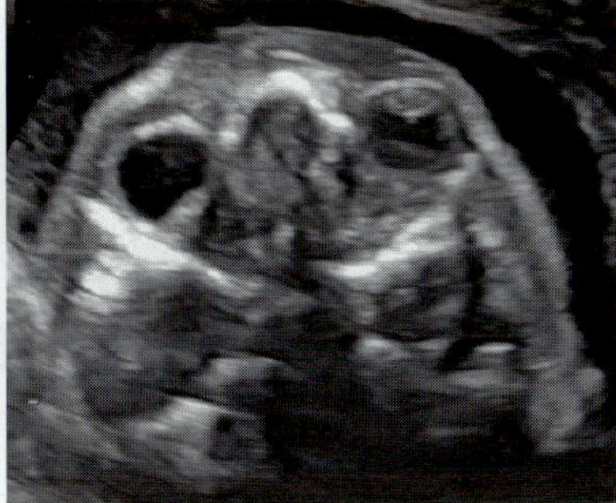

1. **Identify the finding.**
2. **What is the autosomal recessive genetic syndrome associated with this condition?**
3. **This syndrome was earlier called as.................. ?**
4. **What are the associated brain findings in this syndrome?**

Ans.

1. Coronal and axial view of the orbits showing hyperechogenic lens.
2. Walker-Warburg syndrome
3. HARD±E (hydrocephalus, agyria, retinal dysplasia, ±encephalocele) syndrome
4. Type 2 lissencephaly, hydrocephalus, cerebellar malformations (includes vermian and general cerebellar hypoplasia), kinked Z-shaped brainstem with bifid pons and medulla oblongata, posterior encephalocele.

SUGGESTED READING

1. Achiron R, Katorza E, Reznik-Wolf H, Pras E, Kidron D, Berkenstadtt M. Very early in-utero diagnosis of Walker-Warburg phenotype: the cutting edge of technology. Ultrasound Int Open. 2016;2(2):E54-7.
2. Brasseur-Daudruy MV, Vivier PH, Ickowicz V, Eurin D, Verspyck E. Walker-Warburg syndrome diagnosed by findings of typical ocular abnormalities on prenatal ultrasound. Pediatr Radiol. 2012;42(4):488-90.

STATION 16.

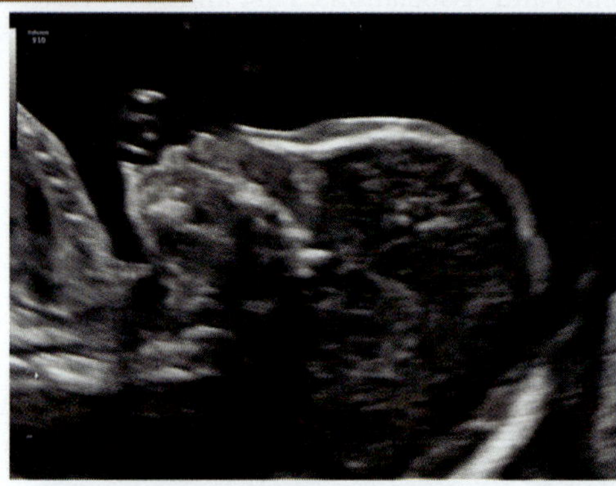

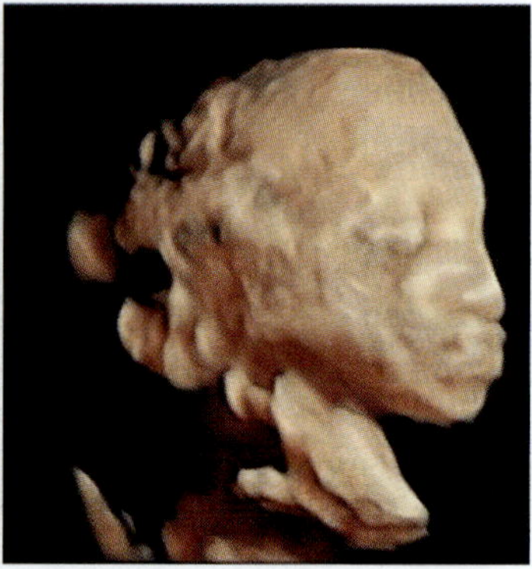

1. **Identify the condition.**
2. **What is the most common association with this phenotype?**
3. **What is the importance of maternal history?**
4. **Name the antibodies which are most often associated with this phenotype.**

Ans.

1. Nasomaxillary hypoplasia with verticalization of nasal bones—binder phenotype.
2. Chondrodysplasia punctata
3. Maternal autoimmune disorders, phenytoin, alcohol, or warfarin intake during pregnancy.
4. Antiribonucleoprotein (RNP) antibodies

SUGGESTED READING

1. Mazzone E, Cos Sanchez T, Persico N, Cannie MM, Jani J. Binder syndrome: a phenotype rather than a definitive diagnosis? Ultrasound Obstet Gynecol. 2019;53(1):131-2.
2. Sabu B, Shenoy D, Vidya Lekshmy R. Binder phenotype—prenatal diagnosis, management, and postnatal outcome: Insights from a station series and updated review of the literature. J Fetal Med. 2024;11(06).

STATION 17.

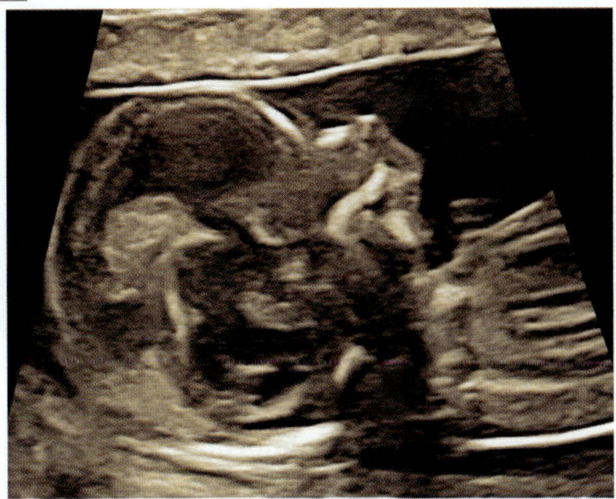

1. **Identify the findings.**
2. **Name the sequence associated with this finding.**
3. **What is the triad associated with this sequence?**
4. **What is the clinical significance of identifying this condition in utero?**

Ans.

1. The midsagittal profile view shows a receding chin suggestive of micrognathia. Absence of superimposed line sign—as the posterior portion of the maxillary line appears single. Presence of amniotic fluid seen anterior to the tip of the tongue in the oral cavity.
2. Pierre Robin sequence
3. Micrognathia, a small posterior cleft of the secondary palate and glossoptosis.
4. Glossoptosis often causes airway obstruction in the immediate neonatal period. Hence, prenatal diagnosis is essential to prepare the multidisciplinary team during the delivery of the fetus to handle early airway emergencies.

SUGGESTED READING

1. Kaufman MG, Cassady CI, Hyman CH, Lee W, Watcha MF, Hippard HK, et al. Prenatal identification of Pierre Robin sequence: a review of the literature and look towards the future. Fetal Diagn Ther. 2016;39(2):81-9.
2. Lakshmy S, Sharmila B, Pawadi P, Ziyaulla T. VP04.08: Ultrasound markers in first trimester diagnosis of Pierre Robin syndrome. Ultrasound Obstet Gynecol. 2020;56:69-69.

STATION 18.

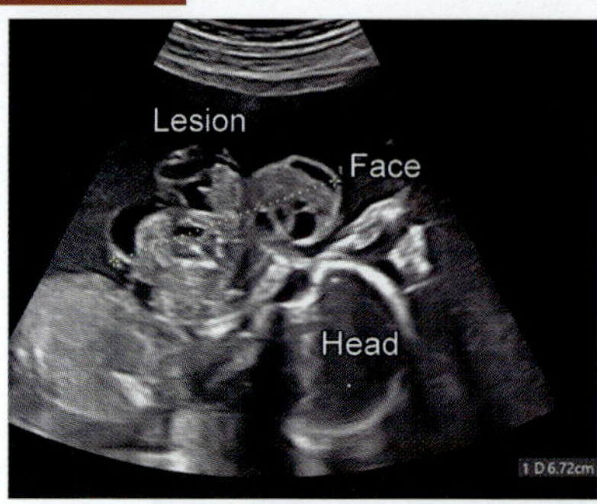

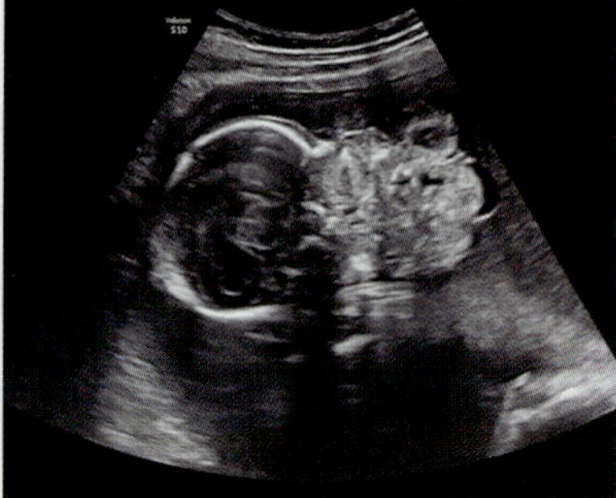

1. **Identify the condition.**
2. **Give two differential diagnoses.**
3. **What is the common liquor abnormality associated with this condition?**
4. **What is the intervention needed in the prenatal period before delivery of this fetus?**

Ans.

1. Heterogeneous mass with solid and cystic components appears protruding from the oral cavity—orofacial teratoma.
2. Lymphangioma, hemangioma
3. Polyhydramnios
4. The airway has to be secured before delivery of this fetus and an EXIT procedure may be needed.

SUGGESTED READING

1. Narayan R, Ahmad Sr MS, Kumar A. Fetal oropharyngeal teratoma: Prenatal diagnosis and imaging characteristics. Cureus. 2020;12(11):e11329.

STATION 19.

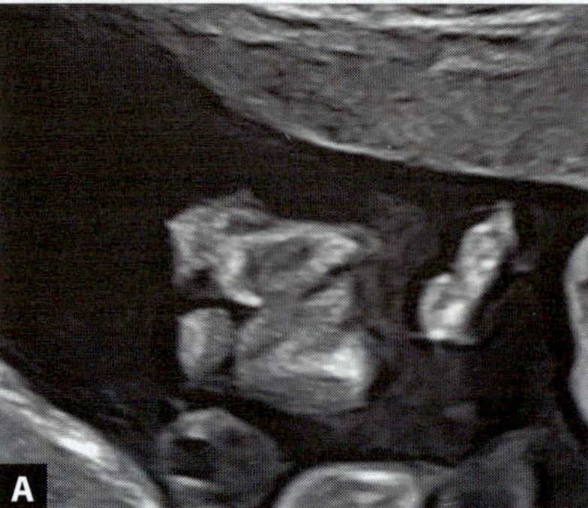

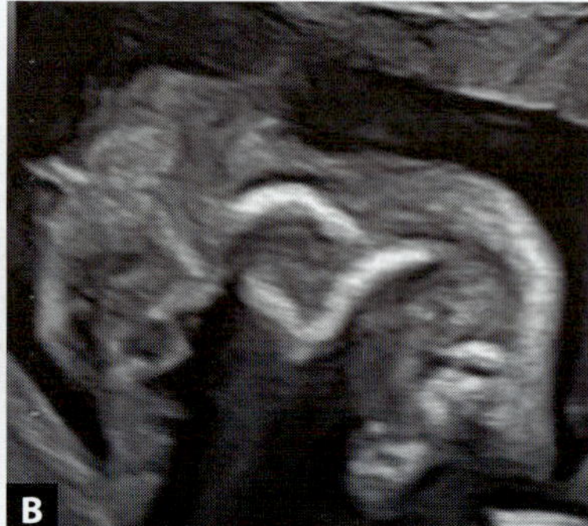

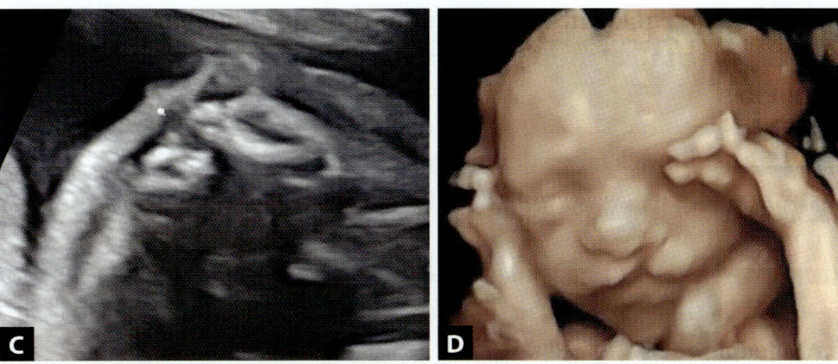

1. **Identify the diagnosis.**
2. **Enumerate the findings leading to the diagnosis.**
3. **Is the premaxillary triangle intact?**
4. **Will the midsagittal view show an abnormality in this case?**

Ans.

1. Unilateral labio-alveolar cleft.
2. Nose chin view shows lateralized defect in the upper lip with intact philtrum and flattening of ipsilateral alae nasi **(Fig. A)**.
3. Yes. The base of the premaxillary triangle is intact **(Fig. B)**.
4. No. The midsagittal profile will be normal in cases of unilateral cleft lip.

SUGGESTED READING

1. Selvaraj LR, Ziyaullah T. Syndromes and Associations. First and Mid Trimester Ultrasound Diagnosis of Orofacial Clefts: An Atlas and Guide. Singapore: Springer; 2021. pp. 155-67.

STATION 20.

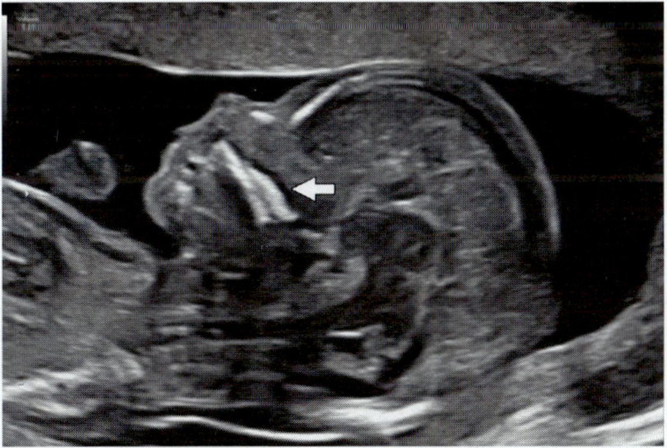

1. **Identify the sign marked by the arrow.**
2. **What constitutes superimposed line sign?**

3. **What is the significance of this sign?**
4. **What is the clinical utility of evaluating this sign?**

Ans.

1. Midsagittal view of face showing superimposed line sign.
2. The cranial line is formed by the vomer and the caudal line by the secondary palate.
3. In cleft of the secondary palate, the line formed by the palate is absent and hence only the vomer bone is visualized, creating a single line instead of the normal superimposed double line.
4. The superimposed line sign can help to identify isolated cleft of the secondary palate and also extension of the cleft into the secondary palate in cases of cleft lip and palate.

SUGGESTED READING

1. Lakshmy SR, Rose N, Masilamani P, Umapathy S, Ziyaulla T. Absent 'superimposed-line' sign: novel marker in early diagnosis of cleft of fetal secondary palate. Ultrasound Obstet Gynecol. 2020;56(6):906-15.

CHAPTER 7

Abnormalities of Thorax

Chanchal, Neha Gupta, Vrunda Appannagari

STATION 1.

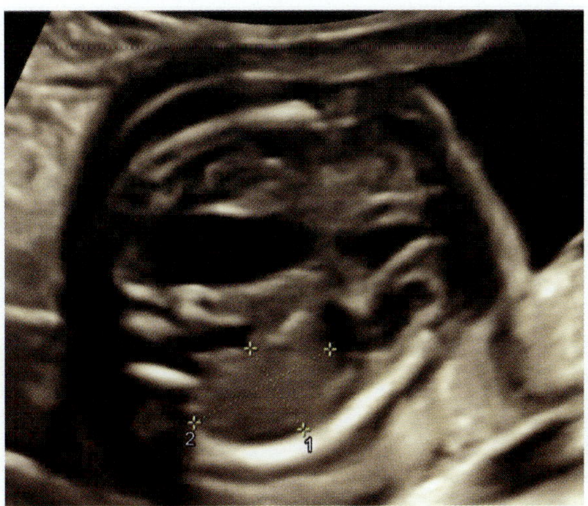

1. **Review the ultrasound image and identify the abnormality.**
2. **Which sided abnormality is more common and what are the most common contents?**
3. **Name two aneuploidies and two syndromes associated with this condition.**
4. **What is the ratio used to assess severity and prognosis of this condition?**
5. **Classify the severity on the basis of the ratio.**

Ans.

1. Congenital diaphragmatic hernia.
2. Left-sided congenital diaphragmatic hernia (CDH) is seen in >80% of cases, contents, stomach, and bowel loops.
3. a. Trisomy 18 and Trisomy 13.
   b. Pallister–Killian syndrome, Fryns syndrome.
4. Assessment of severity is by observed/expected lung-to-head ratio (O/E LHR).
5. CDHs are classified as severe if the O/E LHR ratio is <25%, moderate if 26–45%, and mild if >45%.

SUGGESTED READING

1. Alfaraj MA, Shah PS, Bohn D, Pantazi S, O'Brien K, Chiu PP, et al. Congenital diaphragmatic hernia: lung-to-head ratio and lung volume for prediction of outcome. Am J Obstet Gynecol. 2011;205(1):43.e1-8.
2. Jani J, Nicolaides KH, Keller RL, Benachi A, Peralta CF, Favre R, et al. Observed to expected lung area to head circumference ratio in the prediction of survival in fetuses with isolated diaphragmatic hernia. Ultrasound Obstet Gynecol. 2007;30(1):67-71.

STATION 2.

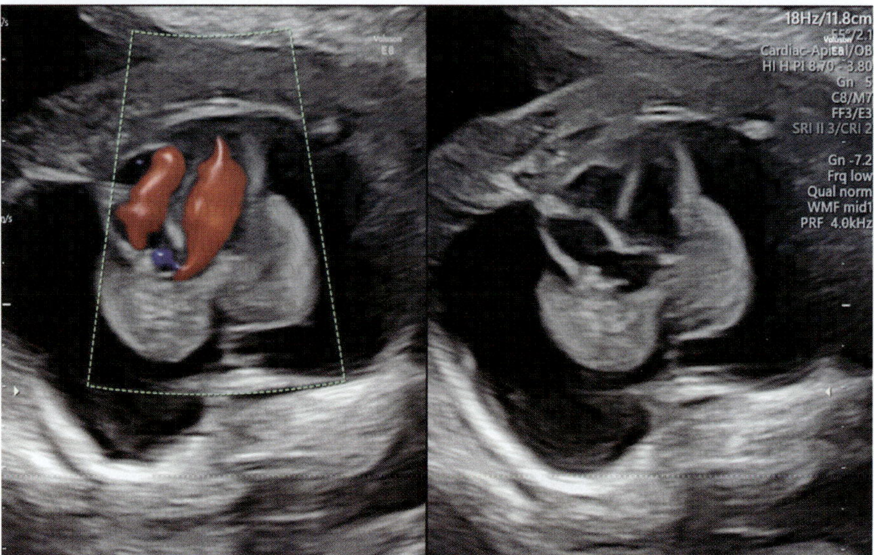

1. **Identify the abnormality.**
2. **Name two chromosomal abnormalities and one syndrome associated with this condition.**
3. **What further investigations do you counsel the patient in isolated cases?**
4. **Name two fetal therapies that can be offered in this condition.**

Ans.

1. Pleural effusion
2. a. Trisomy 21, Monosomy X (seen in 10% of cases)
   b. Noonan's syndrome (seen in 5% of cases)
3. Invasive testing for fetal fluorescence in situ hybridization (FISH)/ quantitative fluorescent polymerase chain reaction (QFPCR), microarray, and exome sequencing.
4. Thoraco-amniotic shunt, pleurodesis.

SUGGESTED READING

1. Abbasi N, Ryan G. Fetal primary pleural effusions: Prenatal diagnosis and management. Best Pract Res Clin Obstet Gynaecol. 2019;58:66-77.
2. Klam S, Bigras JL, Hudon L. Predicting outcome in primary fetal hydrothorax. Fetal Diagn Ther. 2005;20(5):366-70.

STATION 3.

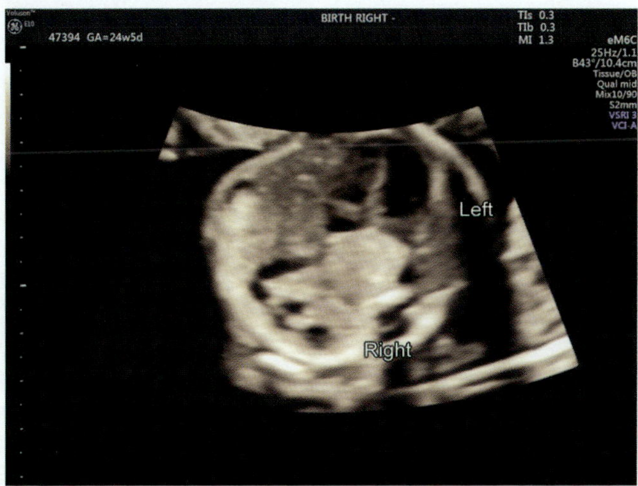

1. **Identify the abnormality in this ultrasound image showing an axial view of fetal thorax.**
2. **Name two complications associated with this abnormality.**
3. **Name the ratio which is a sonographic indicator that has been proposed for the evaluation of fetuses at risk of complications and possible intervention and how is the ratio obtained/calculated.**
4. **What value signifies the risk of development of complications?**

Ans.

1. Congenital cystic/congenital pulmonary adenomatoid malformation (CCAM/CPAM)
2. Hydrops fetalis and mediastinal shift
3. CPAM volume ratio (CVR). The CVR is obtained by dividing the CPAM volume by the head circumference (measured in cm). CVR = (Length × Height × Width × 0.52)/Head circumference.
4. CVR >1.6 signifies the risk of developing hydrops.

SUGGESTED READING

1. Crombleholme TM, Coleman B, Hedrick H, Liechty K, Howell L, Flake AW, et al. Cystic adenomatoid malformation volume ratio predicts outcome in prenatally diagnosed cystic adenomatoid malformation of the lung. J Pediatr Surg. 2002;37(3):331-8.

2. Zhu P, Cheng K, He M, Wang Y, Shen P, He K, et al. Diagnostic value of congenital pulmonary airway malformation volume ratio for fetal hydrops due to congenital lung malformations: a systematic review and meta-analysis. Orphanet J Rare Dis. 2022;17(1):213.

STATION 4.

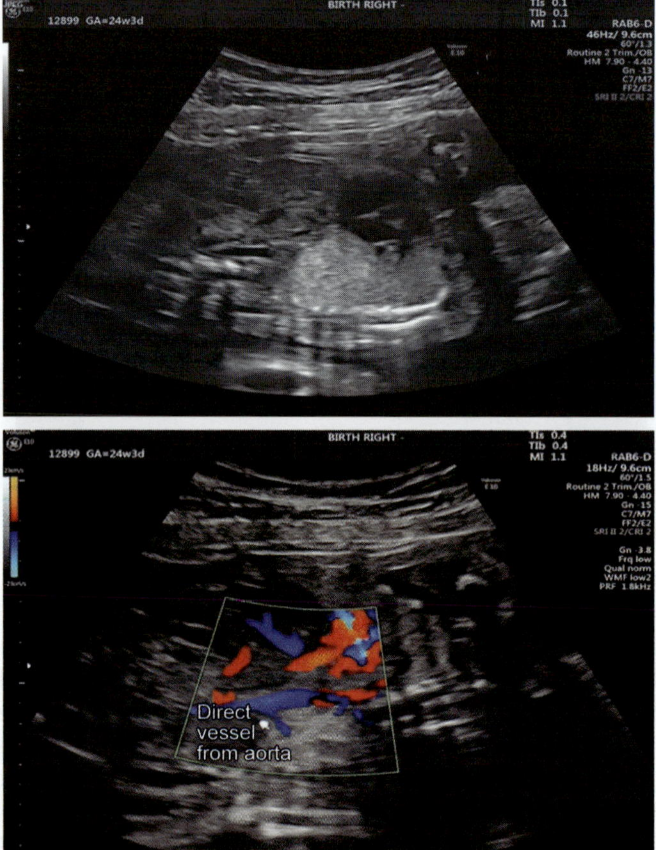

1. **Identify the echogenic mass within the fetal thorax. How do you differentiate it from CPAM?**
2. **Name two different types of this abnormality and the most common structural abnormality associated with them.**
3. **How will you counsel the patient?**
4. **What are the therapeutic options available for this lesion in severe cases?**

Ans.

1. Bronchopulmonary sequestration. Color Doppler demonstrates a feeding vessel that arises from the descending aorta which differentiates it from CPAM.

2. *Intralobar* in 75% of cases located inside the pleura of functioning lung. In 25% of cases it is *extralobar*, located outside the normal lung with its own visceral pleura. Associated anomalies are diaphragmatic hernia, cardiac or vertebral anomalies which are found in up to 50% of cases with extralobar sequestration.
3. Regression occurs in 30% of cases by third trimester. Four weekly ultrasound follow-up to monitor growth of the lesion and to look for development of hydrothorax or hydrops.
4. Ultrasound-guided laser coagulation of feeding vessel if severe hydrothorax or hydrops.

SUGGESTED READING

1. Savic B, Birtel F, Tholen W, Funke H, Knoche R. Lung sequestration: report of seven cases and review of 540 published cases. Thorax. 1979;34(1):96-101.

STATION 5.

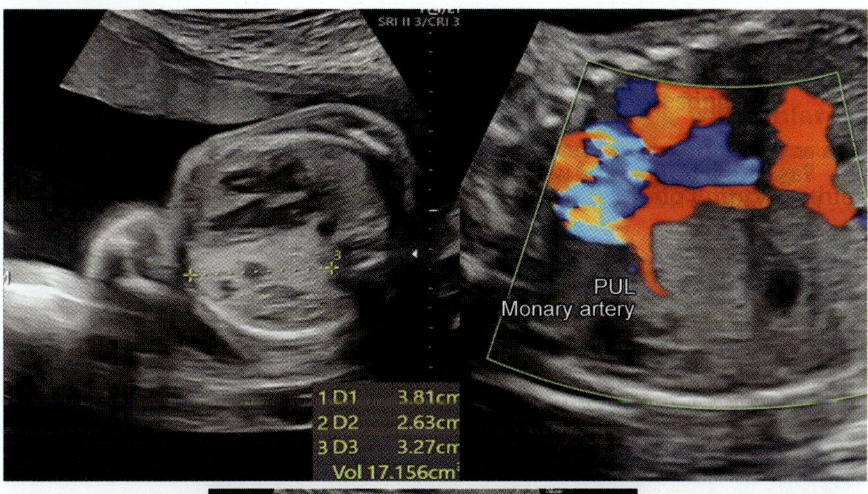

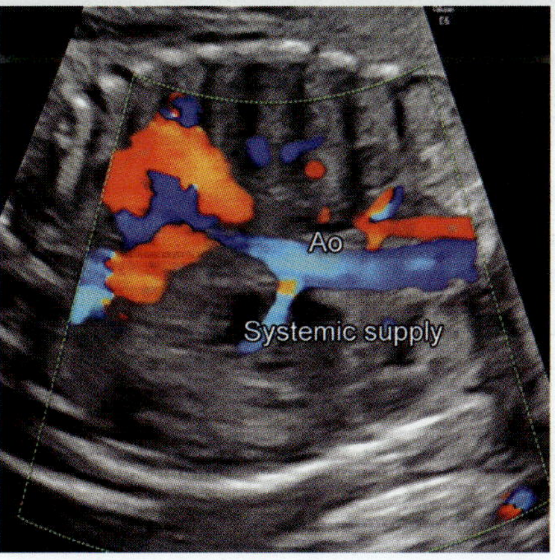

1. **Identify the abnormality in the first gray scale image.**
2. **What are the color Doppler images telling us about the lesion?**
3. **What is the association with chromosomal abnormalities and genetic syndromes?**
4. **What is the suggested follow-up for this abnormality?**

Ans.

1. Bronchopulmonary anomaly—mixed (solid cystic) appearance with mediastinal shift. The possibilities are CCAM/CPAM or bronchopulmonary sequestration or both (hybrid lesion).
2. Color Doppler shows that the lesion has dual supply—both from pulmonary artery and aorta. Hence, this is a hybrid lesion.
3. The incidence of chromosomal abnormalities and genetic syndromes is not increased.
4. Ultrasound scans every 4 weeks to monitor growth of the lesion and hydrothorax or hydrops.

SUGGESTED READING

1. Kane SC, Da Silva Costa F, Crameri JA, Reidy KL, Kaganov H, Palma-Dias R. Antenatal assessment and postnatal outcome of fetal echogenic lung lesions: a decade's experience at a tertiary referral hospital. J Matern Fetal Neonatal Med. 2019;32(5):703-9.

STATION 6.

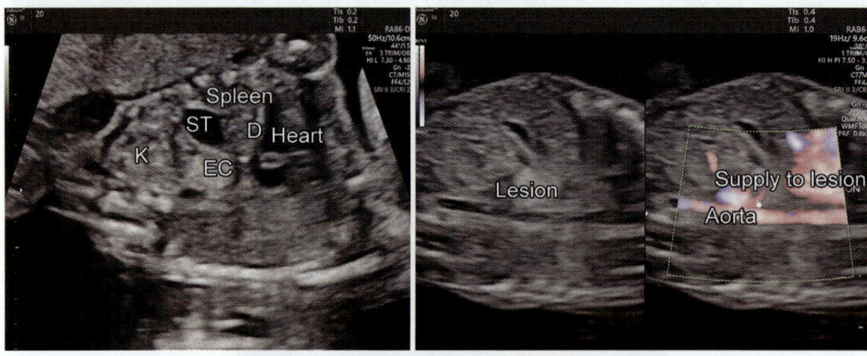

1. **Identify the abnormality in the first image?**
2. **What does the power Doppler image signify?**
3. **What are the differentials of this echogenic mass?**
4. **How will you counsel?**

Ans.

1. An echogenic lesion seen on the left side below the diaphragm above the kidney in a paravertebral location.
2. It shows a feeder vessel from the intra-abdominal portion of the aorta.

3. Extralobar-bronchopulmonary sequestration (ELS), left-sided adrenal mass.
4. Magnetic resonance imaging (MRI) helps in further categorization. 4 weekly ultrasound to monitor the lesion. 30% may show regression or disappearance during third trimester, if it is ELS. Postnatal evaluation.

SUGGESTED READING

1. Houda el M, Ahmed Z, Amine K, Amina BS, Raja F, Chiraz H. Antenatal diagnosis of extralobar pulmonary sequestration. Pan Afr Med J. 2014;19:54.

STATION 7.

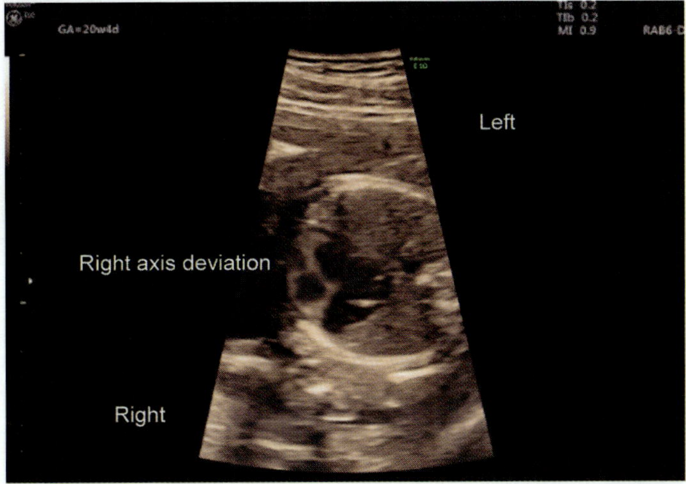

1. **Identify the abnormality.**
2. **Describe Scimitar syndrome.**
3. **Describe types of pulmonary hypoplasia with two examples for each.**
4. **Name two postnatal complications in cases of pulmonary hypoplasia.**

Ans.

1. Right pulmonary hypoplasia
2. Hypoplastic right lung with hypoplastic right pulmonary artery and partial pulmonary venous drainage of right lung into inferior vena cava is referred to as Scimitar syndrome.
3. *Primary pulmonary hypoplasia:* Congenital acinar dysplasia, hypoplastic lung in genetic disorders like trisomy 21. Secondary pulmonary hypoplasia is due to fetal lung compression secondary to underlying anomalies affecting the thoracic cavity or amniotic fluid volume, e.g., CDH, CPAM, skeletal dysplasia, oligohydramnios due to renal agenesis.
4. Acute respiratory failure, tracheomalacia, persistent pulmonary hypertension, pneumothorax.

SUGGESTED READING

1. Delgado-Peña YP, Torrent-Vernetta A, Sacoto G, de Mir-Messa I, Rovira-Amigo S, Gartner S, et al. Pulmonary hypoplasia: An analysis of cases over a 20-year period. An Pediatr (Barc). 2016;85(2):70-6.
2. Laudy JA, Wladimiroff JW. The fetal lung. Pulmonary hypoplasia. Ultrasound Obstet Gynecol. 2000;16(5):482-94.

STATION 8.

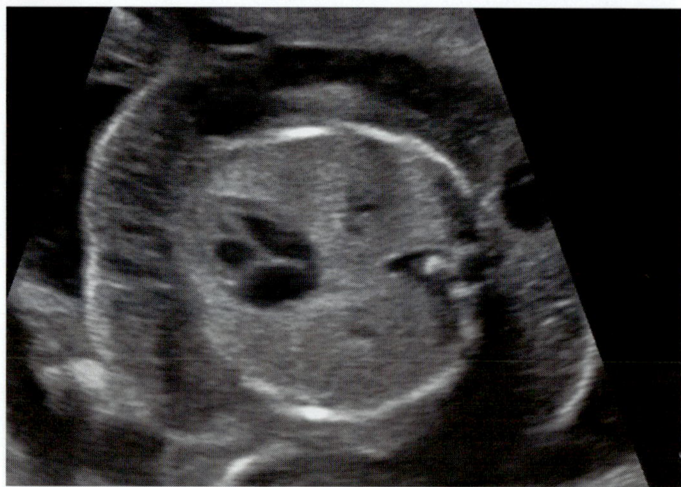

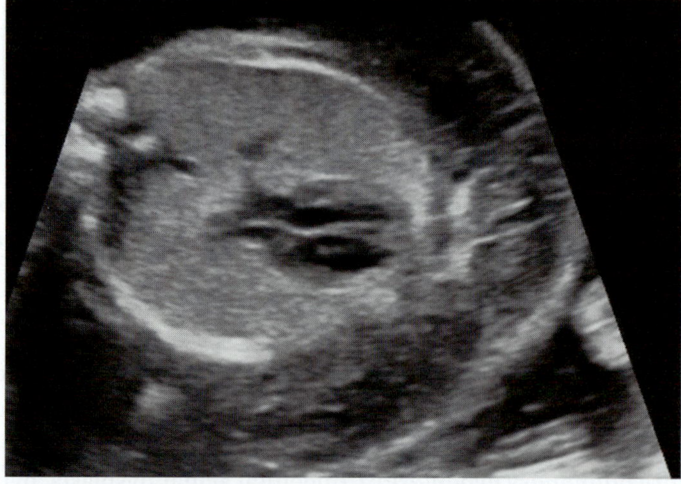

1. **Identify the abnormality.**
2. **Name two causes due to which the abnormality occur.**
3. **Describe the characteristic ultrasound findings of this abnormality.**
4. **Which is the most common associated genetic disorder with this abnormality?**

Ans.

1. CHAOS/congenital high airway obstruction syndrome with subcutaneous edema (cystic hygroma).
2. It is a rare congenital anomaly, caused by laryngeal or tracheal atresia, tracheal stenosis, obstructing laryngeal cysts, and obstructing tumors of the oropharynx and the cervical region.
3. Prenatal ultrasound findings include highly echogenic, enlarged lungs, dilated trachea and bronchi, inverted hemidiaphragms, small and compressed heart, and ascites.
4. Fraser's syndrome. It is an autosomal recessive syndrome with tracheal or laryngeal atresia, renal agenesis, microphthalmia, and syndactyly or polydactyly.

SUGGESTED READING

1. D'Eufemia MD, Cianci S, Di Meglio F, Di Meglio L, Di Meglio L, Vitale SG, et al. Congenital high airway obstruction syndrome (CHAOS): discussing the role and limits of prenatal diagnosis starting from a single-center case series. J Prenat Med. 2016;10(1-2):4-7.
2. Sanford E, Saadai P, Lee H, Slavotinek A. Congenital high airway obstruction sequence (CHAOS): a new case and a review of phenotypic features. Am J Med Genet A. 2012;158A(12):3126-36.

STATION 9.

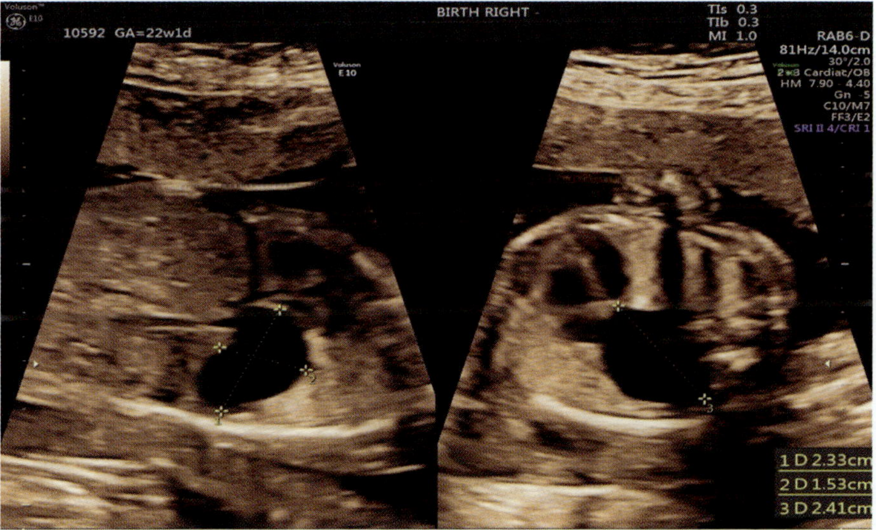

1. **2D ultrasonography (USG) image showing fetal thorax at 22 weeks. What is the differential diagnoses?**
2. **Name any two other cystic lesions seen in the fetal thorax.**

3. **Write the prognostic factors of these cysts which can be determined on prenatal ultrasound and which can be useful in planning postnatal treatment.**
4. **What additional investigation and follow-up would you explain to the couple if the cyst is larger than 5 cm and causing compression of surrounding structures?**

Ans.

1. Mediastinal cyst most likely bronchogenic cyst.
2. Pericardial cyst and thymic cyst.
3. The prognostic factors of fetal mediastinal cysts are the size, location, the adjacent relationship with the surrounding tissues, volume, and the gestational age at which it presents.
4. Fetal MRI may be helpful to delineate the type of lesion and assess its relation with the structures it is compressing. Four weekly ultrasound follow-up and a pediatric surgeon consultation is recommended.

SUGGESTED READING

1. Ma B, He Y, Zhang M, Wang Y, Nie F. Analysis of the prenatal ultrasound diagnostic value and prognostic factors of fetal mediastinal cysts. Quant Imaging Med Surg. 2024;14(5):3643-54.

STATION 10.

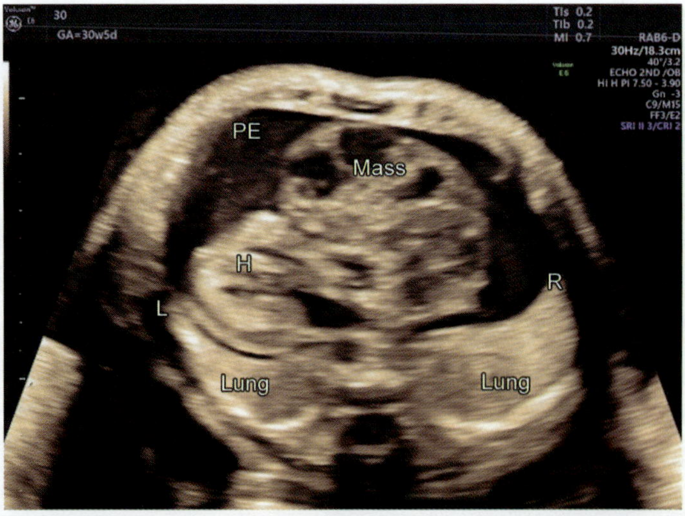

1. **How would you identify whether this is pleural or pericardial effusion?**
2. **Identify the findings in the image. What is the most probable diagnosis?**
3. **What are the other types of tumors like these?**
4. **What other procedure or investigation can be considered?**
5. **How will you follow-up this patient?**

Ans.

1. This is pericardial effusion as lungs are pushed backward toward the spine. In pleural effusion, the heart and the lungs are in center surrounded by the fluid.
2. The image shows pericardial effusion. A large mass is attached to the right side of the heart. Due to the mass, there is deviation of the heart to the left side (levorotation) of the heart. The mass has a solid cystic appearance. There is compression of the heart. The most probable diagnosis is fetal primary cardiac tumor with pericardial effusion. Most likely teratoma.
3. Fetal primary cardiac tumors can be cardiac or pericardial. Majority are benign. Rhabdomyomas are the most common followed by teratoma, fibroma, hemangioma, and myxoma.
4. Pericardiocentesis can be considered here to relieve the cardiac compression. Fetal MRI for further categorization of the lesion.
5. 2–4 weekly ultrasound. Review with pediatric cardiologist.

SUGGESTED READING

1. Gupta N, Dash P, Marwah A. Fetal cardiac teratoma and pericardiocentesis: a case report. Prenat Diagn. 2024;44(6-7):876-8.

STATION 11.

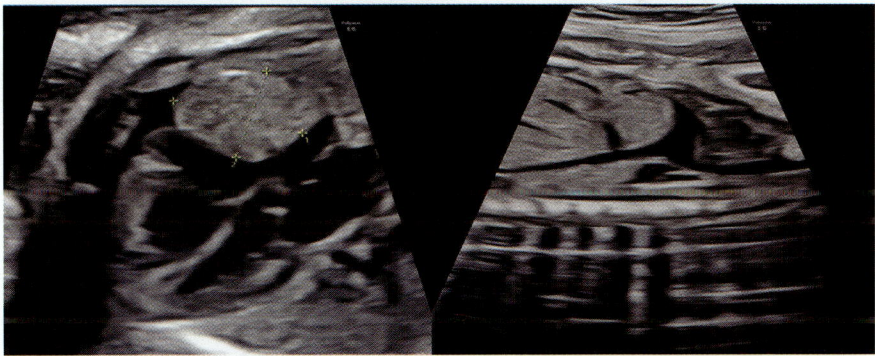

1. **2D USG images showing axial and sagittal sections of fetal thorax are shown above. What is the differential diagnosis for the marked mass?**
2. **How would you follow-up this fetus?**
3. **Name a possible fetal complication that may arise due to this.**
4. **Does this finding impact antenatal management?**

Ans.

1. There is a solid, echogenic mass located in the anterior mediastinum toward the right side near the right atrium which is likely a mediastinal tumor. Differential diagnoses include thymic mass and lymphangioma.

2. 4 weekly USG surveillance should be done.
3. Nonimmune hydrops.
4. No, the mother should receive standard antenatal care with an aim to deliver at term followed by postnatal evaluation of the newborn.

SUGGESTED READING

1. Biko DM, Lichtenberger JP 3rd, Rapp JB, Khwaja A, Huppmann AR, Chung EM. mediastinal masses in children: radiologic-pathologic correlation. Radiographics. 2021;41(4):1186-207.

STATION 12.

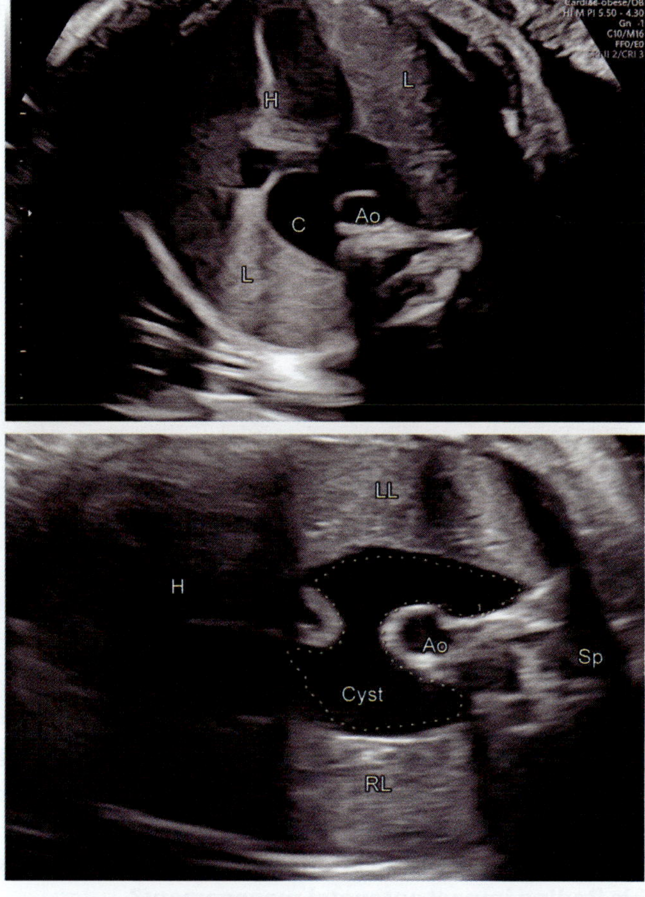

(H: heart, L: lung, Ao: aorta, C: cyst, Sp: spine)

1. **Explain the findings in the scan. What is the most probable diagnosis?**
2. **What are the differentials of the cyst in this location?**
3. **What further investigations can be done?**
4. **How will you follow-up?**

Ans.

1. A clear fluid-filled collection is seen in the posterior mediastinum in between the lungs behind the heart encircling aorta. This is a posterior mediastinal cyst.
2. Differentials are neurogenic cyst, lymphangioma, bronchogenic cyst, and esophageal duplication cyst.
3. Fetal MRI may be helpful to delineate the type of lesion and assess its relation with the structures it is compressing.
4. 4 weekly ultrasound surveillance and pediatric surgery consultation is recommended.

SUGGESTED READING

1. Biko DM, Lichtenberger JP 3rd, Rapp JB, Khwaja A, Huppmann AR, Chung EM. mediastinal masses in children: radiologic-pathologic correlation. Radiographics. 2021;41(4):1186-207.

STATION 13.

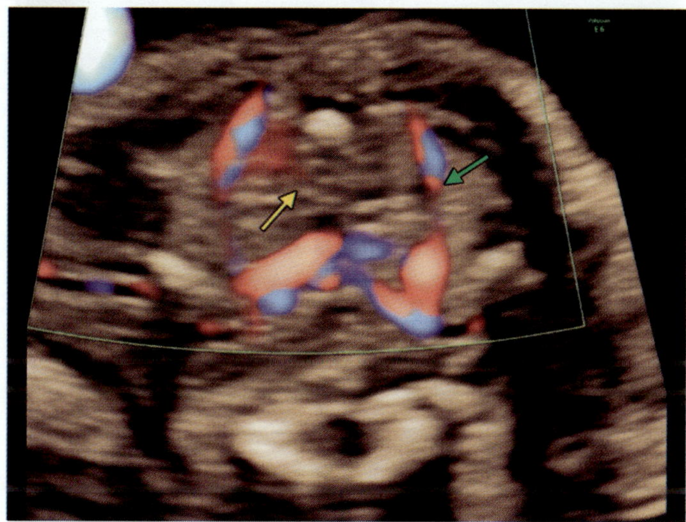

1. **This is a 2D with color Doppler axial image of fetal thorax. Identify the structure labeled with yellow arrow.**
2. **Identify the structure marked with green arrow.**
3. **What are the boundaries of the structure labeled with yellow arrow?**
4. **Name the ratio that has been suggested as a possible way of identifying a genetic syndrome.**

Ans.

1. Thymus
2. Internal mammary artery

3. The "Thy box" is bound anteriorly by the sternum, laterally by internal mammary arteries, and posteriorly by the left brachiocephalic vein.
4. A low thymic thoracic (TT) ratio has been suggested as a simple way of identifying fetuses at high risk for 22 q deletion syndrome.

SUGGESTED READING

1. Chaoui R, Heling K-S, Sarut Lopez A, Thiel G, Karl K. The thymic-thoracic ratio in fetal heart defects: a simple way to identify fetuses at high risk for microdeletion 22q11. Ultrasound Obstet Gynecol. 2011;37(4):397-403.
2. Paladini D. How to identify the thymus in the fetus: the thy box. Ultrasound Obstet Gynecol. 2011;37(4):488-92.

STATION 14.

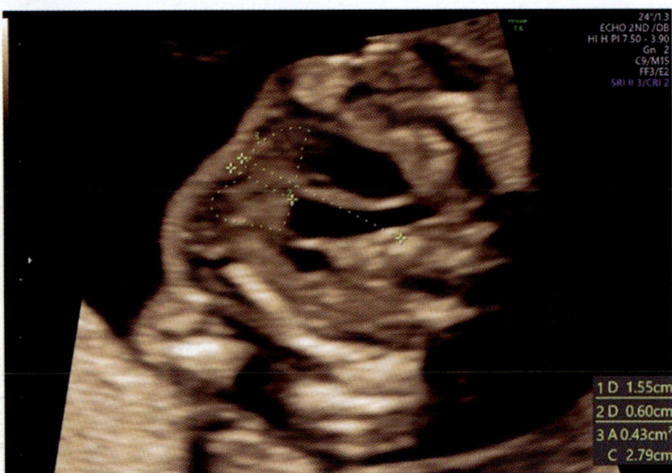

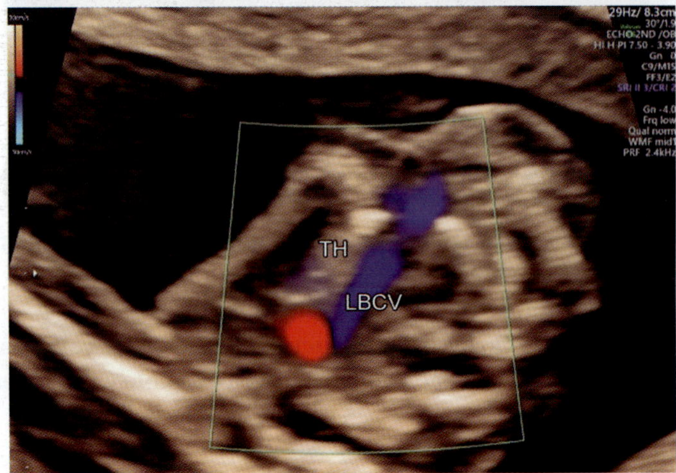

1. **Identify the abnormality in the given image.**
2. **What is thymic-thoracic ratio?**

3. What is the impact of gestational age on the thymic-thoracic ratio?

4. Name two abnormalities associated with the condition shown above.

Ans.

1. Hypoplastic thymus
2. Ratio of anterior-posterior thymic to the intrathoracic mediastinal diameter.
3. The thymic-thoracic ratio is dependent on gestational age.
4. Di George syndrome, Trisomy 21.

SUGGESTED READING

1. Chaoui R, Heling K-S, Sarut Lopez A, Thiel G, Karl K. The thymic–thoracic ratio in fetal heart defects: a simple way to identify fetuses at high risk for microdeletion 22q11. Ultrasound Obstet Gynecol. 2011;37(4):397-403.

STATION 15.

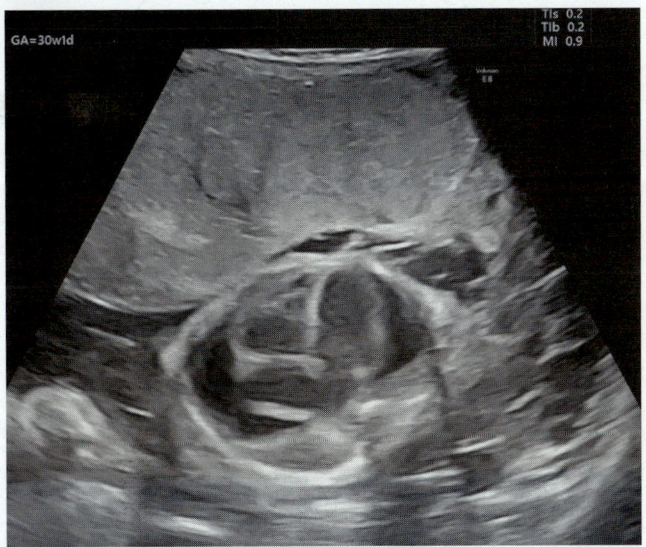

1. Identify the abnormality.

2. Name two possible etiologies.

3. Name two maternal investigations that should be advised.

4. Name two fetal investigations that should be done.

Ans.

1. Pericardial effusion
2. Fetal infection, fetal anemia
3. TORCH (Toxoplasmosis, Rubella, Cytomegalovirus, or Herpes) immunoglobulin (Ig)M, IgG, and indirect Coombs test (ICT)
4. Middle cerebral artery peak systolic velocity (MCA PSV), fetal echo.

SUGGESTED READING

1. Slesnick TC, Ayres NA, Altman CA, Bezold LI, Eidem BW, Fraley JK, et al. Characteristics and outcomes of fetuses with pericardial effusions. Am J Cardiol. 2005;96(4):599-601.

STATION 16.

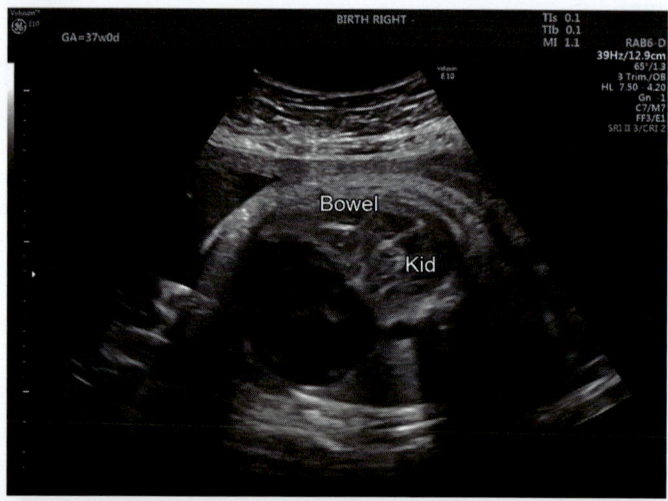

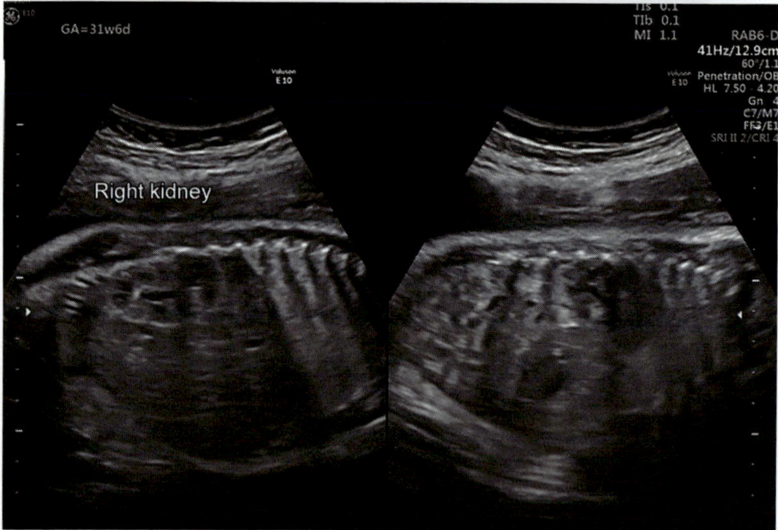

1. **Low-risk primigravida with normal nuchal and anomaly scans comes for routine growth scan. USG images of fetal thorax and abdomen are shown above. Identify the abnormality.**
2. **What is the clue to the diagnosis?**
3. **What are the prognostic indicators?**
4. **How would you follow-up this pregnancy?**

Ans.

1. Left-sided congenital diaphragmatic hernia.
2. Cardiac axis deviation, empty left renal fossa.
3. The O/E LHR is the most important prognostic indicator.
4. 2–3 weekly ultrasound surveillance.

SUGGESTED READING

1. Singh C, Shahnaz G, Handa R, Gupta NP, Sundar J. A missing kidney and a hidden congenital diaphragmatic hernia. J Clin Ultrasound. 2021;49(4):401-4.

CHAPTER 8 Congenital Abnormalities of the Heart: Structural Defects and Arrhythmias

Bijoy K Balakrishnan, Alok Varshney

STATION 1.

1. **Identify the vessel shown in the diagram.**
2. **Which chamber of the heart does this vessel drain blood into?**
3. **Name the cardiac condition which is commonly associated with it.**
4. **Name the feature suggestive of coarctation of aorta shown in image B below.**

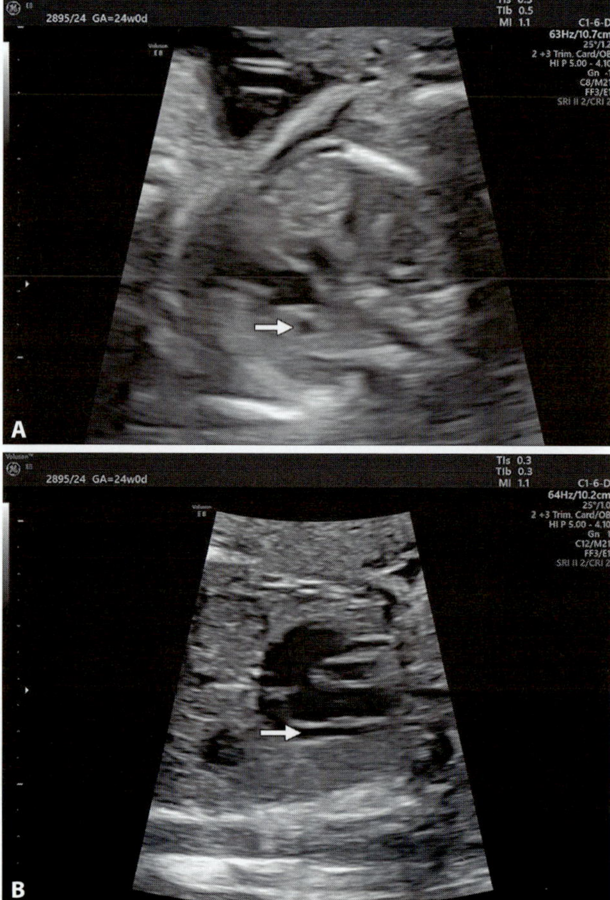

Ans.

1. Persistent left superior vena cava
2. Right atrium
3. Coarctation of aorta
4. Tobacco pipe sign

SUGGESTED READING

1. Abuhamad AZ, Chaoui R. A practical guide to fetal echocardiography: Normal and abnormal hearts, 4th edition. Gurugram: Wolters Kluwer; 2021.

STATION 2.

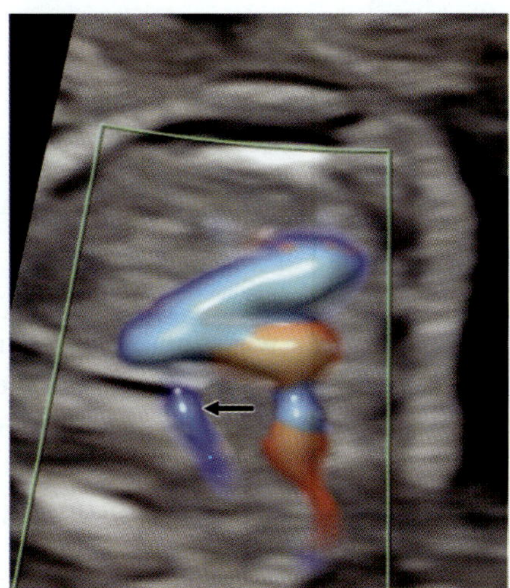

1. **Identify the vessel shown in the image.**
2. **Mention the aneuploidy which is commonly associated with this condition.**
3. **Which is the best plane to visualize this vessel while fetal echo?**
4. **What is the likelihood ratio of this marker as an isolated finding in the presence of all other soft markers being absent?**

Ans.

1. Aberrant right subclavian artery (ARSA)
2. Trisomy 21
3. Three-vessel trachea (3vT) view. ARSA courses behind the trachea and esophagus from the left posterior thoracic side to the right arm.
4. 3.94

SUGGESTED READING

1. Abuhamad AZ, Chaoui R. A practical guide to fetal echocardiography: Normal and abnormal hearts, 4th edition. Gurugram: Wolters Kluwer; 2021.

2. Agathokleous M, Chaveeva P, Poon LC, Kosinski P, Nicolaides KH. Meta-analysis of second-trimester markers for trisomy 21. Ultrasound Obstet Gynecol. 2013;41(3):247-61.

STATION 3.

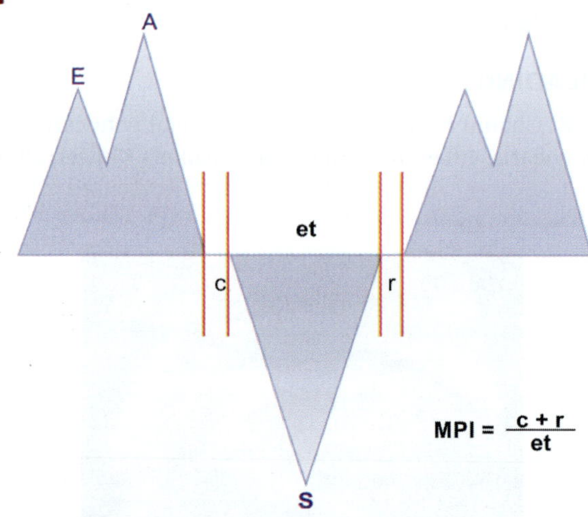

1. **In the image of the Doppler waveform kept across the tricuspid valve, the "A" wave corresponds to which part of the cardiac cycle?**
2. **What is the name of the parameter used to calculate cardiac performance?**
3. **As per ISUOG guidelines, what is the optimal gestational age for performing cardiac screening in a fetus?**
4. **What are the recommended planes for fetal echocardiography as per the ISUOG guidelines?**

Ans.

1. Atrial systole
2. Myocardial performance index or Tei index
3. Between 18 and 22 weeks of gestation
4. Five planes are as follows:
   a. Axial plane at the level of upper abdomen, showing fetal stomach, cross-section of descending aorta (dAo) and inferior vena cava, spine, and liver.
   b. Four-chamber view of fetal heart, showing right and left ventricles and atria, foramen ovale, and pulmonary veins to right and left of dAo.
   c. Left ventricular outflow-tract view, showing proximal ascending aorta (Ao), left ventricle (LV), right ventricle (RV), left atrium (LA), and right atrium (RA), and cross-section of dAo.

d. Right ventricular outflow-tract view showing main pulmonary artery and bifurcation into right and left pulmonary arteries and cross-sections of aorta.

e. Three-vessel-and-trachea view, showing superior vena cava, main pulmonary artery, ductus arteriosus, transverse aortic arch (from proximal Ao to dAo), and trachea.

SUGGESTED READING

1. Abuhamad AZ, Chaoui R. A practical guide to fetal echocardiography: Normal and abnormal hearts, 4th edition. Gurugram: Wolters Kluwer; 2021.
2. Carvalho JS, Axt-Fliedner R, Chaoui R, Copel JA, Cuneo BF, Goff D, et al. ISUOG practice guidelines (updated): fetal cardiac screening. Ultrasound Obstet Gynecol. 2023;61(6):788-803.

STATION 4.

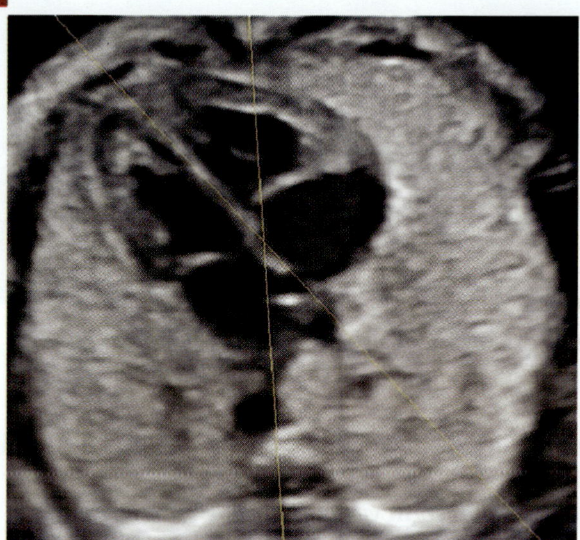

1. **Identify the parameter which is measured in the image.**
2. **What is the normal range of the parameter that is measured?**
3. **Name two conditions associated with an exaggerated left axis deviation on echocardiography.**
4. **What is situs solitus?**

Ans.

1. Cardiac axis
2. 45 ± 15
3. Absent pulmonary valve, aortic stenosis, atrial septal defect (ASD), pulmonary atresia, tetralogy of Fallot (TOF).

4. Situs solitus is defined when liver is on the right side and the stomach on the left side, with the inferior and the superior vena cava connecting to the systemic right atrium on the right side.

SUGGESTED READING

1. Abuhamad AZ, Chaoui R. A practical guide to fetal echocardiography: Normal and abnormal hearts, 4th edition. Gurugram: Wolters Kluwer; 2021.

STATION 5.

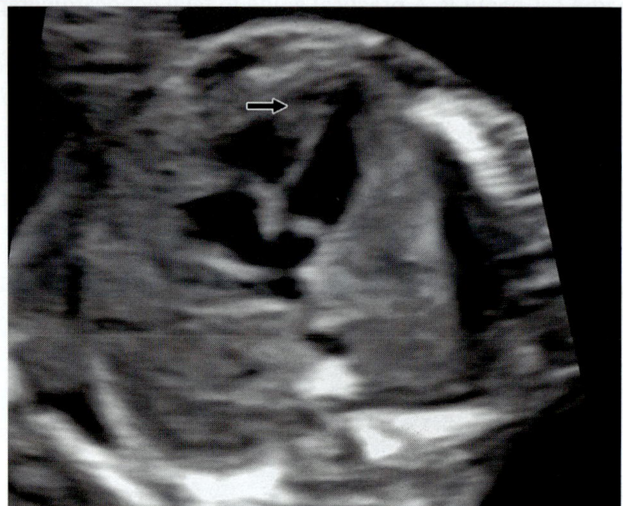

1. **Identify the cardiac chamber shown in the above image.**
2. **Mention one of the main ultrasound characteristics of this cardiac chamber.**
3. **Name two conditions in which the apex is formed by the right ventricle of the heart.**
4. **Name two causes of right ventricle enlargement in utero.**

Ans.

1. Right ventricle
2. Coarse trabeculation with presence of moderator band.
3. Hypoplastic left heart syndrome (HLHS), dextrocardia
4. - *Cardiac*
     - Hypoplastic left heart syndrome
     - Interrupted aortic arch
     - Aortic coarctation

- Ventricular septal defect
- Congenital pulmonary stenosis: wall hypertrophy > chamber dilatation
- Dilated fetal cardiomyopathy

- *Extracardiac*
    - Fetal growth restriction

SUGGESTED READING

1. Abuhamad AZ, Chaoui R. A practical guide to fetal echocardiography: Normal and abnormal hearts, 4th edition. Gurugram: Wolters Kluwer; 2021.
2. Gallafrio CC, Lianza AC, Afonso TR, Sawamura KSS, Rodrigues ACT, Tavares GMP. Isolated dilation of right heart chambers in fetal echocardiography: Correlation with postnatal findings in a quarterly hospital. Austin J Clin Case Rep. 2022;9(4):1255.

STATION 6.

1. **Which is the most reliable criteria to determine fetal situs?**
2. **Name a condition associated with abnormal situs.**
3. **What are the chief characteristics of right atrial isomerism?**
4. **What is the usual prognosis of right atrial isomerism?**

Ans.

1. Position of the aorta and inferior vena cava below the diaphragm are the most reliable criteria for the determination of situs. dAo is seen on the left and inferior vena cava is on the right.
2. Kartagener syndrome.
3. Three lobed lungs on both sides, pyramidal atrial appendages bilaterally, midline liver, and asplenia. There is no left atrium to receive pulmonary venous drainage, and total anomalous pulmonary venous drainage into a systemic vein is seen in >50% of cases. Cardiac defects include transposition of great arteries (TGA), common atrioventricular (AV) valve, ventricular hypoplasia or single ventricle physiology, pulmonary atresia, and pulmonary vein obstruction.
4. Right atrial isomerism is usually associated with severe cyanotic heart disease in infancy. Death in the first year of life is common, especially if there are pulmonary atresia and anomalous pulmonary venous return.

SUGGESTED READING

1. Abuhamad AZ, Chaoui R. A practical guide to fetal echocardiography: Normal and abnormal hearts, 4th edition. Gurugram: Wolters Kluwer; 2021.
2. Routhu M, Mohammad IA. Prenatal evaluation of heterotaxy syndrome by fetal echocardiography and correlating with autopsy. Ultrasound. 2019;27(2): 111-21.

STATION 7.

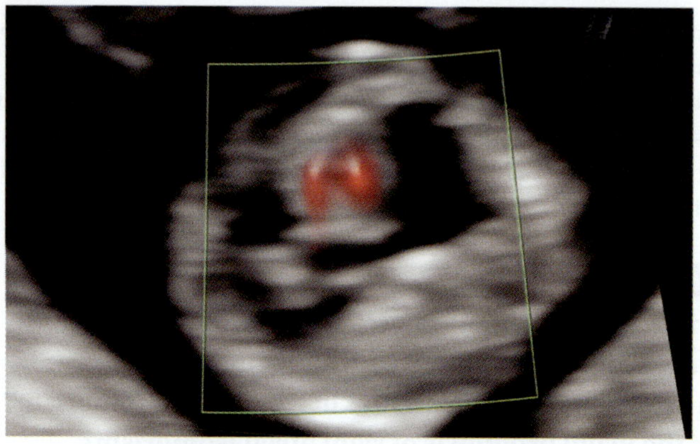

1. **Identify the condition given in the image.**
2. **When is the collection of fluid in pericardial cavity said to be abnormal?**
3. **Which are the most common cardiac conditions associated with nonimmune hydrops?**
4. **Mention four congenital cardiac conditions associated with normal four chamber view of the heart.**

Ans.

1. Pericardial effusion
2. When it is >2 millimeters.
3. Rhythm abnormalities including tachyarrhythmias and heart blocks, structural malformations including valvular heart defects most commonly tricuspid regurgitation, and cardiac tumors most commonly rhabdomyomas.
4. Tetralogy of Fallot, TGA, double-outlet right ventricle, small ventricular septal defects, common arterial trunk, and aortic arch abnormalities.

SUGGESTED READING

1. Abuhamad AZ, Chaoui R. A practical guide to fetal echocardiography: Normal and abnormal hearts, 4th edition. Gurugram: Wolters Kluwer; 2021.
2. Di Salvo DN, Brown DL, Doubilet PM, Benson CB, Frates MC. Clinical significance of isolated fetal pericardial effusion. J Ultrasound Med. 1994;13(4):291-3.

3. Khairudin D, Alfirevic Z, Mone F, Navaratnam K. Non-immune hydrops fetalis: a practical guide for obstetricians. Obstet Gynecol. 2023;25:110-20.

STATION 8.

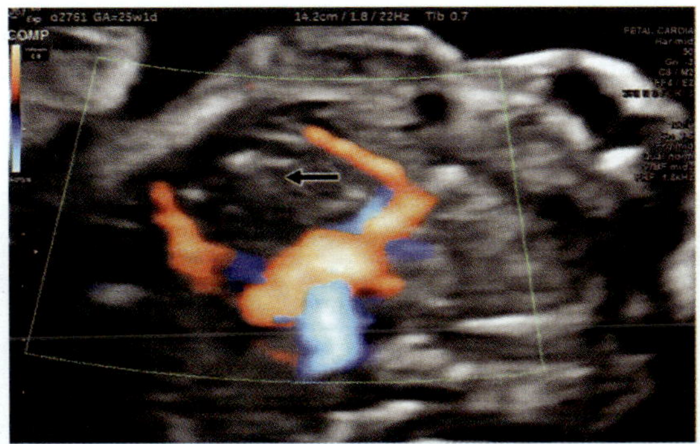

1. **Identify the gland shown in the image.**
2. **Name the artery which forms the boundary of this gland.**
3. **Enumerate any two conditions associated with the hypoplasia of this structure.**
4. **Which ration can be employed to assess this structure objectively?**

Ans.

1. Thymus
2. Internal mammary artery
3. Di George syndrome, trisomy 18 and 21, fetal growth restriction
4. Thymic thoracic ratio. Normal value is 0.44.

SUGGESTED READING

1. Abuhamad AZ, Chaoui R. A practical guide to fetal echocardiography: Normal and abnormal hearts, 4th edition. Gurugram: Wolters Kluwer; 2021.
2. Monteiro M, Aires T, Pimental K, Pedrosa K, Lima S, Aquino M, et al. "Ultrasonographic evaluation of the fetal thymic-thoracic ratio and its association with conotruncal heart defects." J Gynecol Obstet Human Reprod. 2022;51(2):102281.

STATION 9.

1. **On ultrasound, the foramen ovale flap opens into which cardiac chamber.**
2. **Apex of the heart is normally formed by which chamber of the heart.**
3. **Which atrioventricular valve has insertion close to apex of heart?**
4. **Name one fetal cardiac condition in which the direction of flow across the foramen ovale is reversed?**

Ans.

1. Left atrium
2. Right ventricle

3. Tricuspid valve
4. Aortic stenosis/atresia

SUGGESTED READING

1. Abuhamad AZ, Chaoui R. A practical guide to fetal echocardiography: Normal and abnormal hearts, 4th edition. Gurugram: Wolters Kluwer; 2021.

STATION 10.

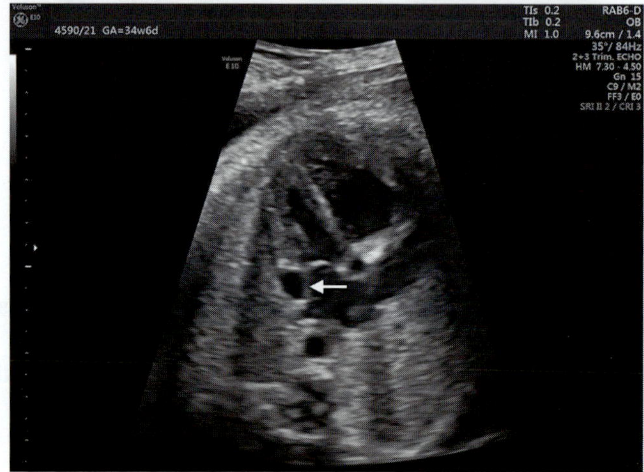

1. **Identify the structure given in the image.**
2. **What is the plane in which this condition can be identified?**
3. **Which structure does this drain into?**
4. **Name two conditions associated with dilatation of this structure.**

Ans.

1. Coronary sinus
2. Posterior plane of the four-chamber view. The coronary sinus is identified at posterior left atrioventricular groove.
3. It drains into the right atrium.
4. Persistent left superior vena cava which typically drains into the coronary sinus and through it into the right atrium. Cardiac type of total anomalous pulmonary venous connection in which the pulmonary veins drain into the coronary sinus and thence into the right atrium.

SUGGESTED READING

1. Abuhamad AZ, Chaoui R. A practical guide to fetal echocardiography: Normal and abnormal hearts, 4th edition. Gurugram: Wolters Kluwer; 2021.
2. Konduri A, Aggarwal S. Partial and total anomalous pulmonary venous connection. In: StatPearls. Treasure Island (FL): StatPearls Publishing; 2025.

STATION 11.

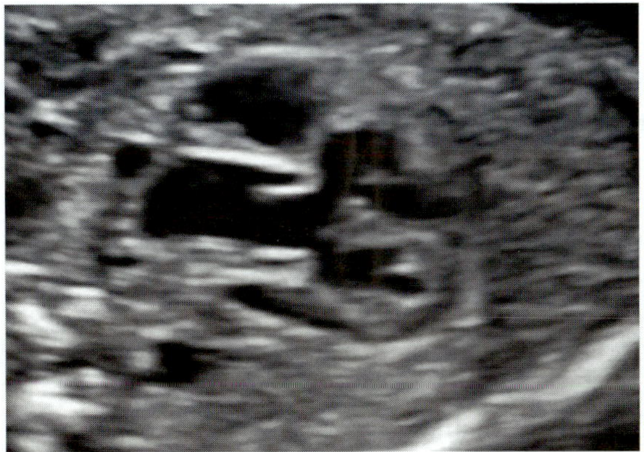

1. **Identify the condition.**
2. **Identify the vessel that is overriding the interventricular septum.**
3. **What is the earliest sign seen in the first trimester for this condition?**
4. **Name two most common chromosomal/genetic associations.**

Ans.

1. Tetralogy of Fallot
2. Aorta
3. Left axis deviation
4. Trisomy 21 and Di Georges'

SUGGESTED READING

1. Abuhamad AZ, Chaoui R. A practical guide to fetal echocardiography: Normal and abnormal hearts, 4th edition. Gurugram: Wolters Kluwer; 2021.

STATION 12.

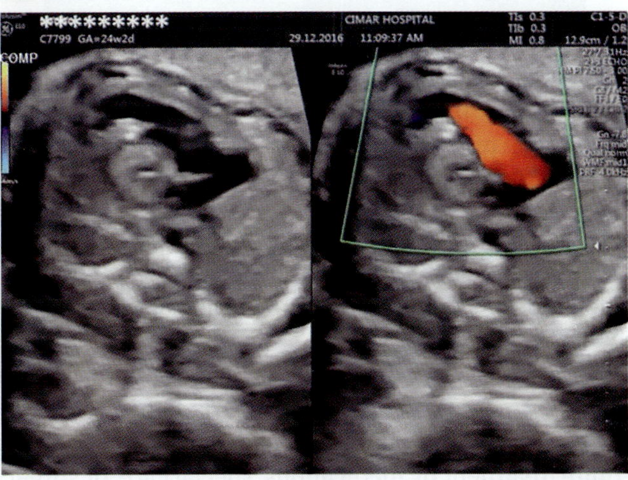

1. **Identify the condition.**
2. **Apex of the heart is formed by which chamber of the heart in this condition.**
3. **Mention two differential diagnoses for the condition given above.**
4. **What is the pathognomonic sign in three vessel trachea view (3vT) view?**

Ans.

1. Hypoplastic left heart syndrome
2. Right ventricle
3. Coarctation of aorta, critical aortic stenosis, mitral valve dysplastic syndrome
4. Reversed flow in aortic arch.

SUGGESTED READING

1. Abuhamad AZ, Chaoui R. A practical guide to fetal echocardiography: Normal and abnormal hearts, 4th edition. Gurugram: Wolters Kluwer; 2021.

STATION 13.

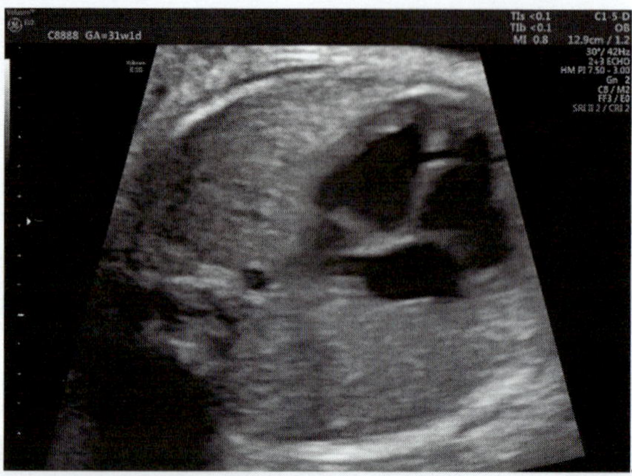

1. **Identify the congenital cardiac anomaly.**
2. **What are the different types of this condition?**
3. **Which is the type most commonly associated with genetic defects?**
4. **Prognosis of isolated ventricular septal defects (VSDs)?**

Ans.

1. VSD
2. Inlet, outlet, muscular, and perimembranous VSD.
3. Deletion of 22q11.2
4. Size, site, and maternal age are prognostic factors for the natural closure of the defect. Muscular isolated VSD is mostly a benign finding, while perimembranous VSD tends to have larger size, lower closure rates, and more likely require treatment by medications, special care, or surgery to thrive.

SUGGESTED READING

1. Abuhamad AZ, Chaoui R. A practical guide to fetal echocardiography: Normal and abnormal hearts, 4th edition. Gurugram: Wolters Kluwer; 2021.
2. Chen X, Zhang Q, Lu M, Feng Q, Qin L, Liao S. Prenatal finding of isolated ventricular septal defect: genetic association, outcomes and counselling. Front Genet. 2024;15:1447216.

STATION 14.

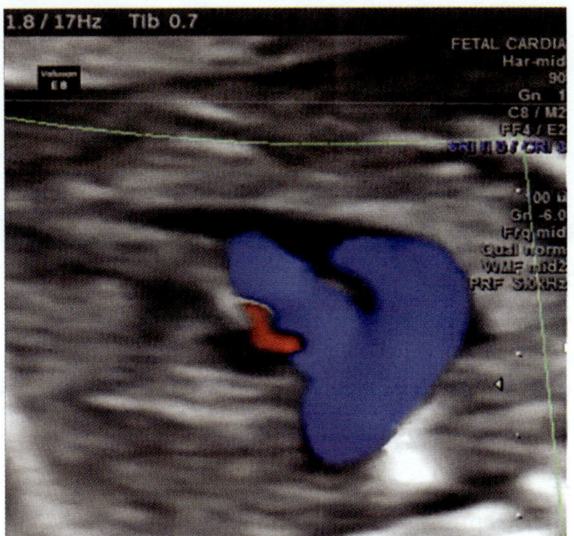

1. **What are the ultrasound findings seen in five-chamber view of this condition?**
2. **Mention two differential diagnoses of this condition.**
3. **What sign is seen in the three vessel trachea view (3vT) view in this condition?**

Ans.

1. In five-chamber view, VSD and origin of both great arteries from the anterior (right) ventricle can be visualized [double-outlet right ventricle (DORV)].
2. Tetralogy of Fallot and transposition of great vessels (TGA)
3. Single vessel in 3vT view.

SUGGESTED READING

1. Abuhamad AZ, Chaoui R. A practical guide to fetal echocardiography: Normal and abnormal hearts, 4th edition. Gurugram: Wolters Kluwer; 2021.
2. Mogra R. Simplifying ultrasound assessment of the fetal heart: Incorporating the complete Three Vessel View into routine screening. Australas J Ultrasound Med. 2013;16(4):168-75.

STATION 15.

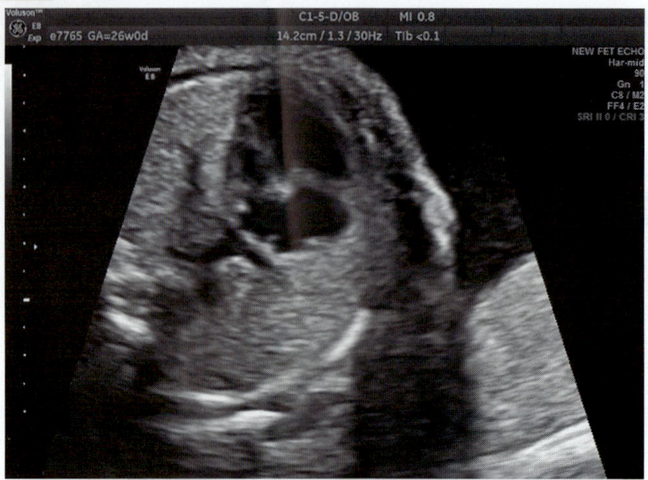

1. **Identify the condition.**
2. **Mention the different types of this condition.**
3. **Which type is associated with dilated coronary sinus?**
4. **Name the sign which is seen in the area behind the heart in this condition.**

Ans.

1. Total anomalous pulmonary venous connection (TAPVC).
2. Type 1—supracardiac type; Type II—cardiac; Type III—infracardiac; and Type IV—mixed.
3. Cardiac type. A dilated coronary sinus in the absence of a left superior vena cava (LSVC) should raise the suspicion for the presence of TAPVC.
4. Twig sign

SUGGESTED READING

1. Abuhamad AZ, Chaoui R. A practical guide to fetal echocardiography: Normal and abnormal hearts, 4th edition. Gurugram: Wolters Kluwer; 2021.
2. Chih WL, Ko H, Chang TY. Prenatal ultrasound markers of isolated total anomalous pulmonary venous return and a sequential approach to reach diagnosis. J Med Ultrasound. 2024;32(2):104-9.

STATION 16.

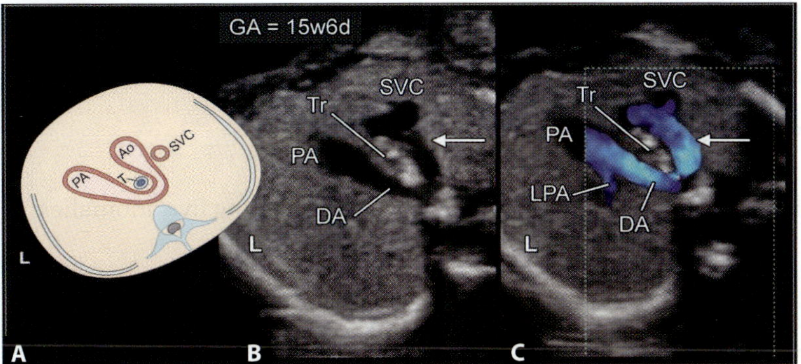

1. **Identify the condition.**
2. **Which is the best plane to demonstrate this condition?**
3. **What is the most common genetic association?**
4. **What is the other organ to be assessed with this condition?**

Ans.

1. Right aortic arch with right ductus arteriosus.
2. Three-vessel trachea view.
3. A microdeletion of chromosome 22q11.2, also known as DiGeorge syndrome in 5% of cases.
4. Thymus gland

SUGGESTED READING

1. Abuhamad AZ, Chaoui R. A practical guide to fetal echocardiography: Normal and abnormal hearts, 4th edition. Gurugram: Wolters Kluwer; 2021.
2. Petrescu AM, Ruican D, Tudorache S, Cernea N, Dobrescu MA, Iliescu DG. Associated chromosomal abnormalities in fetuses diagnosed prenatally with right aortic arch. Curr Health Sci J. 2021;47(2):170-6.

STATION 17.

1. **What is the term used to describe the position of the heart in which the heart is located in the right chest with cardiac axis pointed to the right?**
2. **Mention the anomalies associated with Pentalogy of Cantrell.**

3. **Enumerate two congenital cardiac conditions associated with left axis deviation of the heart.**
4. **Enumerate two congenital cardiac conditions associated with right axis deviation of the heart.**

Ans.

1. Dextroversion
2. Pentalogy of Cantrell is a syndrome encompassing five anomalies:
   a. Midline supraumbilical abdominal defect
   b. Defect of the lower sternum
   c. Defect in the diaphragmatic pericardium
   d. Deficiency of the anterior diaphragm
   e. Intracardiac abnormalities
3. Tetralogy of Fallot, common arterial trunk, coarctation of aorta, and Ebstein's anomaly.
4. Left-sided diaphragmatic hernia, isomerism and situs inversus, inversion of the ventricles (in congenitally corrected transposition or levo-transposition), atrioventricular septal defects, a double-outlet right ventricle, and a common atrium.

SUGGESTED READING

1. Abuhamad AZ, Chaoui R. A practical guide to fetal echocardiography: Normal and abnormal hearts, 4th edition. Gurugram: Wolters Kluwer; 2021.
2. Jeanty P, Chaoui R, Tihonenko I, Grochal F. Review of findings in fetal cardiac section drawings Part 1: The 4-chamber view. J Ultrasound Med. 2007;26(11):1601-10.

STATION 18.

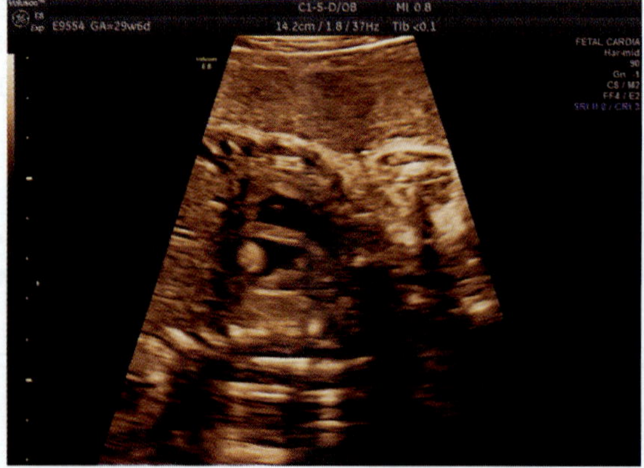

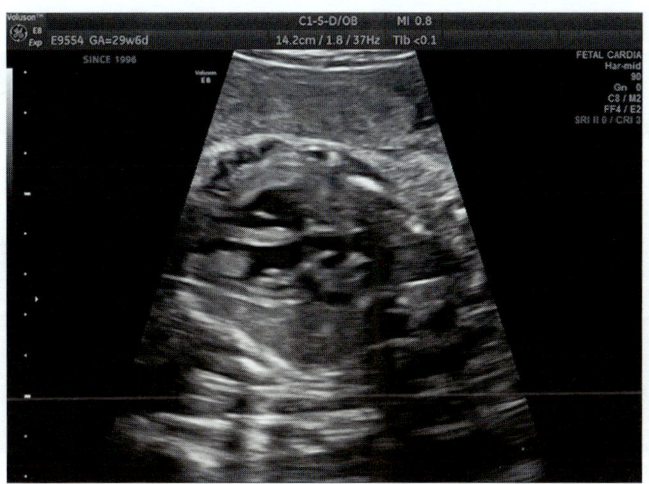

1. **Identify the lesion.**
2. **Mention a condition associated with this lesion.**
3. **Enumerate the most common site of origin of this lesion in the heart.**
4. **Write the inheritance pattern associated with this condition.**
5. **What other structure should be assessed when this condition is encountered?**

Ans.

1. Rhabdomyoma
2. Tuberous sclerosis
3. It can occur within the cardiac walls, interventricular septum, cardiac apex, and outflow conus.
4. When associated with the tuberous sclerosis complex, the inheritance is autosomal dominant. TSC1 and two genes should be investigated.
5. Hamartomas in multiple organ systems including the brain, heart, skin, lungs, and kidneys.

SUGGESTED READING

1. Abuhamad AZ, Chaoui R. A practical guide to fetal echocardiography: Normal and abnormal hearts, 4th edition. Gurugram: Wolters Kluwer; 2021.
2. Zhen L, Yang YD, He Y, Pan M, Han J, Yang X, et al. "Prenatal genetic diagnosis of cardiac rhabdomyoma: A single-center experience." Eur J Obstet, Gynecol, Reprod Biol. 2020;249:7-10.

STATION 19.

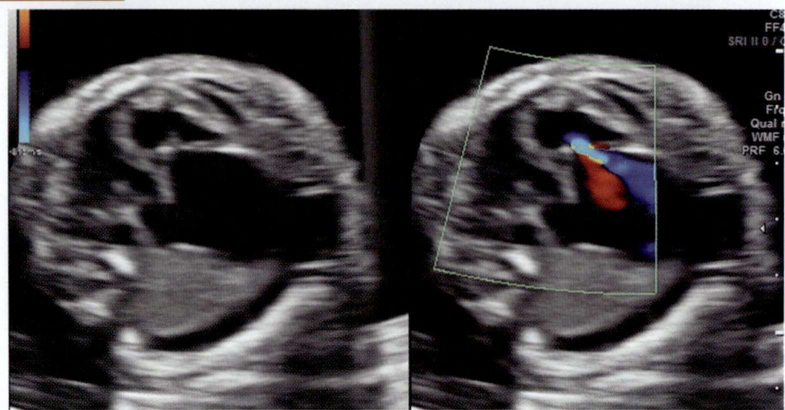

1. **Identify the condition.**
2. **Which valve is apically displaced in this condition?**
3. **Name the echocardiographic prognostic score which is used to predict the outcome of fetuses with this anomaly.**
4. **What is the most common cardiac pathology associated with this condition?**

Ans.

1. Ebstein's anomaly
2. Septal and posterior leaflet of tricuspid valve is apically displaced.
3. Celermajer index—in this the ratio of the combined area of the RA and atrialized RV to that of the functional RV and left heart in a four-chamber view at end diastole is calculated. A score below 0.5 predicts a favorable outcome, whereas a score greater than 1.5 correlates with very poor outcome.
4. Tricuspid regurgitation and pulmonary stenosis

SUGGESTED READING

1. Abuhamad AZ, Chaoui R. A practical guide to fetal echocardiography: Normal and abnormal hearts, 4th edition. Gurugram: Wolters Kluwer; 2021.

STATION 20.

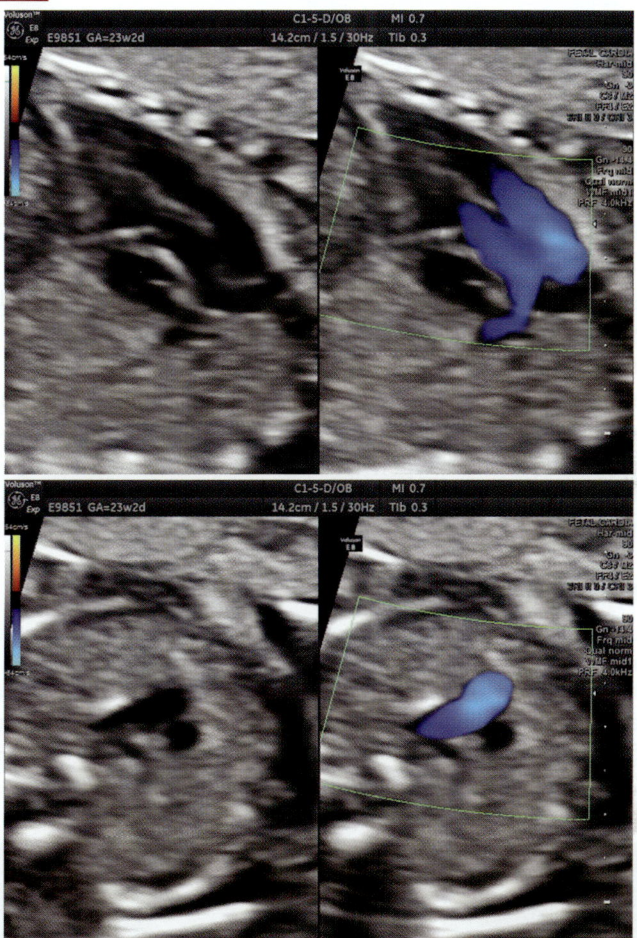

1. Identify the condition.
2. What is the lead sign in diagnosing this condition?
3. Mention two differential diagnoses.
4. What is the prognosis of this condition when isolated?

Ans.

1. Transposition of great arteries.
2. Presence of I sign in three-vessel view.
3. Double outlet right ventricle, corrected TGA.
4. Dextro-transposition of great arteries (D-TGA) is a surgically correctable disease. The most common surgical procedure is the Jatene arterial switch operation (ASO) with a perioperative mortality of about 2–4%, and a high 10-year survival rate—88–97%. However, neurodevelopmental dysfunctions are frequently seen (reduced performance in attention, visual–spatial skills, and executive functions, and anxiety disorders). Delayed brain development in utero possibly increases postnatal susceptibility to acquired white matter injury.

   The I-transposition, however, is less dangerous than a d-transposition because the great arteries are also reversed. This "double reversal" allows the body to still receive oxygen-rich blood and the lungs to still receive the oxygen-poor blood. These patients hence not require surgery often even until adulthood, unless associated cardiac anomalies are present.

SUGGESTED READING

1. Abuhamad AZ, Chaoui R. A practical guide to fetal echocardiography: Normal and abnormal hearts, 4th edition. Gurugram: Wolters Kluwer; 2021.
2. Stancioi-Cismaru AF, Dinu M, Carp-Veliscu A, Capitanescu RG, Pana RC, Sirbu OC, et al. Live-birth incidence of isolated D-transposition of great arteries—The shift in trends due to early diagnosis. Diagnostics. 2024;14(11):1185.

STATION 21.

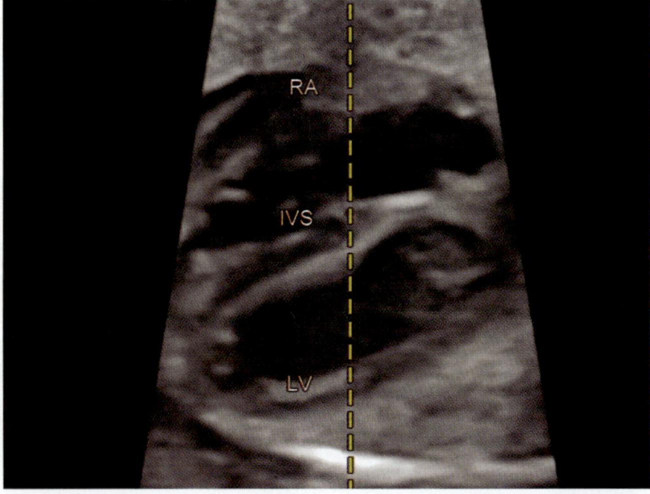

A woman with 24 weeks of gestation is undergoing fetal echocardiography examination. The cardiac rhythm appears intermittently irregular.

1. **Why is M-mode used in the assessment of cardiac rhythm?**
2. **Where should the M-mode sampling line be placed?**

3. **What are the limitations of M-mode?**
4. **How can Pulse-wave Doppler echocardiography supplement M-mode in assessing fetal cardiac rhythm irregularities?**

Ans.

1. M-mode echocardiography can simultaneously measure atrial and ventricular motion through the sampling line. This helps determine the sequence of atrial and ventricular motion, thus inferring electrical events.
2. The M-mode cursor should intersect both an atrium and a ventricle to record the relationship between atrial and ventricular contractions.
3. The onset and peak of atrial and ventricular contractions are not clearly defined in M-mode, limiting its ability to measure atrioventricular (AV) time intervals. Additionally, fetal movements and variable positions may complicate correct placement of the sampling line.
4. Pulse-wave Doppler echocardiography can record blood flow across the mitral valve (atrial contraction) and aortic valve (ventricular contraction) simultaneously. This allows for precise measurement of atrial and ventricular rates as well as the atrial-to-ventricular interval (PR interval), distinguishing normal from abnormal conduction patterns.

SUGGESTED READING

1. Hornberger LK. Echocardiographic assessment of fetal arrhythmias. Heart. 2007;93(11):1331-3.
2. Liao H, Tang C, Qiao L, Zhou K, Hua Y, Wang C, et al. Prenatal management strategy for immune-associated congenital heart block in fetuses. Front Cardiovasc Med. 2021;8:644122.

STATION 22.

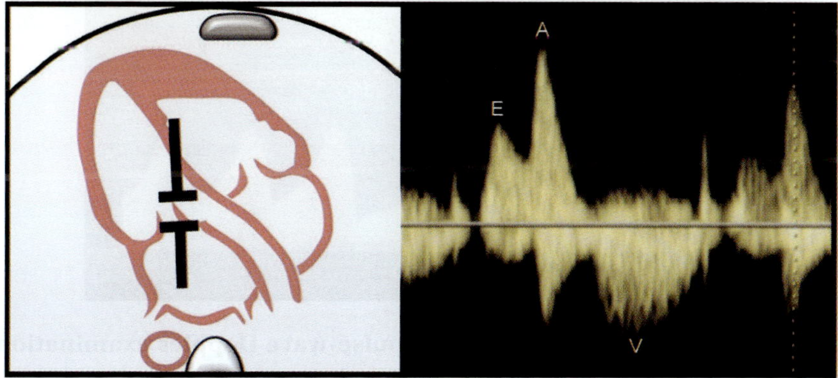

An image is shown from a fetal echocardiographic examination.

1. **Which modality is being used in the image shown above?**
2. **What do E, A, and V represent in the context of the cardiac cycle?**
3. **How is mechanical atrioventricular interval (PR interval) calculated?**
4. **What is the normal range for mechanical PR interval?**

Ans.

1. Pulse-wave Doppler
2. The *E-wave* represents early passive filling of the left ventricle during early diastole when the mitral valve opens. The *A-wave* represents active filling due to atrial contraction during late diastole (atrial systole). The *V-wave* signifies blood flow leaving the left ventricle into the aorta during ventricular systole.
3. Mechanical PR interval is calculated from the start of the A-wave (atrial systole) to the start of the V-wave (ventricular systole).
4. Normal PR interval is 120 + 20 ms. A PR interval >150 ms indicates first-degree heart block.

SUGGESTED READING

1. Hernandez-Andrade E, Benavides-Serralde JA, Cruz-Martinez R, Welsh A, Mancilla-Ramirez J. Evaluation of conventional Doppler fetal cardiac function parameters: E/A ratios, outflow tracts, and myocardial performance index. Fetal Diagn Ther. 2012;32(1-2):22-9.
2. Phoon CKL, Kim MY, Buyon JP, Friedman DM. Finding the "PR-fect" solution: What is the best tool to measure fetal cardiac PR intervals for the detection and possible treatment of early conduction disease? Congenital Heart Disease. 2012;7:349-60.

STATION 23.

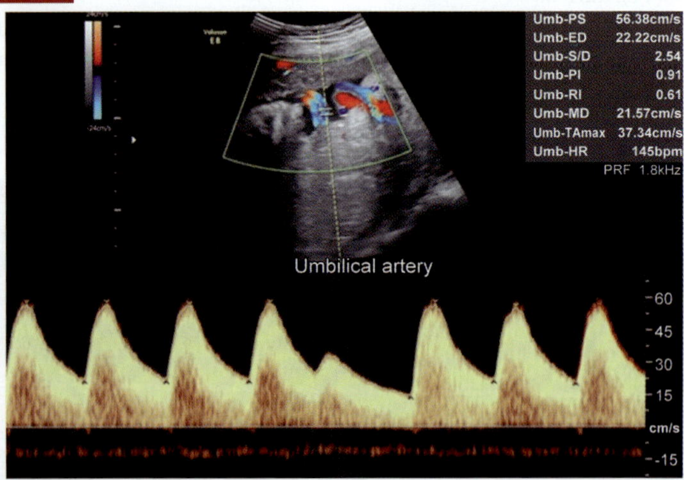

You are performing umbilical artery pulse-wave Doppler examination. You observe the waveform pattern shown above.

1. **Identify the rhythm abnormality.**
2. **How will you confirm your diagnosis?**
3. **What are the risk factors for progression to tachyarrhythmia?**
4. **How to manage the above condition?**

Ans.

1. Premature atrial contraction (PACs). These are the most common fetal arrhythmias, causing irregular cardiac rhythm or skipped beats. The waveform shows a conducted atrial ectopic beat, resulting in early ventricular systole and a smaller umbilical blood flow peak, followed by a compensatory pause, which is characteristic of PACs.
2. Use M-mode echocardiography to simultaneously record atrial and ventricular contractions, determining their relationship and rates.
3. Frequent PACs, PACs occurring in bigeminy, multiple blocked PACs, short runs of supraventricular tachycardia (SVT) associated with PACs, signs of cardiac failure, and the presence of a foramen ovale aneurysm.
4. PACs usually resolve spontaneously without treatment. Advise the mother to avoid caffeine, smoking, alcohol, and certain drugs. Perform fetal echocardiography to rule out structural heart defects or foramen ovale aneurysm. Monitor weekly for the development of SVT. Consider delivery if associated with cardiac dysfunction.

SUGGESTED READING

1. Bet BB, Eijsbroek FC, van Leeuwen E, Linskens IH, Knobbe I, Clur SA, et al. Fetal premature atrial contractions: natural course, risk factors and adverse outcome. Ultrasound Obstet Gynecol. 2024;63(5):650-7.
2. Strasburger JF, Cheulkar B, Wichman HJ. Perinatal arrhythmias: Diagnosis and management. Clin Perinatol. 2007;34(4):627-52.
3. Veduta A, Panaitescu AM, Ciobanu AM, Neculcea D, Popescu MR, Peltecu G, et al. Treatment of fetal arrhythmias. J Clin Med. 2021;10(11):2510.
4. Weber R, Stambach D, Jaeggi E. Diagnosis and management of common fetal arrhythmias. J Saudi Heart Assoc. 2011;23(2):61-6.

STATION 24. During obstetric ultrasound, a fetus shows a heart rate of 95 beats/minute (BPM). No other abnormality is seen.

1. **What is fetal bradycardia?**
2. **What is the most common cause of transient bradycardia in a fetus?**
3. **List three most common causes for fetal bradycardia.**
4. **What is the characteristic feature of sinus bradycardia on fetal echocardiography?**

Ans.

1. Fetal heart rate <110 BPM.
2. Increased vagal stimulation in the fetus, commonly associated with abdominal pressure by the ultrasound probe.
3. Sinus bradycardia, blocked atrial bigeminy/trigeminy, and high-degree atrioventricular (AV) heart block.
4. A 1:1 AV conduction on M-mode or pulse wave echocardiography with a slow atrial rate.

SUGGESTED READING

1. Hornberger LK, Sahn DJ. Rhythm abnormalities of the fetus. Heart. 2007; 93(10):1294-300.
2. Srinivasan S, Strasburger J. Overview of fetal arrhythmias. Curr Opin Pediatr. 2008;20(5):522-31.

STATION 25.

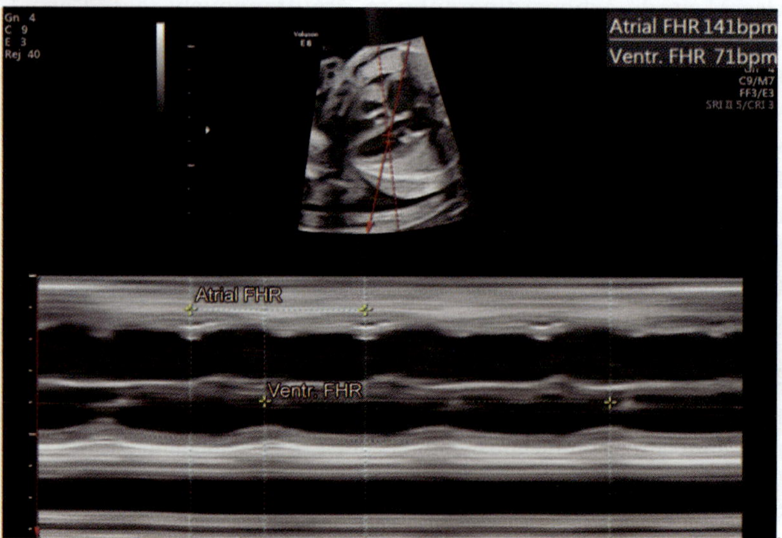

1. **Identify the rhythm abnormality.**
2. **What are the risk factors for this condition?**
3. **What are the complications of this condition?**
4. **Is the above condition reversible?**

Ans.

1. The rhythm abnormality shown in the image is *congenital atrioventricular block (CAVB)*. The atrial rhythm is regular and the rate of 141 BPM is normal. However, the ventricles are beating regularly but at a much slower rate (71 BPM). Moreover, the atria and ventricles are beating independently due to complete interruption of the AV conduction.
2. CAVB can occur in the fetuses with congenital heart defects, especially left atrial isomerism, congenitally corrected TGA or atrioventricular septal defect. Maternal risk factors include metabolic disease (i.e., type 2 diabetes mellitus), medications (i.e., anticonvulsants and retinoic acids), viral infections, and connective tissue disorders causing autoantibodies (e.g., systemic lupus erythematosus and Sjogren's syndrome).
3. Complications include fetal hydrops, impaired left ventricular function, fetal or neonatal death, and late-onset left ventricular cardiomyopathy.

4. CAVB or third-degree AV block is generally irreversible. However, if the block is incomplete (e.g., first or second degree) and detected early, interventions like maternal steroids may help reduce inflammation and prevent progression to complete block.

SUGGESTED READING

1. Hansahiranwadee W. Diagnosis and management of fetal autoimmune atrioventricular block. Int J Womens Health. 2020;12:633-9.
2. Pruetz JD, Miller JC, Loeb GE, Silka MJ, Bar-Cohen Y, Chmait RH. Prenatal diagnosis and management of congenital complete heart block. Birth Defects Res. 2019;111(8):380-8.

STATION 26. A primigravida undergoes fetal echocardiography at 22 weeks of gestation. On scanning, a CAVB is detected with fetal heart rate of 50 BPM. No other congenital malformation is detected in the fetal heart. The physical examination of the mother reveals rashes on the nose and both cheeks.

1. **What is the most probable cause of *CAVB* in this case?**
2. **Which tests should be advised to confirm diagnosis?**
3. **How can this case be treated?**
4. **What is the prognosis of the fetus in such cases?**

Ans.

1. The rash on the mother's nose and cheeks suggests a condition like *systemic lupus erythematosus (SLE)* or a related autoimmune disorder such as *Sjogren's syndrome.* These conditions are often linked to specific autoantibodies. These antibodies can cross the placenta and attach to the fetal heart's conduction system, leading to inflammation and scarring, which ultimately causes CAVB.
2. To confirm the diagnosis, a blood test for *anti-Ro (SSA)* and *anti-La (SSB)* antibodies in the mother is essential. Additional tests, such as the *antinuclear antibody (ANA)* test and *anti-double-stranded DNA (dsDNA) antibodies,* can help confirm SLE.
3. Treatment includes fluorinated steroids (e.g., betamethasone or dexamethasone) and intravenous immunoglobulin (IVIG) to reduce inflammation, and/or β-sympathomimetic drugs (e.g., salbutamol or terbutaline) to increase the heart rate and cardiac output. However, the consensus on an effective treatment protocol is lacking.
4. CAVB detected during pregnancy is usually permanent because the heart's conduction system becomes scarred. Severe fetal bradycardia caused by CAVB can lead to complications like *hydrops fetalis.* Fetal demise occurs in about *22%* of cases, and neonatal mortality ranges from *11 to 16%.* However, the children who survive the neonatal period generally have a good prognosis with appropriate care, including *pacemaker implantation* when needed.

SUGGESTED READING

1. Brito-Zerón P, Izmirly PM, Ramos-Casals M, Buyon JP, Khamashta MA. The clinical spectrum of autoimmune congenital heart block. Nat Review Rheumatol. 2015;11:301-12.
2. Hansahiranwadee W. Diagnosis and management of fetal autoimmune atrioventricular block. Int J Womens Health. 2020;12:633-9.

STATION 27. A 25-year-old woman, G2P1, presents to her obstetrician at 18 weeks of gestation. She has a history of Sjogren's syndrome and a previous pregnancy complicated by fetal CAVB.

1. **How will you screen the fetus for immune-mediated CAVB?**
2. **After what gestational age can immune-mediated fetal arrhythmias be present?**
3. **What is the role of assessing maternal antibody titer in such cases?**
4. **Can any prophylactic treatment be advised?**

Ans.

1. Screening for heart block can be performed by evaluation of the mechanical PR interval, measured by spectral Doppler on serial fetal echocardiograms, between 16 and 28 weeks of gestation. Normal PR interval is 120 + 20 ms. If the PR interval is > 140 ms, more frequent fetal echocardiography should be considered. If PR interval is >150 ms, first-degree heart block should be diagnosed.
2. Circulating maternal antibodies cross the placenta starting from 12 weeks of gestation. Most cases of immune-mediated CAVB are detected between 18 and 25 weeks of gestation.
3. Titers above 100 U/mL are associated with an 85% risk of CAVB.
4. Hydroxychloroquine (HCQ) an anti-inflammatory and immunomodulatory drug that reduces the activity of maternal autoantibodies that cross the placenta. HCQ reduces the recurrence of congenital heart block (CHB) by >50%. In the absence of adverse events, HCQ administration could be recommended until delivery.

SUGGESTED READING

1. Hansahiranwadee W. Diagnosis and management of fetal autoimmune atrioventricular block. Int J Womens Health. 2020;12:633-9.
2. Liao H, Tang C, Qiao L, Zhou K, Hua Y, Wang C, et al. Prenatal management strategy for immune-associated congenital heart block in fetuses. Front Cardiovasc Med. 2021;8:644122.

STATION 28.

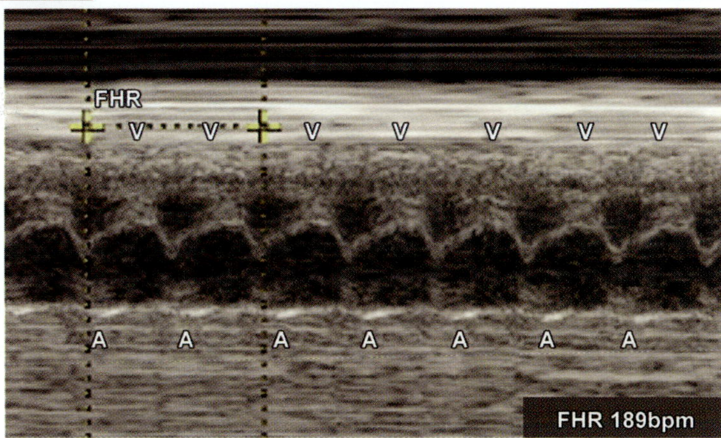

Shown above is an M-mode tracing of a fetal cardiac rhythm.

1. **What is the normal fetal heart rate?**
2. **What is the most likely diagnosis inferred from the above tracing?**
3. **What are the common etiologies for the diagnosis inferred from the tracing?**
4. **What is the treatment for the same?**

Ans.

1. The normal fetal heart rate (FHR) is gestational-age-dependent but has generally been defined as a rate between 120 and 160 BPM. However, the fetal cardiologists consider FHR between 110 and 180 BPM as normal.
2. An FHR > 180 BPM but < 200 BPM with 1:1 AV conduction is considered as *sinus tachycardia*. FHR > 200 BPM is likely to be *SVT.*
3. Etiologies include maternal fever, maternal hyperthyroidism, fetal thyrotoxicosis, myocarditis, anemia, hypoxia, acidosis, and exposure to maternal stimulants, e.g., caffeine and drugs.
4. Treatment involves addressing the underlying cause.

SUGGESTED READING

1. Irish Medical Journal. Uncomplicated Fetal Tachycardia in Labour: Dilemmas and Uncertainties. [online] Available from https://imj.ie/uncomplicated-fetal-tachycardia-in-labour-dilemmas-and-uncertainties [Last accessed May, 2025].
2. Killen S a. S, Strasburger JF. Diagnosis and management of fetal arrhythmias in the current era. J Cardiovasc Dev Dis. 2024;11(6):163.

STATION 29.

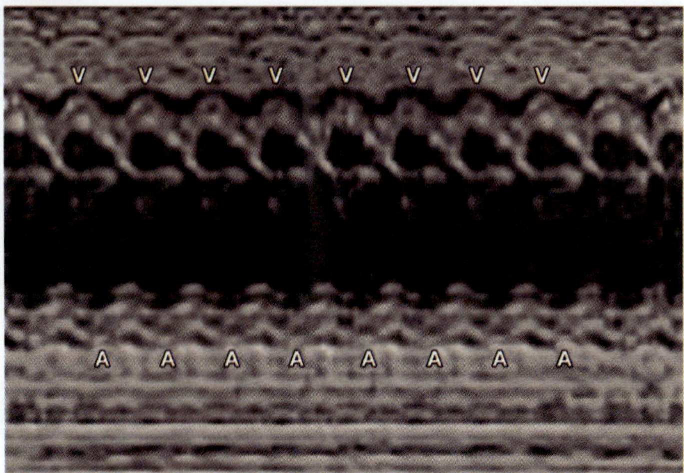

M-mode fetal echocardiography of a fetus of 28 weeks gestational age is shown above. The heart rate is 230 BPM.

1. **Identify the above condition.**
2. **What are its diagnostic characteristics?**
3. **What are the complications of the above condition?**
4. **How is it treated?**

Ans.

1. Fetal supraventricular tachycardia.
2. Heart rate > 200 BPM, with 1:1 of atrioventricular conduction, a monotonous fetal heart rate with lack of atrial or ventricular rate variability.
3. High output cardiac failure, hydrops, cerebrovascular thromboembolism, in utero demise, and preterm delivery.
4. If near term, consider delivery. Otherwise, all pregnant women with sustained fetal tachycardia or intermittent tachycardia with signs of fetal compromise, like hydrops should receive pharmacological treatment. Digoxin is the first choice of drug for the treatment. However, if hydrops is present, maternal side effects or if the SVT is refractory to Digoxin, a second-line drug such as Sotalol or Flecainide can be added. Preterm delivery should be considered in refractory cases or in fetuses with signs of compromise.

SUGGESTED READING

1. Killen S a. S, Strasburger JF. Diagnosis and management of fetal arrhythmias in the current era. J Cardiovasc Dev Dis. 2024;11(6):163.
2. Purkayastha S, Weinreich M, Fontes JD, Lau JF, Wolfe DS, Bortnick AE. Fetal supraventricular tachycardia: What the adult cardiologist needs to know. Cardiol Review. 2022;30(1):31-7.

STATION 30.

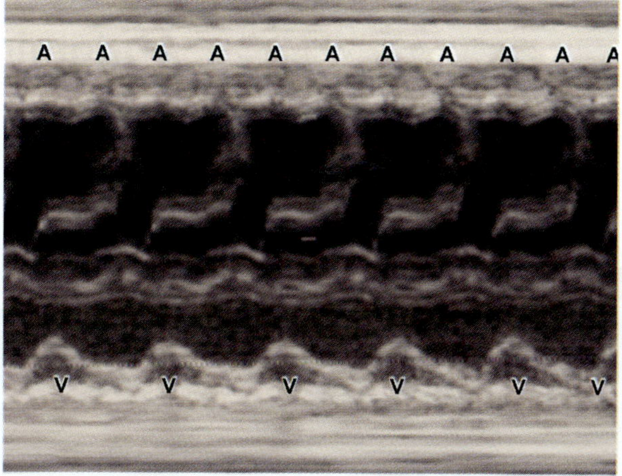

M-mode fetal echocardiography of a fetus of 34 weeks gestational age is shown above. The atrial rate is 400 BPM. The ventricular rate is 200 BPM.

1. **Identify the above condition.**
2. **What are its diagnostic characteristics?**
3. **What are the complications of the above condition?**
4. **How is it treated?**

Ans.

1. Fetal atrial flutter
2. Defined as a rapid regular atrial rate of 300–600/min, accompanied by variable atrioventricular conduction, resulting in slower ventricular rates.
3. High output cardiac failure, hydrops, cerebrovascular thromboembolism, in utcro demise, and preterm delivery.
4. Pharmacological treatment includes Digoxin as the first choice of drug as Sotalol or Flecainide can also be added to control the heart rate.

SUGGESTED READING

1. Killen S a. S, Strasburger JF. Diagnosis and management of fetal arrhythmias in the current era. J Cardiovas Dev Dis. 2024;11(6):163.
2. Krapp M. Review of diagnosis, treatment, and outcome of fetal atrial flutter compared with supraventricular tachycardia. Heart. 2003;89(8):913-7.

Congenital Abnormalities of the Gastrointestinal Tract and Abdominal Wall

Tulika Ranjan Joshi

STATION 1.

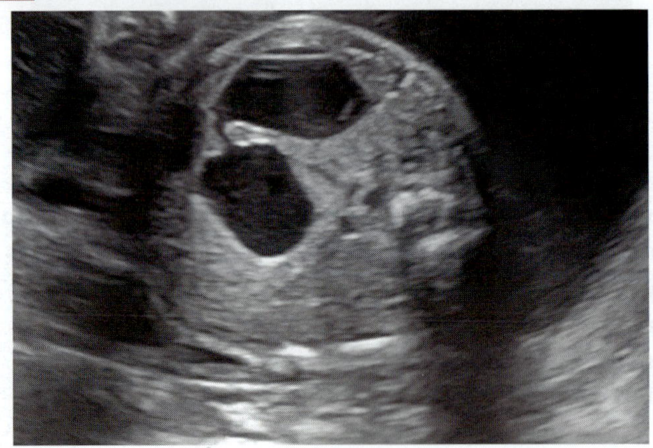

1. **Identify the sonographic sign seen in figure above.**
2. **Identify the anatomic abnormality shown.**
3. **Which genetic malformation is seen most commonly associated with this condition?**
4. **Which anatomic malformation is most commonly associated with this condition?**

Ans.

1. Double bubble sign
2. Duodenal atresia
3. Trisomy 21 (Down's syndrome) 40–50% cases
4. Other gastrointestinal malformations like gut malrotations 40%.

SUGGESTED READING

1. Bishop JC, McCormick B, Johnson CT, Miller J, Jelin E, Blakemore K, et al. The double bubble sign: duodenal atresia and associated genetic etiologies. Fetal Diagn Ther. 2020;47(2):98-103.

STATION 2.

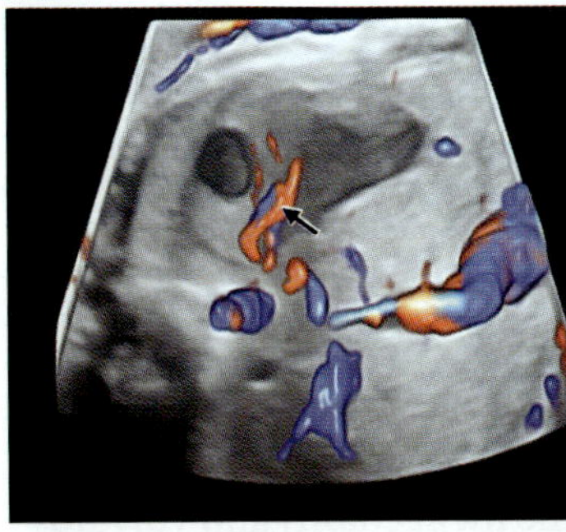
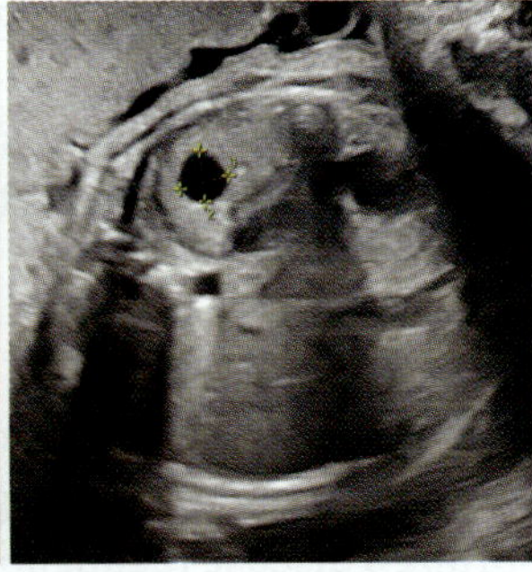

1. **Identify the abnormality in this 31-week fetus.**
2. **Identify the vessel anterior to the structure (arrow).**
3. **Name three differential diagnoses of this condition.**
4. **What is antenatal course of such lesions?**
5. **What will be your prenatal advice and postnatal follow-up plan?**

Ans.

1. Splenic cyst
2. Splenic artery originating from celiac trunk.
3. Pancreatic cyst, adrenal cyst, and double bubble sign of duodenal atresia.
4. Most of the splenic cysts remain stable during antenatal period but rarely enlargement, hemorrhage, infection, and rupture may occur.
5. Periodic follow-up scans 4 weekly followed by postnatal ultrasound evaluation.

SUGGESTED READING

1. Venkataraman D. Fetal splenic cyst: antenatal diagnosis and outcome. BMJ Case Rep. 2009;2009:bcr0920080843.

STATION 3.

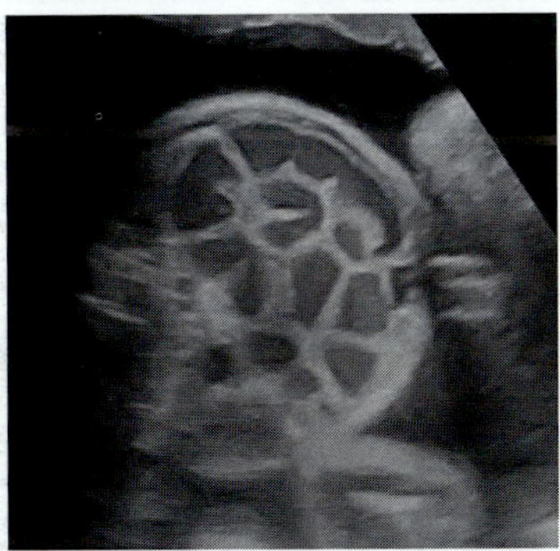

1. **Identify the pathology in 32-week 5-day fetus.**
2. **What is the cutoff value to diagnose small bowel dilation in second/third trimester?**
3. **What is the differential diagnosis of this condition?**
4. **Name two prognostic factors with reasons.**

Ans.

1. Small bowel dilatation/atresia
2. A dilated small bowel with a diameter of ≥7 mm and length greater than 15 mm during the mid to late stages of pregnancy.
3. Hirschsprung's disease (aganglionic megacolon) and volvulus
4. Meconium peritonitis (risk of cystic fibrosis 90%) and polyhydramnios (high risk of delayed anastomosis and increased surgical complications).

SUGGESTED READING

1. Iacobelli BD, Zaccara A, Spirydakis I, Giorlandino C, Capolupo I, Nahom A, et al. Prenatal counselling of small bowel atresia: watch the fluid. Prenat Diagn. 2006;26(3):214-17.

STATION 4.

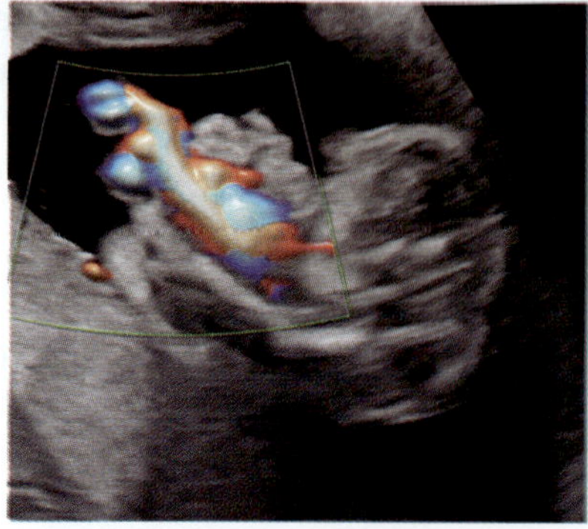

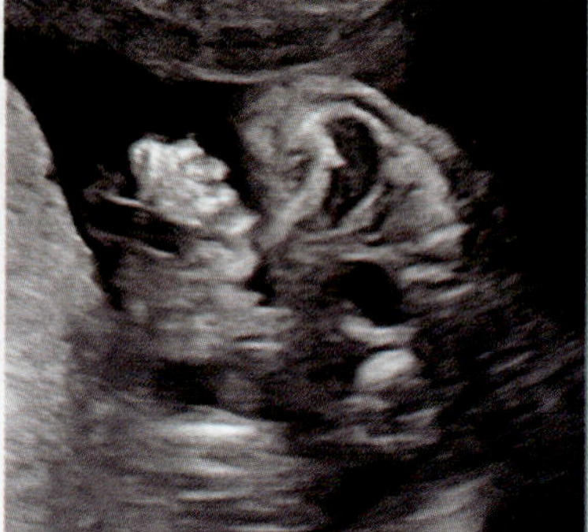

1. **Identify the abnormality in this 23-week 4-day fetus.**
2. **Give a differential diagnosis of this condition and explain how to differentiate between the two conditions.**
3. **What is the risk of genetic/syndromic associations with this abnormality?**
4. **What are the poor prognostic factors?**

Ans.

1. Gastroschisis
2. Omphalocele. Free floating bowel loop with cord insertion lateral to the herniated bowel (paraumbilical defect).
3. Very low
4. Intestinal wall edema with bowel dilatation.

SUGGESTED READING

1. Lao OB, Larison C, Garrison MM, Waldhausen JH, Goldin AB. Outcomes in neonates with get a gastroschisis in US children's hospitals. Am J Perinatol. 2010;27(1):97-101.

STATION 5.

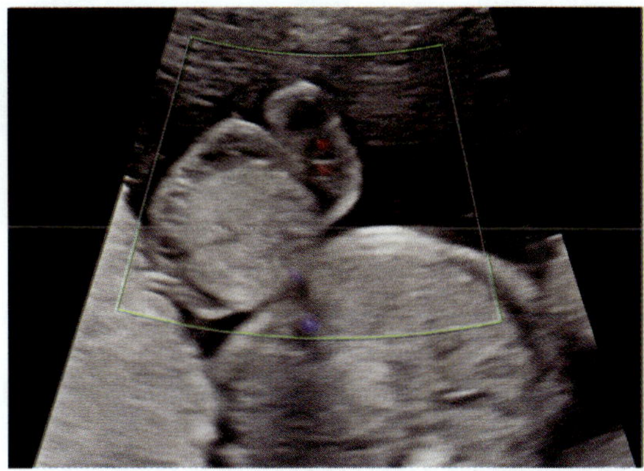

1. **Describe and identify the condition shown in this 24-week fetus.**
2. **What is the risk of genetic/chromosomal abnormalities associated with this condition and what are the ultrasound markers which predict a higher risk?**
3. **Name two polymalformative syndromes associated with this pathology.**
4. **What is the poor prognostic factor in terms of postnatal therapy?**

Ans.

1. Midline ventral abdominal wall defect with cord insertion at the convexity of the defect with herniated abdominal viscera (liver and bowel loops)—omphalocele.
2. There is 40–70% risk of chromosomal abnormalities (mainly trisomy 18 followed by 13). Small omphaloceles have higher risk of chromosomal abnormalities as compared to larger ones with liver in second trimester. Increased nuchal translucency (NT) in first trimester also indicates a higher risk.
3. Pentalogy of Cantrell and OEIS (omphalocele-exstrophy-imperforate anus-spinal defects) syndrome.
4. Large omphaloceles with mostly herniated liver indicate need of delayed closure and increased chances of sepsis.

SUGGESTED READING

1. Poaty H, Pelluard F, Diallo MS, Ondima IPL, Andre G, Silou-Massaba JF. Omphalocele: a review of common genetic etiologies. Egypt J Med Hum Genet. 2019;20:37.

STATION 6.

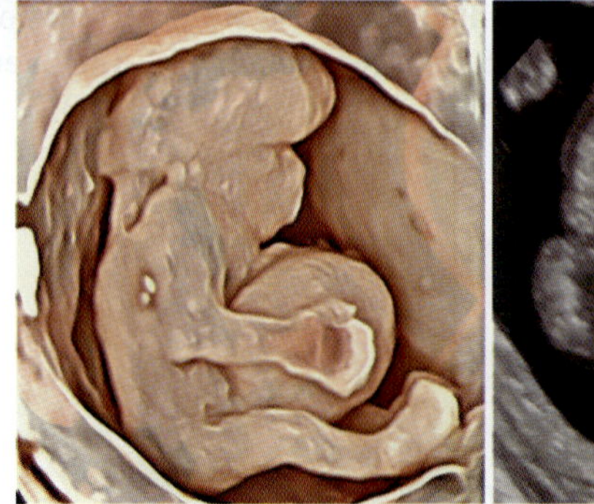

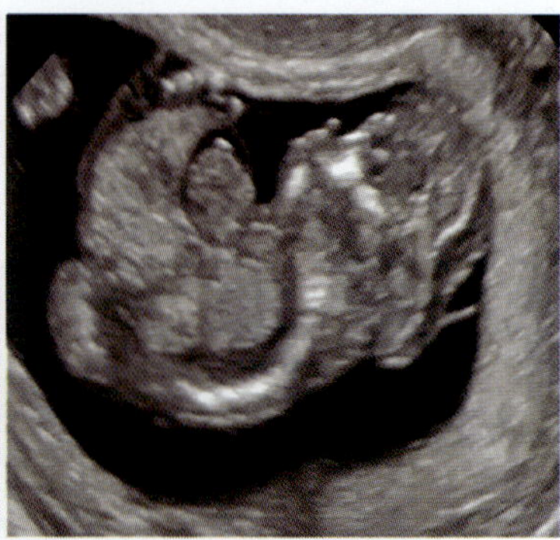

1. **Identify the abnormality and name its components.**
2. **Which embryonic structure's failure of development leads to this pathology?**
3. **Which cardiac defects are most commonly seen with this poly-malformative syndrome?**
4. **Name another structural defect/s seen in this image.**

Ans.

1. Pentalogy of Cantrell, Components—A midline anterior ventral wall defect, a diaphragmatic defect, a cleft distal sternum, a defect of the apical pericardium with communication into the peritoneum, and an intracardiac defect.
2. Septum transversum
3. Ventricular septal defects and Fallot's tetralogy
4. Acrania—exencephaly and cleft palate (maxillary gap sign)

SUGGESTED READING

1. Williams AP, Marayati R, Beierle EA. Pentalogy of Cantrell. Semin Pediatr Surg. 2019;28(2):106-10.

STATION 7.

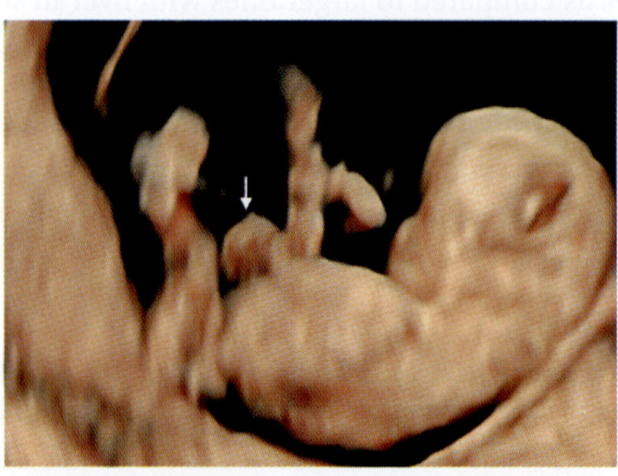

1. **Identify the condition in this 10-week fetus (arrow).**
2. **At which gestational age is this condition seen and by which gestational age it disappears?**
3. **What is the degree of rotation of primary intestinal loop and in which direction?**

Ans.

1. Physiological midgut herniation
2. Physiological gut rotation starts at 6th embryonic week. Sonographically, it can be seen from 9th to 10th week. The condition disappears by 12th week.
3. The primary intestinal loop rotates to 270° in counter clockwise direction.

SUGGESTED READING

1. Sadler TW, Langman J. Third month to birth: The fetus and placenta. In: Sadler TW (Ed). Langman's Medical Embryology, 12th edition. Philadelphia, PA: Lippincott Williams & Wilkins; 2012. pp. 96-116.

STATION 8.

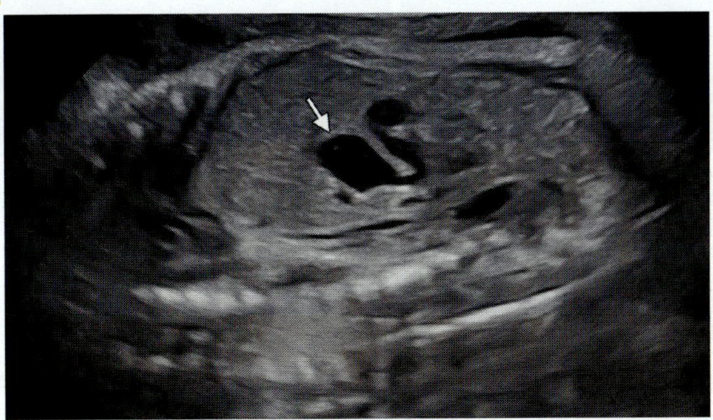

1. **Identify the anechoic cystic lesion in right upper quadrant of a 31-week fetus.**
2. **What is the differential diagnosis of fetal right upper quadrant cystic lesion?**
3. **In how many types choledochal cyst is classified and which one is the most common?**
4. **What are the early and long-term complications of this lesion?**

Ans.

1. Fetal choledochal cyst
2. Cystic biliary atresia, hepatic cysts, gallbladder duplication, ovarian cysts, and enteric duplication cysts.
3. It is classified in five major types by the portion of the biliary tree affected. Cystic dilatation of the common bile duct (type 1) comprises 80–90% of the cysts.

4. In affected newborns, 70% have jaundice after birth and a palpable abdominal mass is seen in 25% of cases. In untreated patients' risk of recurrent cholangitis, pancreatitis, liver cirrhosis, portal hypertension, and malignant transformation is high.

SUGGESTED READING

1. Lata I, Mandelia A, Mandal K. Successful antenatal diagnosis and management of a rare case of congenital fetal choledochal cyst. Maternal-Fetal Medicine. 2021;3(3):225-8.

STATION 9.

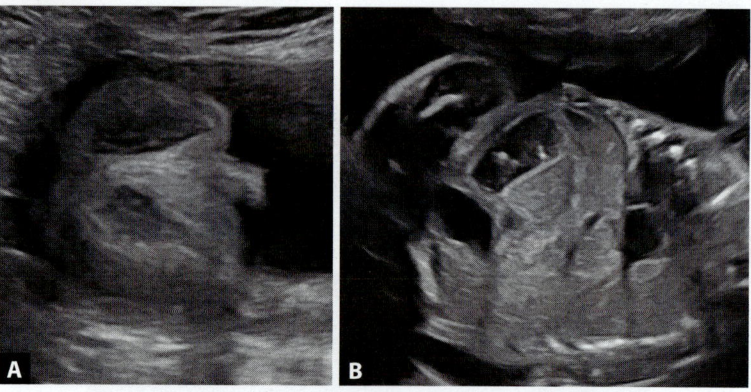

1. **Describe the findings and identify the pathology in a 26-week fetus shown in above images A and B.**
2. **Name two chromosomal anomalies frequently associated with this condition.**
3. **Name two polymalformative syndromes associated with this condition.**
4. **Fill up the blanks:**
   The urorectal septum develops between ________ and hindgut. It fuses with the perineal body by _____ week of embryonic development thereby forming ______ anteriorly and the hindgut posteriorly.

Ans.

1. Absence of target sign in perinium with dilatation of rectosigmoid colon. The features are suggestive of anorectal malformation spectrum.
2. It has a high risk of trisomy 18 and 21.
3. *VACTERL:* look for ► anorectal malformation + vertebral anomalies + cardiac defects + esophageal atresia (EA) [tracheoesophageal (TE) fistula] + renal agenesis + limb anomalies. And *Caudal regression syndrome*:

look for ► anorectal malformation + renal agenesis + sacral agenesis + lumbar vertebral anomalies + femoral hypoplasia + talipes.

4. Allantois, 7th, urogenital sinus

SUGGESTED READING

1. Sadler TW, Langman J. Third month to birth: The fetus and placenta. In: Sadler TW (Ed). Langman's Medical Embryology, 12th edition. Philadelphia, PA: Lippincott Williams & Wilkins; 2012. pp. 96-116.

STATION 10.

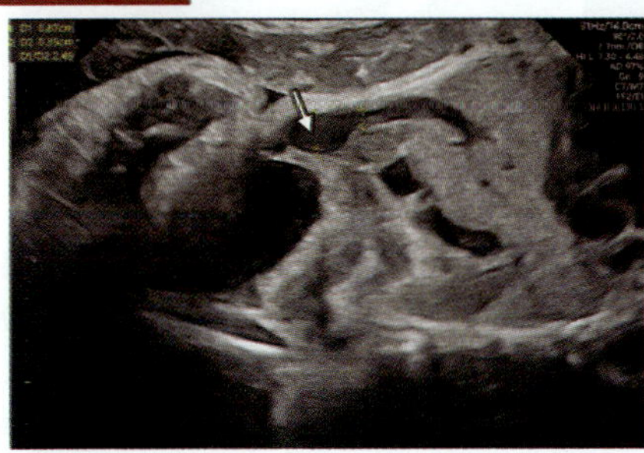
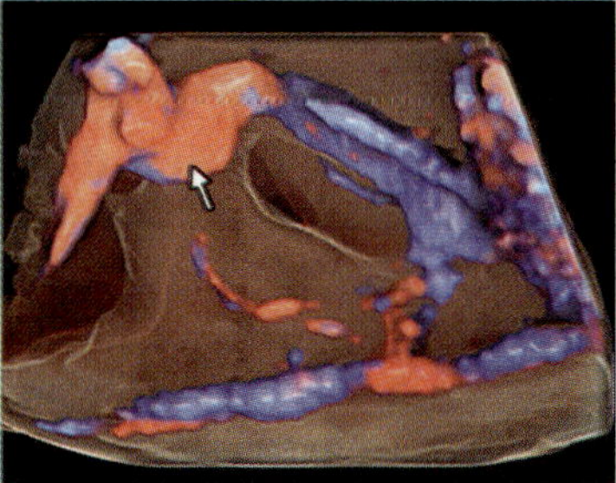

1. **Identify the intrabdominal vascular cystic mass (arrow) in a 34-week fetus.**
2. **Name any two diagnostic criteria.**
3. **What complications may be seen in this condition with advancing gestation?**
4. **What is the common chromosomal abnormality reported with this condition especially in nonisolated cases?**

Ans.

1. Fetal intra-abdominal umbilical vein varix (FIUVV)
2. If the diameter of the umbilical vein was above +2 SD of the reference range for gestational-age and the diameter of subhepatic part of umbilical vein 1.5 times its intrahepatic portion (other—the diameter of FIUVV is >9 mm in term fetus, the diameter of the subhepatic segment of the upper umbilical vein exceeding 50% the diameter of the intrahepatic segment at any time during gestation).
3. Fetal growth restriction, thrombus formation, major dilatation (>12 mm), turbulence, fetal hydrops, and intrauterine fetal death (IUFD).
4. Trisomy 21 (20% cases) followed by deletion 22q.

SUGGESTED READING

1. Alam K, Goswami P, Joshi T. FIUVV: Associations and outcome. J Fetal Med. 2022;9:91-9.

STATION 11.

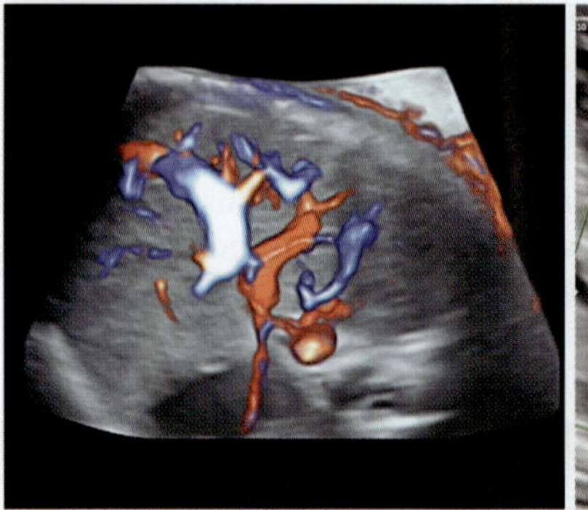

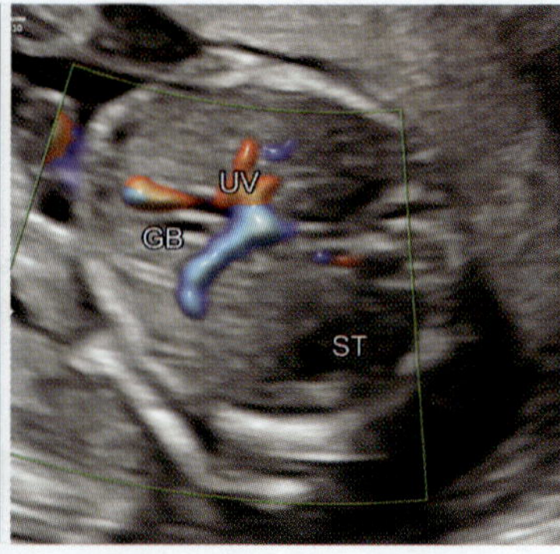

1. **Identify the condition in this 25-week fetus.**
2. **Fill up the blanks:**
   Embryologically, the ______ branch of the initially paired umbilical veins (UV) begins to become obliterated within the ______ week of gestation and tends to completely disappear by the ______ week.
3. **What are the different types of this condition and which one is associated with poor prognosis?**
4. **What is the prognosis in isolated types?**

Ans.

1. Persistent right umbilical vein (PRUV)
2. Right, 4th, and 7th
3. Intrahepatic and extrahepatic and supernumerary. Extrahepatic is associated with poor fetal outcome due to agenesis of the ductus venosus
4. Prognosis is normal in isolated types.

SUGGESTED READING

1. Weichert J, Hartge D, Germer U, Axt-Fliedner R, Gembruch U. Persistent right umbilical vein: a prenatal condition worth mentioning? Ultrasound Obstet Gynecol. 2011;37(5):543-8.

STATION 12.

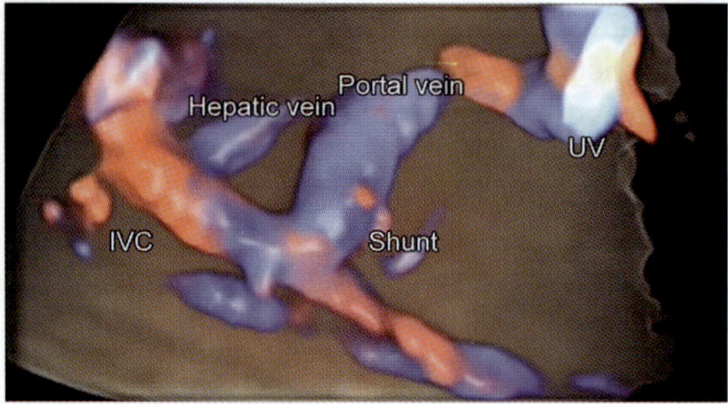

(IVC: inferior vena cava; UV: umbilical veins)

1. **Identify the abnormality in this 23-week fetus.**
2. **What are the two different routes of umbilical venous return in this condition?**
3. **Name common chromosomal abnormalities associated with the condition.**
4. **Name a syndrome associated with this abnormality.**

Ans.

1. Extrahepatic agenesis of the ductus venosus (ADV)
2. a. *Extrahepatic umbilical venous drainage by passing the liver:* The UV directly connects to the iliac vein/the inferior vena cava/the renal vein/the right atrium/the coronary sinus.
   b. *Intrahepatic umbilical venous drainage without liver bypass:* The UV connects to the portal system in its usual way without giving rise to the DV.
3. Trisomy 21, 18, or Turner's syndrome
4. Noonan syndrome (ADV with cystic hygroma with heart defects with facial abnormalities).

SUGGESTED READING

1. Nagy RD, Cernea N, Dijmarescu AL, Manolea MM, Zorilă GL, Drăgușin RC, et al. Ductus venosus agenesis and portal system anomalies-association and outcome. Biology (Basel). 2022;11(4):548.

STATION 13.

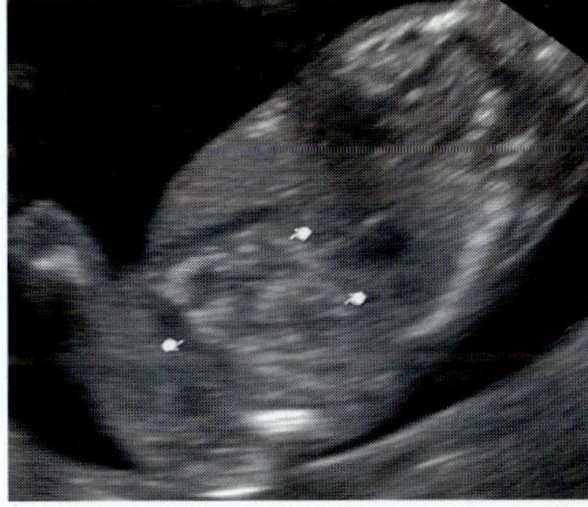

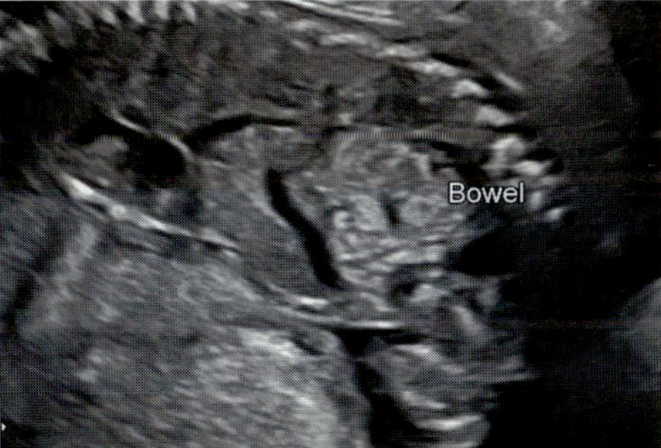

1. **Identify the condition in this 19-week fetus.**
2. **Describe the etiopathogenesis.**
3. **What is likelihood ratio (LR) of this condition for trisomy 21?**
4. **Which genetic tests would you recommend for this fetus if the couple has consanguineous marriage, history of (h/o) multiple transfusions in past and h/o previous multiple pregnancy losses due to fetal hydrops?**

Ans.

1. Echogenic bowel
2. Etiopathogenesis
   - Reduction of microvillar enzymes leads to constipation and thickened calcified meconium (T21 and cystic fibrosis).
   - Mesenteric ischemia due to hemodynamic redistribution [fetal growth restriction (FGR)].
   - Increased fluid inside/outside the bowel lumen (fetal infections).
3. Echogenic bowel has an LR of 11.4 for trisomy 21.
4. *HBB* gene sequencing to rule out α-thalassemia.

SUGGESTED READING

1. Krishnan P, Singh M. Echogenic Bowel. In: StatPearls. Treasure Island (FL): StatPearls Publishing; 2024.

STATION 14.

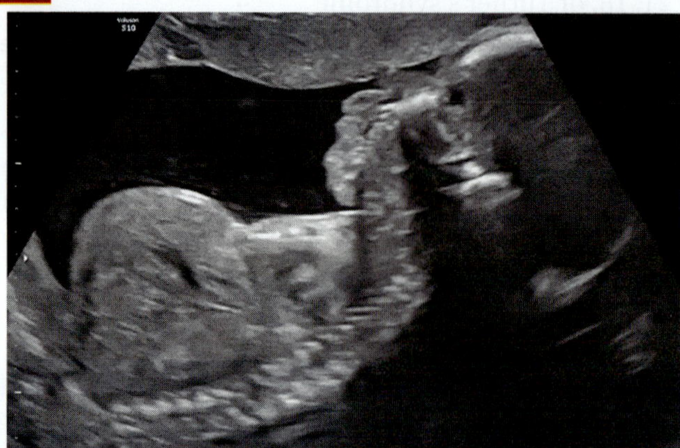

1. **Identify the anomaly in this 20-week fetus.**
2. **What are the causes of this abnormality in the fetus?**
3. **What are other abdominal signs of fetal infection?**
4. **Name two syndromes associated with this condition.**

Ans.

1. Hepatomegaly
2. Fetal infections, storage diseases, congestive heart failure/venous congestion in the fetus, and fetal hepatic tumors (hemangioma/hepatoblastoma).
3. Splenomegaly, ascites, echogenic bowel
4. Beckwith-Wiedemann syndrome and Zellweger syndrome

SUGGESTED READING

1. Jensen KK, Oh KY, Patel N, Narasimhan ER, Ku AS, Sohaey R. Fetal hepatomegaly: Causes and associations. Radiographics. 2020;40(2):589-604.

STATION 15.

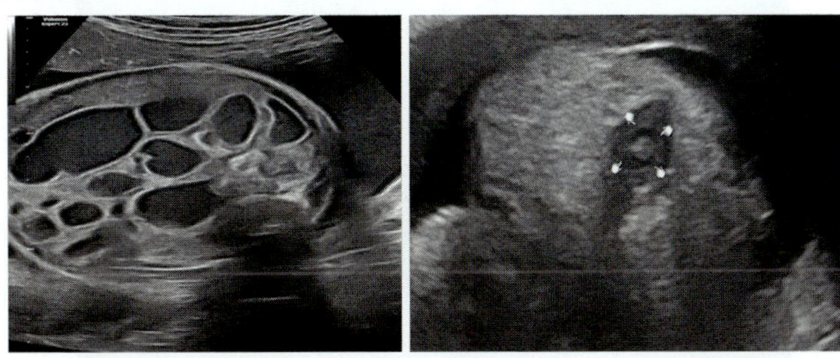

Courtesy: CCD image by Dr Dinesh Prakash Singh, Consultant Fetal Medicine, Prakash Ultrasound, Giridih, Jharkhand.

1. **What are the causes of late-onset bowel dilatation and polyhydramnios in this 37-week fetus?**
2. **Define target sign.**
3. **What are the red flags to start investigations for congenital chloride diarrhea (CCD) in this fetus?**
4. **What is the mode of inheritance of CCD?**
5. **What is the maximal large bowel diameter at term?**

Ans.

1. Anorectal atresia, Hirschsprung's disease, volvulus and meconium plug syndrome, and congenital chloride diarrhea.
2. On ultrasound examination of the perinium on axial section, a normal fetal anus is seen as of hypoechoic anal sphincter musculature surrounding the echogenic bowel mucosa (Target).
3. Positive familiar anamnesis for consanguinity with prenatal evidence of dilated bowel loops at the end of the second trimester, polyhydramnios, prematurity, and low birth weight.
4. CCD is an autosomal recessive inherited disorder.
5. The largest colon diameter at term reaches 18 mm.

SUGGESTED READING

1. Di Meglio L, Castaldo G, Mosca C, Paonessa A, Gelzo M, Esposito MV, et al. Congenital chloride diarrhea clinical features and management: a systematic review. Pediatr Res. 2021;90(1):23-9.
2. Nyberg DA, Mack LA, Patten RM, Cyr DR. Fetal bowel. Normal sonographic findings. J Ultrasound Med. 1987;6(1):3-6.

STATION 16.

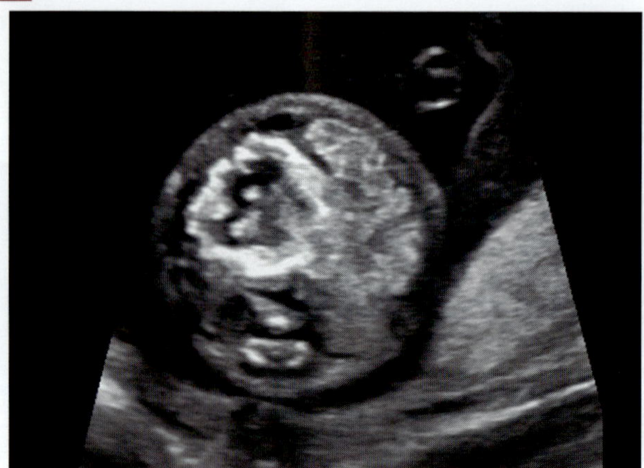

Courtesy: Image by Dr Saumya Shrivastav, Consultant Fetal Medicine, Sansrishti Maternal Fetal Medicine clinic, Hazaribagh, Jharkhand.

1. **Identify the findings in this 19-week fetus.**
2. **What could be the probable causes of this condition?**
3. **What other ultrasonographic findings would you look for to prognosticate this fetus?**
4. **Which genetic tests would you recommend for this fetus if the couple has consanguineous marriage and h/o death of siblings with lower respiratory tract infection and failure to thrive?**
5. **How does this cyst progress with advancing gestation?**

Ans.

1. Meconium pseudocyst
2. Chromosomal abnormalities, congenital infections, and cystic fibrosis
3. External genitalia, anal pit [perianal muscular complex (PAMC)], ascites, intra-abdominal/hepatic calcifications, signs of infection in fetal brain/heart.
4. Fetal clinical exome sequencing for cystic fibrosis.
5. The cyst may show gradual reduction with simultaneous increase in calcifications, bowel dilatation, and ascites.

SUGGESTED READING

1. Khan SA, Khare M, Dagash H, Kairamkonda V. Meconium pseudocyst presenting as massive ascites in a new-born. Radiol Case Rep. 2018;14(2):235-7.

STATION 17.

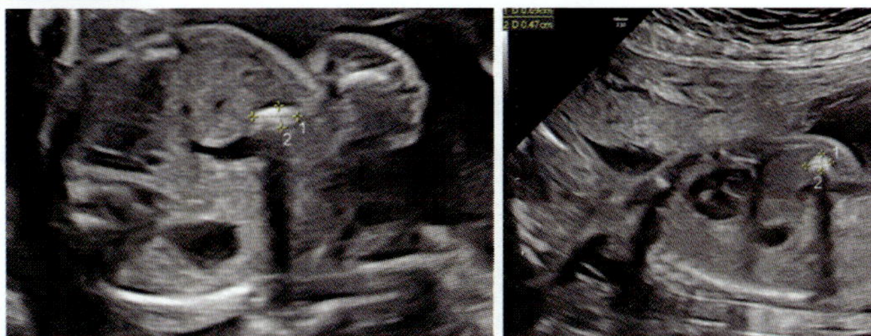

1. **Identify the abnormality in a 22-week fetus.**
2. **What are other extracerebral signs of fetal infection?**
3. **What are the causes of hepatic calcification?**
4. **Name three different patterns of hepatic calcifications.**

Ans.

1. Hepatic calcification
2. Cataract, pleural effusion, myocarditis, echogenic ileus, hepatosplenomegaly (with spleen enlargement prevailing on liver enlargement), thickened placenta, oligohydramnios.
3. Meconium peritonitis, intrauterine fetal infections [rubella, cytomegalovirus (CMV), and herpes simplex virus 2; parvovirus and varicella-zoster virus], fetal tumors, and thromboembolism of hepatic vessels, and chromosomal abnormalities.
4. Peritoneal, parenchymal, and vascular.

SUGGESTED READING

1. Pathak S, Grosu L. Case series of prenatal diagnosis of fetal intrahepatic lesions and postnatal outcome. Ultrasound. 2019;27(2):127-30.

STATION 18.

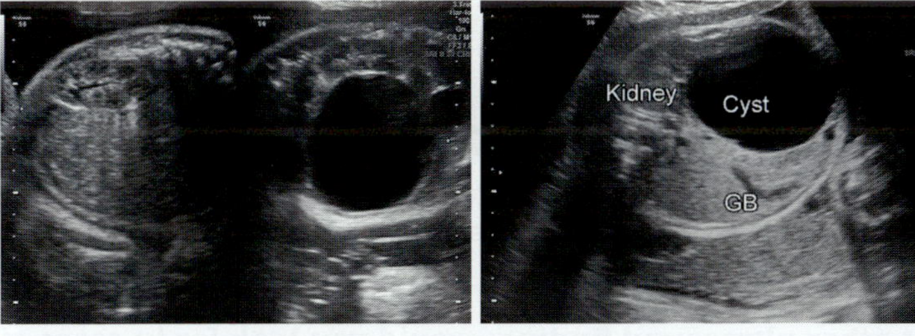

Courtesy: Image by Dr Saumya Shrivastav, Consultant Fetal Medicine, Sansrishti Maternal Fetal Medicine clinic, Hazaribagh, Jharkhand.

1. **Give the differential diagnosis of cystic masses arising from fetal pelvis.**
2. **Give ultrasound characteristic of mesenteric cysts.**
3. **Fetal mesenteric cysts are caused by?**
4. **Enteric duplication cysts are most commonly associated with ____ abnormalities. Why?**

Ans.

1. Fetal gonadal cyst, enteric duplication cyst, mesenteric cyst, meconium pseudocyst, enlarged urinary bladder, hydrometrocolpos, and renal cysts of pelvic kidneys.
2. Thin-walled unilocular/multilocular hypoechoic masses without peristalsis.
3. A mesenteric cyst is caused by impaired lymphatic drainage in the fetal mesentery.
4. Vertebral abnormalities. Enteric duplication cysts are caused by failure of separation of notochord with endoderm.

SUGGESTED READING

1. Cass DL. Fetal abdominal tumors and cysts. Transl Pediatr. 2021;10(5): 1530-41.

STATION 19.

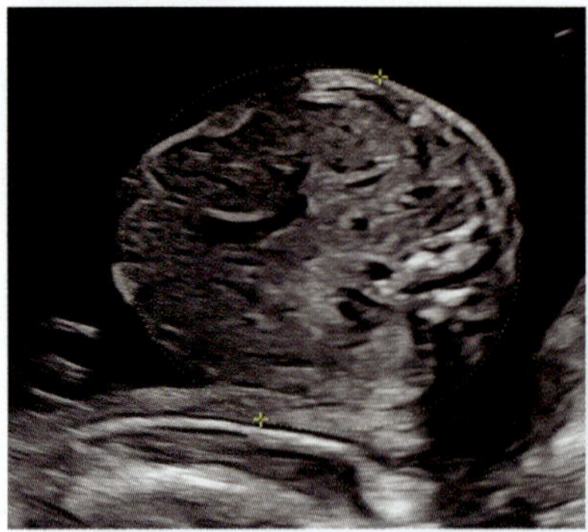

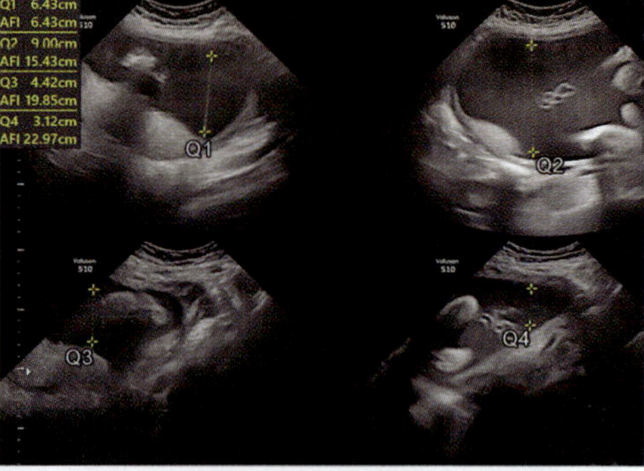

Courtesy: Image by Dr Vivek Krishnan, Clinical Associate Professor and Head, Division of Fetal Medicine & Perinatology, Amrita Center of Excellence in Fetal Care, AIMS, Kochi.

1. **Describe the ultrasound findings in a 36-week fetus.**
2. **What other ultrasound findings would you look for in cases of non-visualization/small stomach bubble?**
3. **What are the different types of esophageal atresia?**
4. **What are the chromosomal abnormalities associated with the condition?**

Ans.

1. Persistent nonvisualization of stomach bubble with polyhydramnios—likely esophageal atresia (EA).
2. Liquor amount (increased or absent), fetal growth, fetal face (facial clefts, microretrognathia), fetal movements [fetal akinesia deformation sequence (FADS)], fetal thorax (congenital diaphragmatic hernia).
3. Five types of EA are recognized, according to the gross classification:
   a. *Type A:* No fistula (7% of cases);
   b. *Type B:* EA with proximal tracheoesophageal fistula (TEF) (2%);
   c. *Type C:* EA with distal TEF (86%);
   d. *Type D:* EA with proximal and distal TEF (1%);
   e. *Type E:* TEF without concomitant EA (4%).
4. Trisomy 21 and trisomy 18

SUGGESTED READING

1. Baldwin DL, Yadav D. Esophageal Atresia. In: StatPearls. Treasure Island (FL): StatPearls Publishing; 2024.

STATION 20.

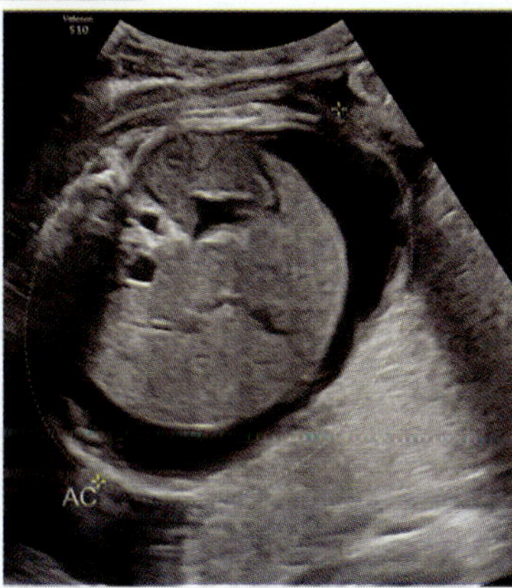

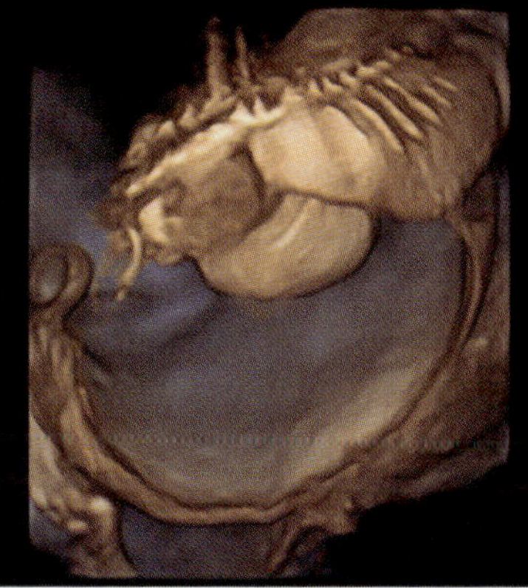

1. **Identify the condition in a 28-week fetus.**
2. **What are the causes of isolated fetal ascites?**
3. **Does fetal paracentesis have any role in improving the prognosis?**
4. **Isolated fetal ascites developing after ___ weeks gestation has a better prognosis than those who are diagnosed earlier.**

Ans.

1. Fetal ascites
2. Fetal abdominal structural abnormalities (genitourinary, gastro-intestinal), fetal infections, cardiac abnormalities, chylous ascites,

metabolic storage disorders, other structural disorders (skeletal dysplasias, CDH, CHAOS), and idiopathic.

3. Apart from chylous ascites fetal paracentesis does not have any role in improving the prognosis of the fetus.
4. 24 weeks

SUGGESTED READING

1. Horgan R, Youssef JA, Levy AT, Berger SI, Dreux S, Brizot ML, et al. Etiology and outcome of isolated fetal ascites: A systematic review. Obstet Gynecol. 2021;138(6):897-904.
2. Sablok A, Sharma A, Gupta R, Thakur S, Kaul A. Isolated fetal ascites: Etiology and Prognosis - A 10-year experience from a tertiary referral care center in India. J Indian Assoc Pediatr Surg. 2021;26(3):162-9.

CHAPTER 10

Congenital Abnormalities of the Kidney and Urinary Tract

Chinmayee Ratha

STATION 1.

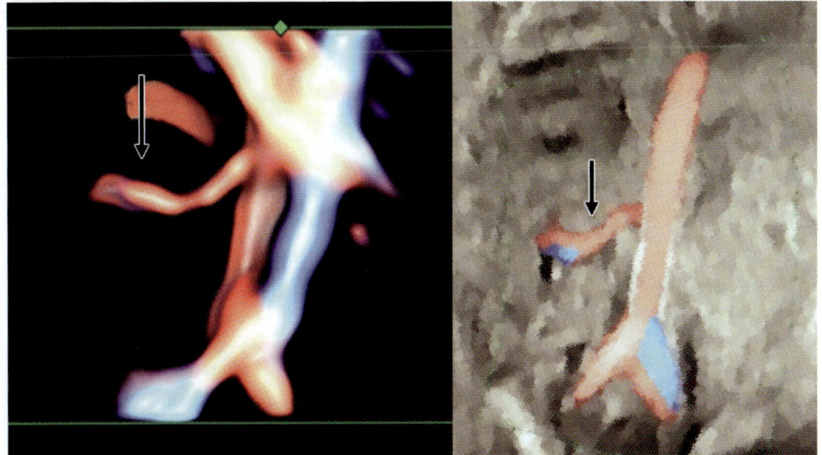

1. **Identify the vessel seen (arrow) arising from the fetal abdominal aorta.**
2. **What does the non-visualization of the contralateral renal artery indicate?**
3. **How do you counsel a couple if the fetus has the above condition?**

Ans.

1. Fetal renal artery
2. Unilateral renal agenesis
3. Prevalence of unilateral renal agenesis is one in 2,000 births and the prognosis is generally normal. Most cases are sporadic and compatible with a normal life.

SUGGESTED READING

1. Society for Maternal-Fetal Medicine (SMFM); Jelin A. Renal agenesis. Am J Obstet Gynecol. 2021;225(5):B28-30.

STATION 2.

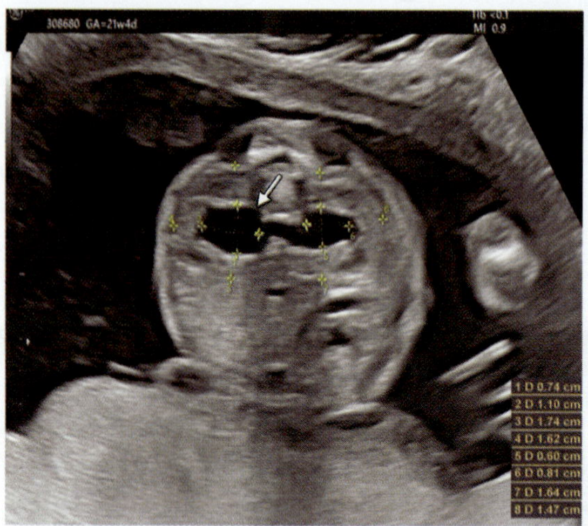

1. **Identify the hypoechoic structure in the picture (arrow).**
2. **What are the features of ultrasound diagnosis of this condition?**
3. **What other investigations are warranted in this condition?**

Ans.

1. Fetal renal pelvis
2. Renal pelviectasis or the dilatation of the collecting system of the kidney observed in the standard transverse view of the abdomen. Based on the anteroposterior diameter of the pelvis the condition is divided into:
    - *Mild (only renal pelvis):* 4–7 mm in the 2nd trimester; 7–9 mm in the 3rd.
    - *Moderate (pelvis and calyces):* 8–10 mm in the 2nd trimester; 10–15 mm in the 3rd.
    - *Severe (cortical thinning):* >10 mm in the 2nd trimester; >15 mm in the 3rd.
3. Detailed ultrasound examination (especially of the contralateral kidney) and to rule out any other congenital anomalies. Fetal karyotyping should be offered only if other markers are present.

SUGGESTED READING

1. Nguyen HT, Phelps A, Coley B, Darge K, Rhee A, Chow JS. 2021 update on the urinary tract dilation (UTD) classification system: clarifications, review of the literature, and practical suggestions. Pediatr Radiol. 2022;52(4):740-51.

STATION 3.

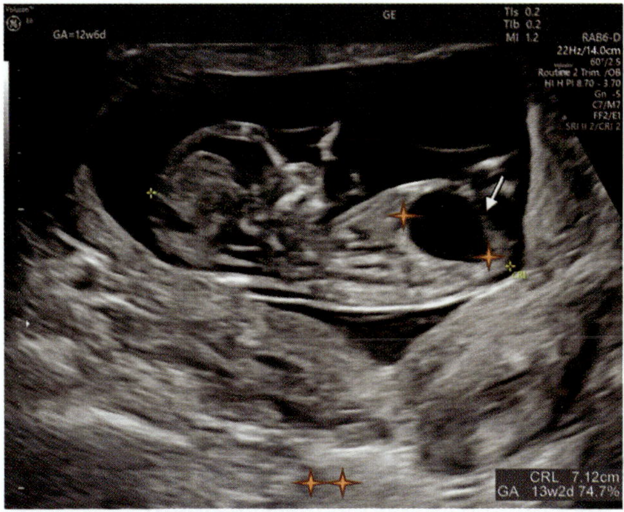

1. **Identify the hypoechoic structure (arrow).**
2. **Is this appearance normal? How do you define "normal" at this gestation?**
3. **What are the clinical implications?**

Ans.

1. Fetal bladder in first trimester
2. No, this appearance is not normal as the fetal bladder appears enlarged for this gestation—also known as "megacystis". The longitudinal diameter of the bladder should be <7 mm in the first trimester—megacystis is diagnosed when this diameter is >7 mm.
3. Megacystis in first trimester could be due to relaxant effects of maternal hormones or due to bladder outlet obstruction. Mild dilatation (7–15 mm) is usually due to muscle relaxation - either a normal variant or due to hypotonia associated with aneuploidies such as Down syndrome or it could be initial stages of obstructive uropathies. Severe dilation (>15 mm) is usually associated with lower urinary tract obstruction or genetic pathologies such as the prune belly syndrome.

SUGGESTED READING

1. Fontanella F, Maggio L, Verheij JBGM, Duin LK, Adama Van Scheltema PN, Cohen-Overbeek TE, et al. Fetal megacystis: a lot more than LUTO. Ultrasound Obstet Gynecol. 2019;53(6):779-87.

STATION 4.

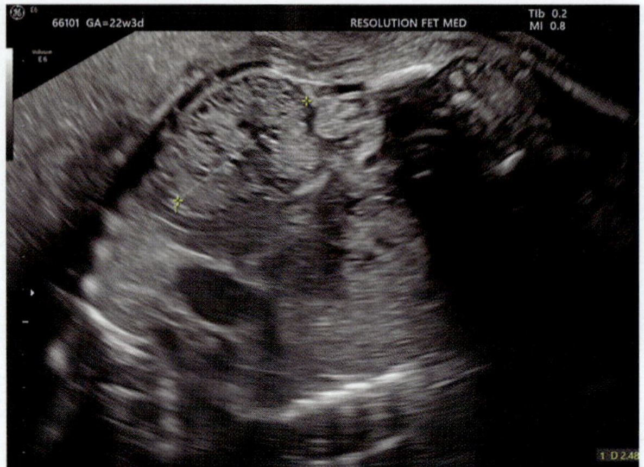

1. **What types of fetal kidneys are shown in the picture?**
2. **What is the common etiology of this condition?**
3. **What is the recurrence risk of this condition?**

Ans.

1. Enlarged, polycystic kidneys
2. The etiology is usually genetic, and the disease is caused by mutations in the *PKD1* gene on chromosome 6p21 or on 16p13.13 and *PKD2* gene (15% of cases) on chromosome 4q13.23.
3. Isolated fetal-onset bilateral polycystic kidney disease usually follows the autosomal recessive (ARPKD) pattern of inheritance. In this condition, assuming that both parents are heterozygous carriers of this gene defect, a 25% recurrence risk is allocated in future pregnancies.
   Some cases may be due to autosomal dominant PKD (a small proportion of these may present in the fetal period)—and the recurrence risk here is about 50% in future pregnancies. Once the molecular diagnosis is confirmed, prenatal diagnosis by chorionic villus sampling (CVS) can be offered.

SUGGESTED READING

1. Suh KW, Jeong JE, Hong SY, Bae JY. Prenatal Diagnosis of a Fatal Case of Fetal Autosomal Dominant Polycystic Kidney Disease. Perinatology. 2023;34(1): 28-35.

STATION 5. **Please read the clinical scenario and answer the questions that follow:**

You are scanning a fetus of 16 weeks' gestation, and you notice mild oligohydramnios. The fetal kidneys are bilaterally enlarged and polycystic. The fetal head examination reveals a small occipital encephalocele.

1. **What is the diagnosis that comes to your mind in the given clinical scenario? What other aspect of fetal anatomy do you want to assess specifically to reach that diagnosis?**
2. **What is the etiology of this condition?**
3. **How will you plan prenatal diagnosis in future pregnancies?**

Ans.

1. In the given clinical scenario, the most likely diagnosis is "Meckel-Gruber syndrome". We would like to check the fetal hands to look for post axial polydactyly which is also another feature of this condition.
2. This condition is genetic with mutations mapped to six different loci in different chromosomes. It is a rare, lethal autosomal recessive condition characterized by ciliopathies caused by dysfunction of cilia and flagella.
3. Since this is a genetic condition, and a molecular diagnosis is available, definite prenatal diagnosis by CVS at 11–14 weeks can be done. However, as the phenotypic features are seen on the scan and may be detected even in the first trimester, planning an ultrasound-based surveillance is also reasonable. It is important to counsel the parents about the 25% chance of recurrence in future pregnancies.

SUGGESTED READING

1. Parelkar SV, Kapadnis SP, Sanghvi BV, Joshi PB, Mundada D, Oak SN. Meckel Gruber Syndrome: a rare and lethal anomaly with review of Literature. J Pediatr Neurosci. 2013;8(2):154-7.

STATION 6. **Please see the image and answer the questions given below:**

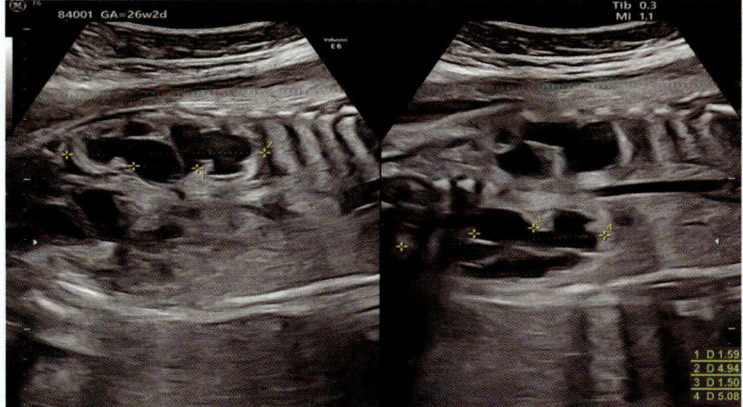

1. **Are these fetal kidneys normal?**
2. **What classification is used for this condition?**
3. **What features should be evaluated in the classification in Question 3 above?**
4. **What is the prognosis in such cases?**

Ans.

1. No—these kidneys appear to have significant pelvicalyceal dilatation—hydronephrosis bilaterally.
2. The UTD (urinary tract dilatation) classification is the current accepted classification which provides values for the diagnosis of UT dilation based on USG imaging.
3. These are stratified based on gestational age at presentation. The renal pelvis is considered not to be dilated when the AP renal pelvis diameter measures <4 mm at <28 weeks gestation, <7 mm at ≥28 weeks, and <10 mm postnatally. In the normal fetus, calyceal dilation is absent, the renal parenchyma has normal thickness and appearance, the ureter is not seen, and the bladder is normal. Additionally, there is no unexplained oligohydramnios. Additional sonographic features that should be evaluated include—calyceal dilation, parenchymal thickness, parenchymal appearance with respect to echogenicity, the presence or absence of cortical cysts and corticomedullary differentiation, bladder abnormalities, the presence of ureterocele or dilated posterior urethra and the presence of otherwise unexplained oligohydramnios on prenatal imaging.
4. The mild cases (UTD A1) generally have a good prognosis and if the etiology is only the relaxant effect of maternal hormones, these may resolve spontaneously or remain asymptomatic after birth too. The prenatal UTD identification allows to stratify into different risk groups based on the possibility of developing uropathy. Thus, if detected in prenatal age, UTD A1 represents the low risk, UTD A2 the intermediate risk and UTD A3 the high risk.

   The severe cases may be associated with pathologies such as vesicoureteric reflux or pelviureteric junction obstruction—which may warrant postnatal interventions and this group should be counselled for postnatal follow-up.

SUGGESTED READING

1. Nguyen HT, Phelps A, Coley B, Darge K, Rhee A, Chow JS. 2021 update on the urinary tract dilation (UTD) classification system: clarifications, review of the literature, and practical suggestions. Pediatr Radiol. 2022;52(4):740-51.

STATION 7. A 26-year-old primigravida, non-consanguineously married, with no known risk factors comes to seek your opinion after the fetal anomaly scan reported "Single live intrauterine fetus with non-visualization of the left fetal kidney."

Please answer the following questions based on the above scenario.

1. **What more information do you want from the scan report?**

2. If despite a second look it is confirmed that there is only one fetal kidney present (unilateral renal agenesis)—and no other fetal anomalies are found—is this anomaly compatible with life?

3. How will you counsel the family?

Ans.

1. The following points need to be clarified in the report:
   a. Status of the right fetal kidney
   b. Amount of liquor
   c. Assessment of the fetal pelvic region to look for an ectopic kidney
   d. Any other fetal anomalies
2. Yes, a single fetal kidney in an otherwise normal fetus is very much compatible with a normal life.
3. In fact, most people with a single functioning kidney have a good quality of life and may remain completely asymptomatic throughout their lives. Patients with a single functional kidney should be periodically evaluated throughout their lifetime for urine protein, blood pressure, and kidney functions. Only some precautions are advised whenever there is any UTI and obviously this person cannot donate his kidney!!

SUGGESTED READING

1. Güngör T, Yazılıtaş F, Çakıcı EK, Ekşioğlu AS, Çelikkaya E, Karakaya D, et al. Retrospective evaluation of children with unilateral renal agenesis. Pediatr Nephrol. 2021;36(9):2847-55.

STATION 8. **A 31-year-old G2P1L1 with 21 + 1 weeks of gestation (non-consanguineous) underwent a targeted imaging for fetal anomalies (TIFFA) scan which revealed a single live intrauterine fetus with fetal growth normal, but the amniotic fluid is significantly reduced for this period of gestation suggestive of severe oligohydramnios. Her quadruple marker test was low risk for aneuploidies.**

Answer the following questions after checking this ultrasound image:

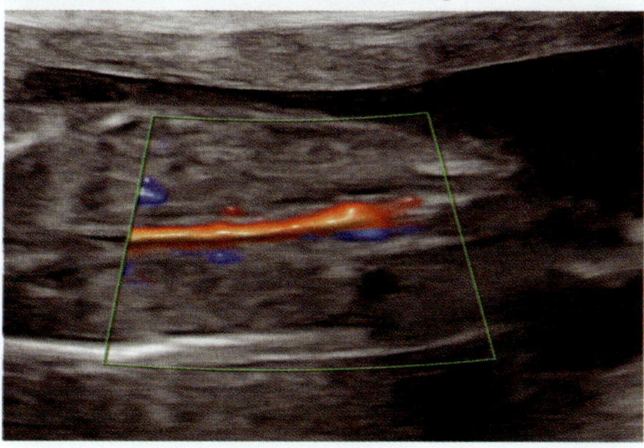

1. **What is the abnormality seen in the image?**
2. **What other anomalies are expected in this fetus?**
3. **How to counsel the couple?**

Ans.

1. Bilateral renal agenesis
2. The fetus can have postural limb abnormalities, severe lung hypoplasia and the characteristic "Potter facies" in addition to the bilateral renal agenesis.
3. The couple should be explained regarding the postnatal lethality of the condition due to pulmonary hypoplasia. The etiology could be sporadic which is most common or chromosomal/genetic.
   In order to establish the exact etiology and to know the recurrence in future the option of invasive testing to be discussed.

SUGGESTED READING

1. Society for Maternal-Fetal Medicine (SMFM); Jelin A. Renal agenesis. Am J Obstet Gynecol. 2021;225(5):B28-30.

STATION 9. **A 27-year-old primigravida with 20 weeks of gestation. First trimester screening—low risk— pregnancy-associated plasma protein A (PAPP-A) - 0.5 MoM (multiple of median).**

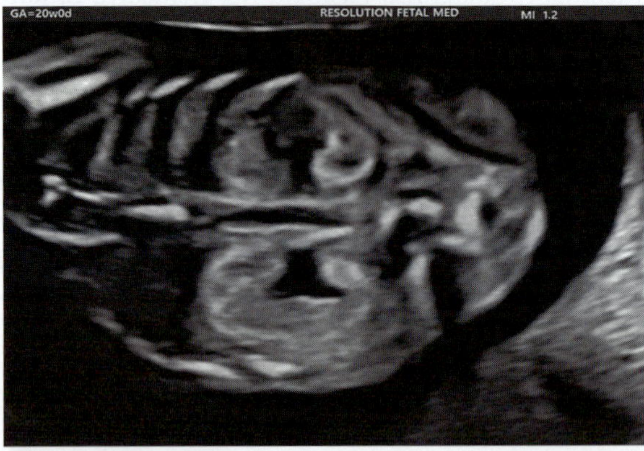

1. **Describe the USG findings.**
2. **What other details should be described in addition to these findings in fetal kidneys?**
3. **How to counsel the couple?**
4. **What is the approach for echogenic kidney?**

Ans.

1. *Scan findings:* Both the fetal kidneys appear to be mildly echogenic.
2. a. Renal cortico-medullary differentiation

b. Measurement of both kidneys
c. Amniotic fluid

3. a. This could be a normal variant and as the pregnancy progresses the echogenicity may resolve and become normal and to look for this, we need to follow up the pregnancy.
   b. It is also known to be associated with dysplastic kidneys with a known genetic etiology which can be confirmed by invasive testing.

4.

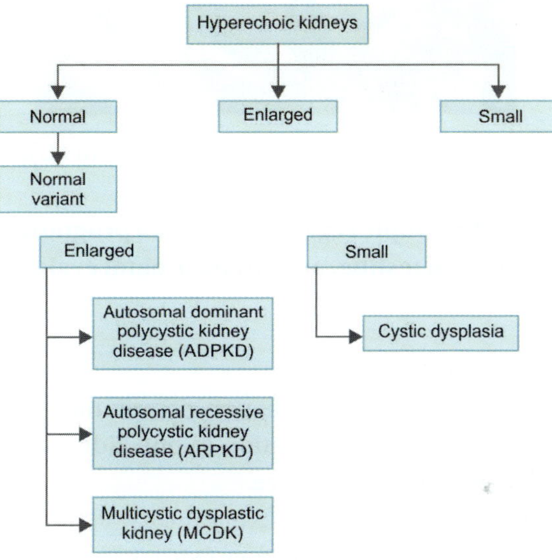

SUGGESTED READING

1. Paladini D, Volpe P. "Urinary tract anomalies". In: Ultrasound of congenital Fetal Anomalies Differential Diagnosis and Prognostic Indicators, 2nd edition. CRC; 2014.

STATION 10. **A 23-year-old primigravida with 19 + 6 weeks of gestation. First trimester screening: Low risk with PAPP-A –0.4 MoM.**

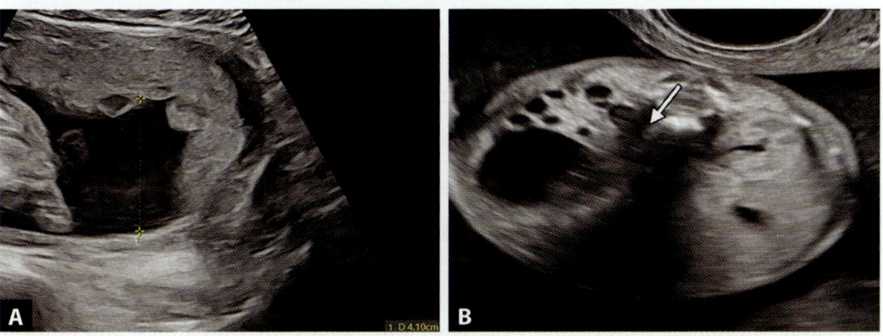

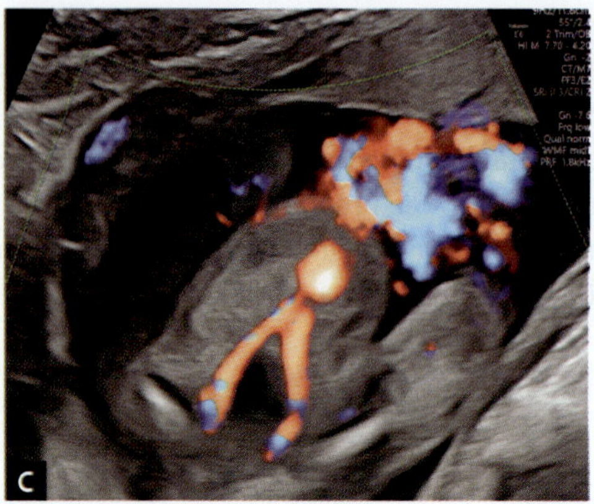

1. **Describe the USG findings in images (A), (B), and (C).**
2. **Identify the condition.**
3. **How to counsel the couple regarding (a) fetal prognosis, (b) follow-up, (c) need for prenatal testing, and (d) post-natal evaluation?**

Ans.

1. a. Single deepest pocket
   b. Echogenic kidney with multiple non-communicating cysts with loss of corticomedullary differentiation in one kidney. The other kidney is normal in echotexture and size.
   c. Fetal bladder
2. Unilateral multicystic dysplastic kidney (MCDK)
3. a. The couple should be counselled that single functioning kidney will have a reasonably good quality of life.
   b. Follow-up should be done to know further progression of the affected kidney and to monitor the functioning of contralateral normal kidney and fetal well-being.
   c. The etiology could be sporadic which is most common or chromosomal/genetic.
   In order to establish the exact etiology and to know the recurrence in future the option of invasive testing to be discussed.
   d. Postnatal evaluation by pediatric nephrologist to plan for further care.

SUGGESTED READING

1. Cai M, Guo C, Wang X, Lin M, Xu S, Huang H, et al. Classifying and evaluating fetuses with multicystic dysplastic kidney in etiologic studies. Exp Biol Med (Maywood). 2023;248(10):858-65.
2. Paladini D, Volpe P. "Urinary tract anomalies". In: Ultrasound of congenital Fetal Anomalies Differential Diagnosis and Prognostic Indicators, 2nd edition. CRC; 2014.

STATION 11.

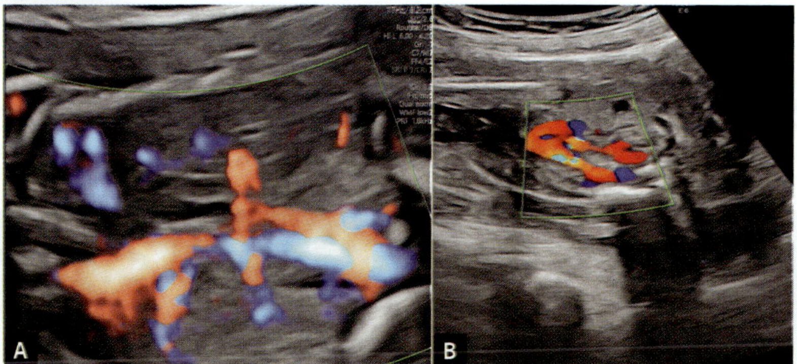

A 26-year-old primigravida with 21 weeks 2 days gestation presents with bilateral dysplastic kidneys with anhydramnios. First trimester screening – low risk.

1. **What are the scan findings in images A and B**
2. **What are the two surrogate markers of renal function?**
3. **How to counsel?**
4. **What is the approach for non-visualization of bladder?**

Ans.

1. a. Bilateral renal vessels present
   b. Fetal bladder is not visualized
2. a. Visualization of the bladder
   b. Liquor
3. Should explain guarded fetal prognosis for this due to the high possibility of pulmonary hypoplasia.
4.

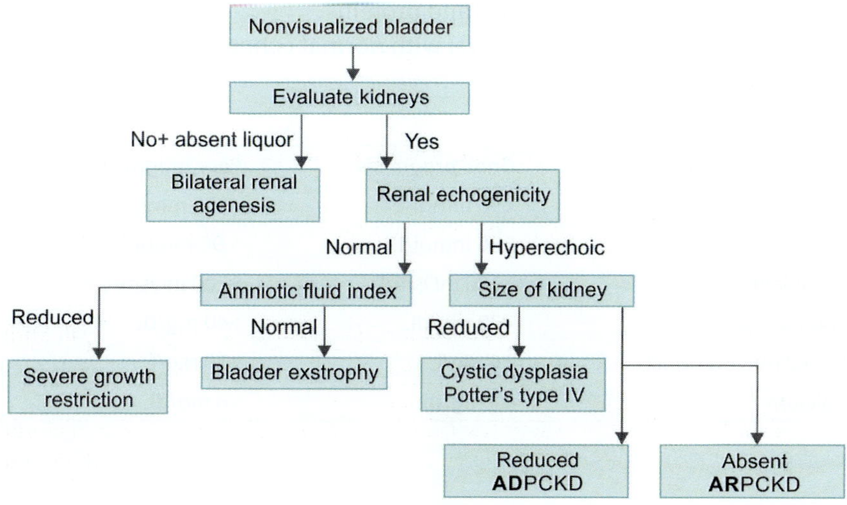

SUGGESTED READING

1. Dias T, Sairam S, Kumarasiri S. Ultrasound diagnosis of fetal renal abnormalities. Best Pract Res Clin Obstet Gynaecol. 2014;28(3):403-15.

STATION 12. A 30-year-old G2P1L1 with 26 weeks 2 days of gestation (non-consanguineous couple) with no screening came to our center for TIFFA scan. Her scan findings are as follows:

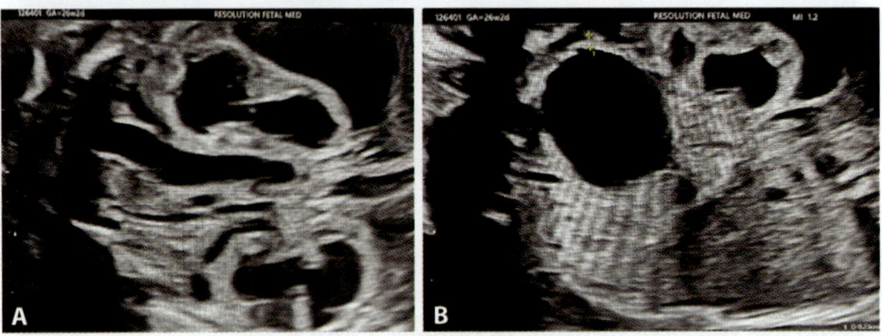

1. **Identify the abnormality in images A and B**
2. **What is the most common syndrome associated with this presentation?**
3. **If the parents are committed to the pregnancy, what are the tests to be done to know the functionality of the fetal kidney.**
4. **Discuss the prognostic criteria of the condition in the scan above.**

Ans.

1. a. Bilateral hydro uretero-nephrosis indicating lower urinary tract obstruction.
   b. An overdistended bladder as suggested by the "keyhole" sign.
2. Prune belly syndrome.
   Sonographic appearance of the kidneys, amniotic fluid volume, and various fetal urine electrolytes and proteins.
3. a. *USG:* Absence of cortical cyst with normal echogenicity
   b. *Biochemical findings:*
4.

Urine electrolytes	*Good prognosis*	*Poor prognosis*
Sodium	<90 mmol/L	>100 mmol/L
Chloride	<80 mmol/L	> 90 mmol/L
Osmolality	<180 mOsm/L	>200 mOsm/L
Total protein	<20 mg/dL	>40 mg/dL
Beta 2 microglobulin	<6 mg/L	>10 mg/L
Calcium	<7 mg/dL	>8 mg/dL

SUGGESTED READING

1. Bianchi DW, Crombleholme TM, D'Alton ME, Malone F. Fetology Diagnosis and Management of the Fetal Patient. 2nd edition. McGraw-Hill Education; 2010.
2. Gupta S, Batra M. SFM Fetal Therapy Practice Guidelines: Fetal Fluid Aspiration. J Fetal Med. 2024;10(04).

STATION 13.

1. What is the full form of CAKUT?

2. What are the two major types of CAKUT?

3. What is the classification of CAKUT?

Ans.

1. Congenital abnormalities of kidney and urinary tract
2. Syndromic and non-syndromic
3.

Anomalies of number
- Renal agenesis
- Bilateral
- Unilateral

Abnormal position, fusion, rotation
- Renal ectopia
- Horseshoe kidney
- Crossed fused ectopia

Dysplasia
- Multicystic dysplastic kidney
- Polycystic dysplastic kidney

Obstruction
- Upper urinary tract obstruction
- Lower urinary tract obstruction

Persistent cloaca
- Genitourinary conundrum

SUGGESTED READING

1. Capone V, Persico N, Berrettini A, Decramer S, De Marco EA, De Palma D, et al. Definition, diagnosis and management of fetal lower urinary tract obstruction: consensus of the ERKNet CAKUT-Obstructive Uropathy Work Group. Nat Rev Urol. 2022;19(5):295-303.

Central and Peripheral Nervous System Abnormalities

Akshatha Prabhu, Anita Kaul

STATION 1.

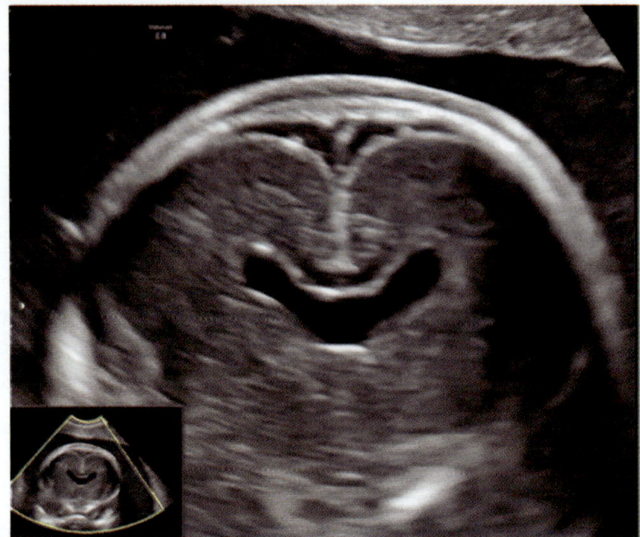

1. **Identify the above ultrasound finding.**
2. **State the differential diagnosis.**
3. **What other structure will you like to document?**
4. **State the important points in counseling.**

Ans.

1. Fused frontal horns
2. Isolated septal agenesis and septo-optic dysplasia
3. Optic chiasma
4. If isolated septal agenesis, usually good outcomes. 25% of these can have septo-optic dysplasia (possible vision and endocrine issues)

SUGGESTED READING

1. Malinger G, Lev D, Kidron D, Heredia F, Hershkovitz R, Lerman-Sagie T. Differential diagnosis in fetuses with absent septum pellucidum. Ultrasound Obstet Gynecol. 2005;25(1):42-9.

STATION 2.

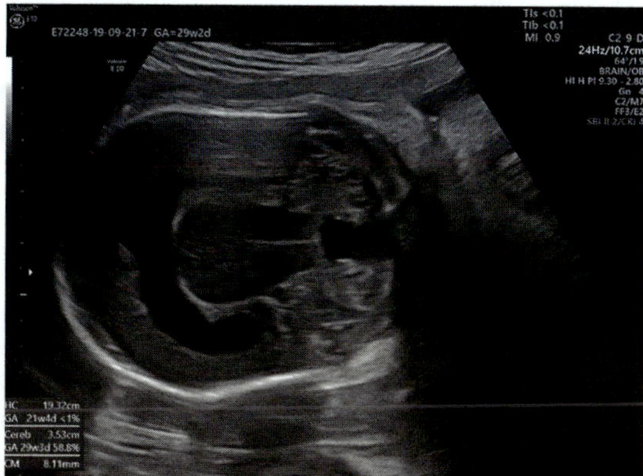

1. **Identify the above ultrasound finding and diagnosis.**
2. **What genetic syndromes are they associated with?**
3. **What is the abnormal pathway of anterior cerebral artery (ACA) in this condition called?**

Ans.

1. Fused cerebral lobes, monoventricle, absence of falx/interhemispheric fissure, and alobar holoprosencephaly
2. Trisomy 18 and 13; occasionally single gene disorders
3. "Snake under the skull" sign of azygous ACA

SUGGESTED READING

1. Bernard JP, Drummond CL, Zaarour P, Molho M, Ville Y. A new clue to the prenatal diagnosis of lobar holoprosencephaly: the abnormal pathway of the anterior cerebral artery crawling under the skull. Ultrasound Obstet Gynecol. 2002;19(6):605-7.
2. Greene MF, Benacerraf BR, Frigoletto FD Jr. Reliable criteria for the prenatal sonographic diagnosis of alobar holoprosencephaly. Am J Obstet Gynecol. 1987;156(3):687-9.

STATION 3.

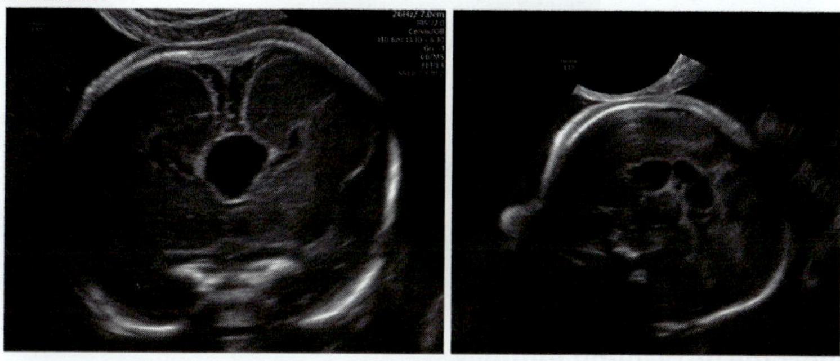

1. **Enumerate the ultrasound findings.**
2. **What is the diagnosis?**
3. **What is the detection rate of genetic abnormalities with chromosomal microarray analysis (CMA) and whole exome sequencing (WES)?**
4. **Name at least two genetic syndromes associated with this condition.**

Ans.

1. Widely separated, pinched frontal horns, interhemispheric cysts, and corpus callosum (CC) not seen
2. Agenesis of corpus callosum
3. About 12.5% can have abnormalities detected in CMA, 47% in WES. In truly isolated agenesis of the corpus callosum (ACC), the yield of WES is 30%.
4. Aicardi syndrome, acrocallosal syndrome, and L1 cell adhesion molecule (L1CAM) mutation

SUGGESTED READING

1. Moutard ML, Kieffer V, Feingold J, Kieffer F, Lewin F, Adamsbaum C, et al. Agenesis of corpus callosum: prenatal diagnosis and prognosis. Childs Nerv Syst. 2003;19:471-6.
2. Tsai P, Shinar S. Agenesis of the corpus callosum: What to tell expecting parents? Prenat Diagn. 2023;43(12):1527-35.

STATION 4.

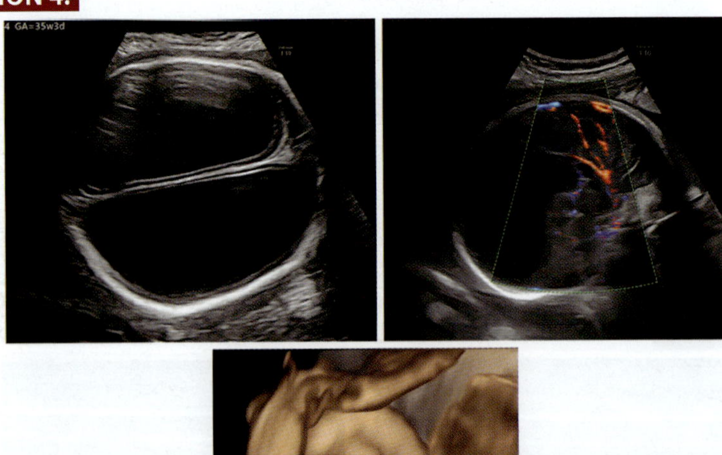

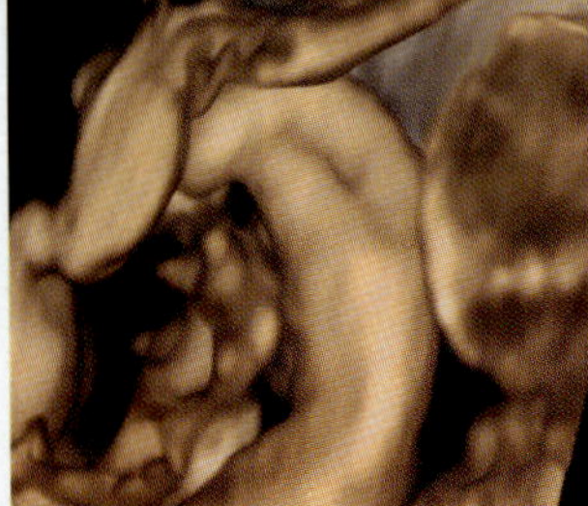

1. **Report the ultrasound findings.**
2. **What is the likely diagnosis with these findings?**

3. **What is the mode of inheritance?**
4. **How is the diagnosis confirmed?**

Ans.

1. Severe ventriculomegaly, dysplastic corpus callosum (evidenced by the abnormal pericallosal course), and adducted thumb
2. L1CAM mutations/MASA syndrome
3. X-linked recessive
4. Amniocentesis for WES/Sanger sequencing

SUGGESTED READING

1. Timor-Tritsch IE, Monteagudo A, Haratz-Rubinstein N, Levine RU. Transvaginal sonographic detection of adducted thumbs, hydrocephalus, and agenesis of the corpus callosum at 22 postmenstrual weeks: the masa spectrum or L1 spectrum. A case report and review of the literature. Prenat Diagn. 1996;16(6):543-8.

STATION 5.

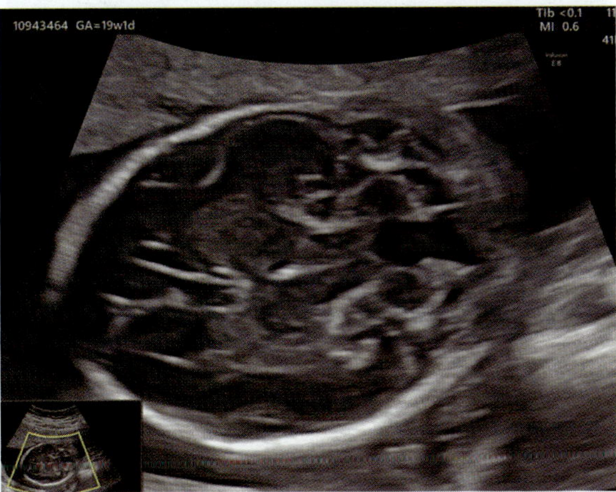

1. **Report the ultrasound findings, what other information would you like to have here?**
2. **What are the differential diagnoses?**
3. **Should prenatal testing be offered?**
4. **How will you counsel?**

Ans.

1. Open fourth ventricle, sagittal views of the brain (a detailed neurosonogram), and MRI after 32 weeks to rule out (r/o) migrational disorders.
2. Blakes pouch cyst, Vermian hypoplasia, mega cisterna magna, and Dandy—Walker malformation
3. Amniocentesis for WES to r/o underlying genetic issues. High association with aneuploidies and genetic syndromes like Walker–Warburg, Meckel–Gruber, Aicardi, Joubert and Neu-Laxova

4. Blakes pouch cyst will have a benign outcome, Vermian hypoplasia will be associated with >30% risk of neurodevelopmental delays, Dandy-Walker malformation will be associated with >50% risk of neurodevelopmental delays.

SUGGESTED READING

1. Guibaud L, des Portes V. Plea for an anatomical approach to abnormalities of the posterior fossa in prenatal diagnosis. Ultrasound Obstet Gynecol. 2006;27(5):477-8.
2. Juan Z, Cuixia G, Yuanjie C, Yan L, Ling Y, Tiejuan Z, et al. Optimal prenatal genetic diagnostic approach for posterior fossa malformation: karyotyping, copy number variant testing, or whole-exome sequencing? Eur J Med Res. 2024;29(1):397.

STATION 6.

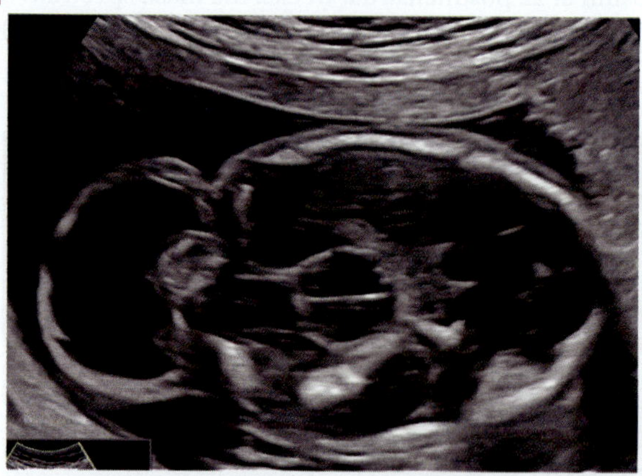

1. **Report the ultrasound findings.**
2. **What is the most common genetic syndrome associated with this finding?**
3. **How will you counsel?**
4. **What is the mode of inheritance?**

Ans.

1. Occipital encephalocele
2. Meckel-Gruber syndrome (occipital encephalocele + multicystic kidneys + polydactyly)
3. Guarded prognosis if associated with Meckel-Gruber syndrome and postnatal surgical intervention
4. Autosomal recessive inheritance—25% recurrence risk in every pregnancy

SUGGESTED READING

1. Liao SL, Tsai PY, Cheng YC, Chang CH, Ko HC, Chang FM. Prenatal diagnosis of fetal encephalocele using three-dimensional ultrasound. J Med Ultrasound. 2012;20(3):150-4.

STATION 7.

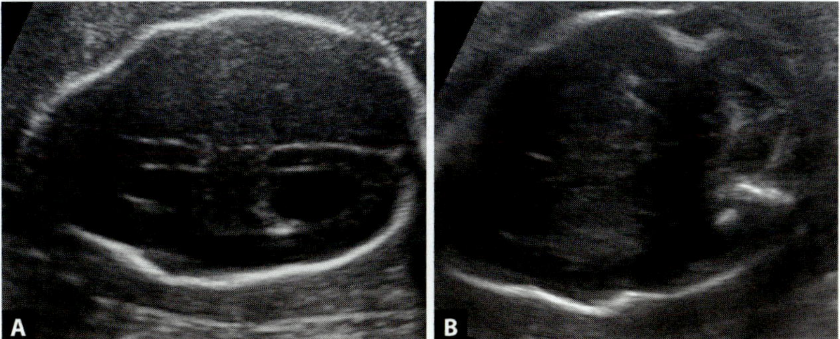

1. **Identify the abnormalities. What are these ultrasound features called?**
2. **Which types of defect are these findings seen?**
3. **How will you counsel?**
4. **Is invasive prenatal testing recommended in these cases?**

Ans.

1. *Image A:* Scalloping of the frontal bones, effacement of cisterna magna, and loss of normal vallecula of the cerebellum
   Image B: Lemon and banana sign/Arnold-Chiari type 2
2. Open neural tube defect (ONTD)
3. Prognosis will depend on the level of involvement of the neural tube, but with brain changes, neurological sequelae are highly likely.
4. As ONTD is usually a sporadic defect, invasive testing not recommended unless associated with other systemic structural abnormalities.

SUGGESTED READING

1. Nicolaides KH, Campbell S, Gabbe SG, Guidetti R. Ultrasound screening for spina bifida: cranial and cerebellar signs. Lancet. 1986;2(8498):72-4.

STATION 8.

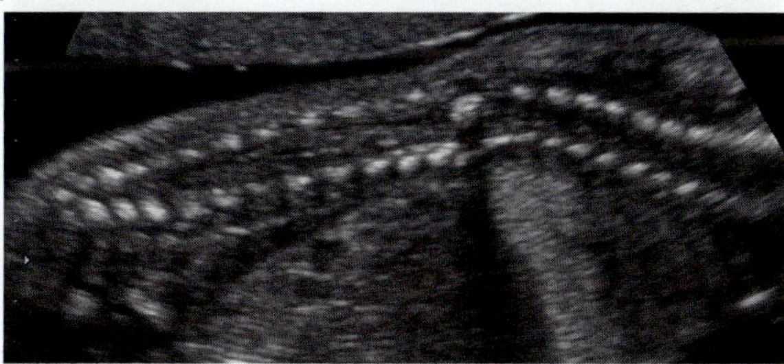

1. **What is the ultrasound diagnosis?**
2. **What type of spinal cord defect is shown above?**
3. **Is this associated with genetic abnormalities?**
4. **What is the prognosis in these cases?**

Ans.

1. Diastematomyelia
2. This is type of spinal dysraphism also known as spina bifida occulta, most commonly seen between L1 and L3. The presence of an extra echogenic focus in the midline between the fetal spinal posterior elements has been described as a reliable sign.
3. No
4. If isolated and timely surgery for tethered cord is done postnatally, prognosis is good.

SUGGESTED READING

1. Allen LM, Silverman RK. Prenatal ultrasound evaluation of fetal diastematomyelia: two cases of type I split cord malformation. Ultrasound Obstet Gynecol. 2000;15(1):78-82.
2. Radiopaedia. (2025). Diastematomyelia. [online] Available from https://radiopaedia.org/articles/diastematomyelia?lang=us [Last accessed April, 2025].
3. Wei Q, Cai A, Wang X, Wang X, Xie L. The Value of Prenatal Ultrasonographic Diagnosis of Diastematomyelia. J Ultrasound Med. 2017;36(6):1129-36.

STATION 9.

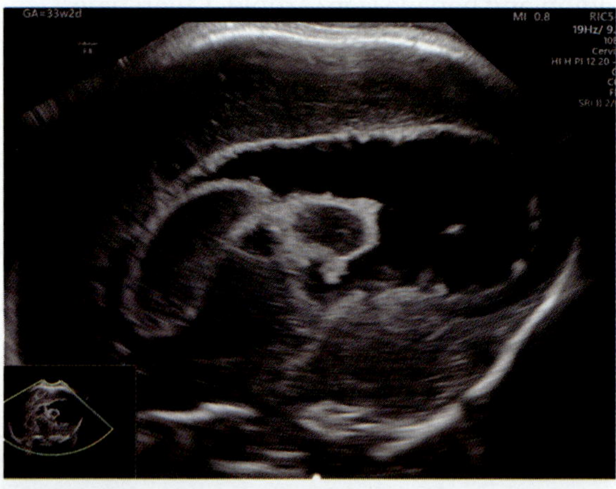

1. **What are the ultrasound findings?**
2. **What is the tentative diagnosis?**
3. **Is this associated with genetic abnormalities?**
4. **What are the other nongenetic causes?**

Ans.

1. Severe ventriculomegaly, echogenic lining of the ventricles with debris noted inside, and echogenic caudothalamic groove
2. *Diagnosis:* Severe ventriculomegaly most likely secondary to a ventricular bleed (type IV)

3. Can be associated—especially with *COL4A1* gene
4. *Maternal:* Trauma, coagulopathy, use of anticoagulants, infections, and seizure disorder.

   Fetal: Thrombocytopenia—neonatal alloimmune thrombocytopenia (NAIT), vascular malformations, tumors, consequence of fetal intervention, complications of monochorionic (MC) twinning.

SUGGESTED READING

1. ISUOG. (2013). Schizencephaly. Schizencephaly. Visual Encyclopedia of Ultrasound in Obstetrics and Gynecology. [online] Available from https://www.isuog.org/education/visuog/obstetrics/brain/cortical-malformations/schizencephaly.html [Last accessed April, 2025]
2. Putbrese B, Kennedy A. Findings and differential diagnosis of fetal intracranial haemorrhage and fetal ischaemic brain injury: what is the role of fetal MRI? Br J Radiol. 2017;90(1070):20160253.

STATION 10.

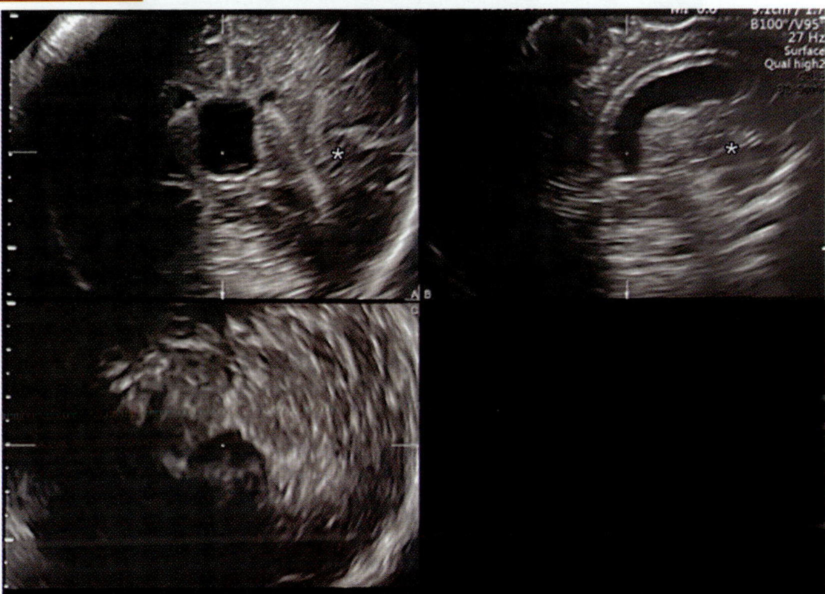

1. **What is the structure marked with the star called?**
2. **What is the outcome?**

Ans.

1. It is an enlarged cavum vergae which is essentially a posterior extension of a cavum septum pellucidum (CSP).
2. Cavum vergae is a common variant—an enlarged, stable cavum vergae is usually associated with normal outcomes.

SUGGESTED READING

1. Gaillard F, Walizai T, Weerakkody Y, et al. Cavum vergae. Reference article, Radiopaedia.org
2. Siala S, Homen D, Smith B, Guimaraes C. Imaging of the septum pellucidum: normal, variants and pathology. Br J Radiol. 2023;96(1151):20221058. doi: 10.1259/bjr.20221058. Epub 2023 May 24. PMID: 37194993; PMCID: PMC10607410.

STATION 11.

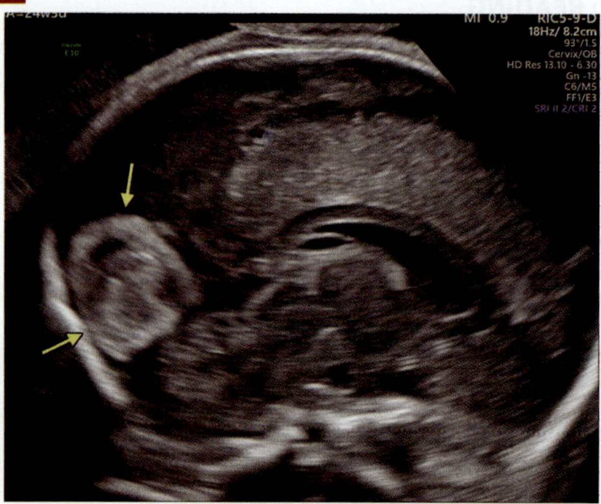

1. **What is the lesion seen and the likely diagnosis?**
2. **Would you order an invasive testing?**
3. **How will you manage this case?**

Ans.

1. Dural sinus thrombus at the torcular Herophili
2. No, it is not known to be associated with genetic syndromes.
3. Usually, expectant management as the outcomes are good in >80% as long as the thrombus is stable and not associated with dural sinus malformations/fistula.

SUGGESTED READING

1. Laurichesse Delmas H, Winer N, Gallot D, Lopes K, Perrotin F, Fluncker S, et al. Prenatal diagnosis of thrombosis of the dural sinuses: report of six cases, review of the literature and suggested management. Ultrasound Obstet Gynecol. 2008;32(2):188-98.

STATION 12.

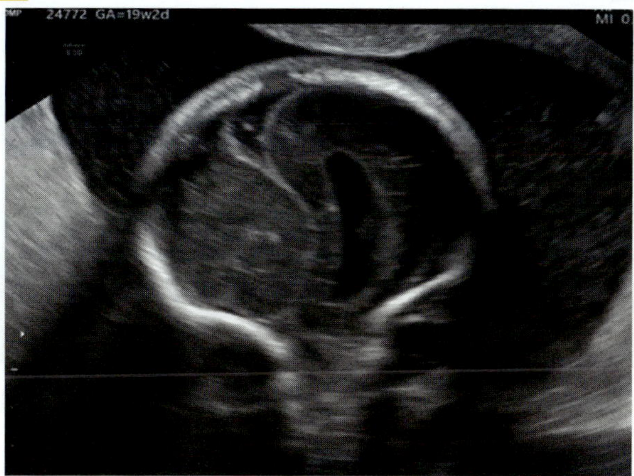

1. **What is the abnormality seen?**
2. **State the differential diagnosis.**
3. **What is the clinical significance?**
4. **Is prenatal testing recommended?**

Ans.

1. Deviated midline, discrepant hemispheres, discrepant ventricles, and premature sulcations
2. Hemimegalencephaly and tubulinopathy
3. As associated abnormalities of sulcation are usually present including agyria, pachygyria, or polymicrogyria, postnatally there is severe neurodevelopmental delay and intractable seizure. Hence, the prognosis is very poor.
4. Yes, the risk of chromosomal abnormalities is not increased but genetic syndromes like Proteus and Klippel–Trenaunay syndromes have to be excluded.

SUGGESTED READING

1. Sepulveda W, Sepulveda F, Schonstedt V, Stern J, Diaz-Serani R. Neuroimaging Findings in Fetal Hemimegalencephaly: Case Study and Review. Fetal Diagn Ther. 2024;51(2):133-44.
2. The Fetal Medicine Foundation. FMF certification: Fetal abnormalities. [online] Available from https://fetalmedicine.org/fmf-certification-2/fetal-abnormalities-1 [Last accessed April, 2025].

STATION 13.

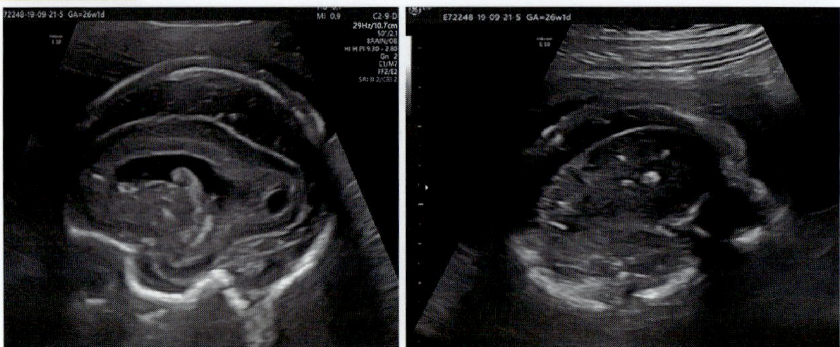

1. **Enumerate the ultrasound findings in this fetus at 26 weeks.**
2. **What is the most likely diagnosis/differential diagnosis?**
3. **What are the extracranial features that may be present?**
4. **How will you confirm your diagnosis?**

Ans.

1. Parenchymal calcifications, ventricular halo, germinolytic cysts, and delayed sulcations
2. Cytomegalovirus (CMV) infection/Aicardi–Goutières syndrome
3. Hepatosplenomegaly, fetal growth restriction, oligohydramnios/polyhydramnios, echogenic bowel, and serositis
4. Amniocentesis [CMV/*Toxoplasma* polymerase chain reaction (PCR)]—if negative WES

SUGGESTED READING

1. Khalil A, Sotiriadis A, Chaoui R, da Silva Costa F, D'Antonio F, Heath PT, et al. ISUOG Practice Guidelines: role of ultrasound in congenital infection. Ultrasound Obstet Gynecol. 2020;56(1):128-51.

STATION 14.

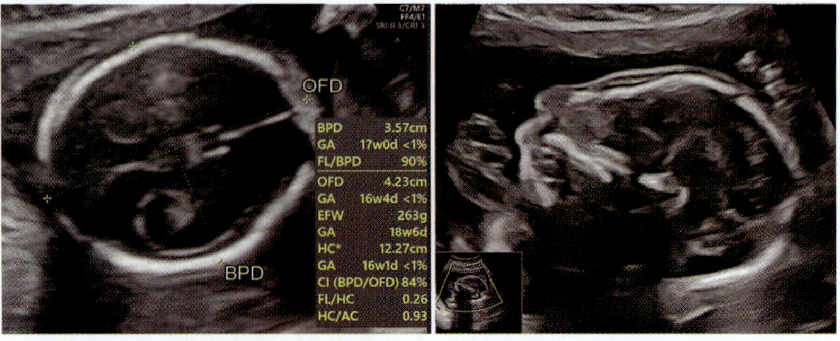

This is a 20 weeks fetus.

1. **Describe the ultrasound features and the probable diagnosis.**
2. **Which charts do you use to establish microcephaly?**

3. **Enumerate the possible causes.**
4. **How will you approach such cases?**

Ans.

1. Head circumference (HC) first centile, delayed sulcations, increased pericerebral space, and sloping forehead. Probable diagnosis: Microcephaly if the HC <-3 standard deviation (SD) on Chervenak's charts
2. Chervenak's charts
3. TORCH (toxoplasmosis, other infections, rubella, cytomegalovirus, herpes simplex) infections, Zika virus infection, and genetic syndromes
4.

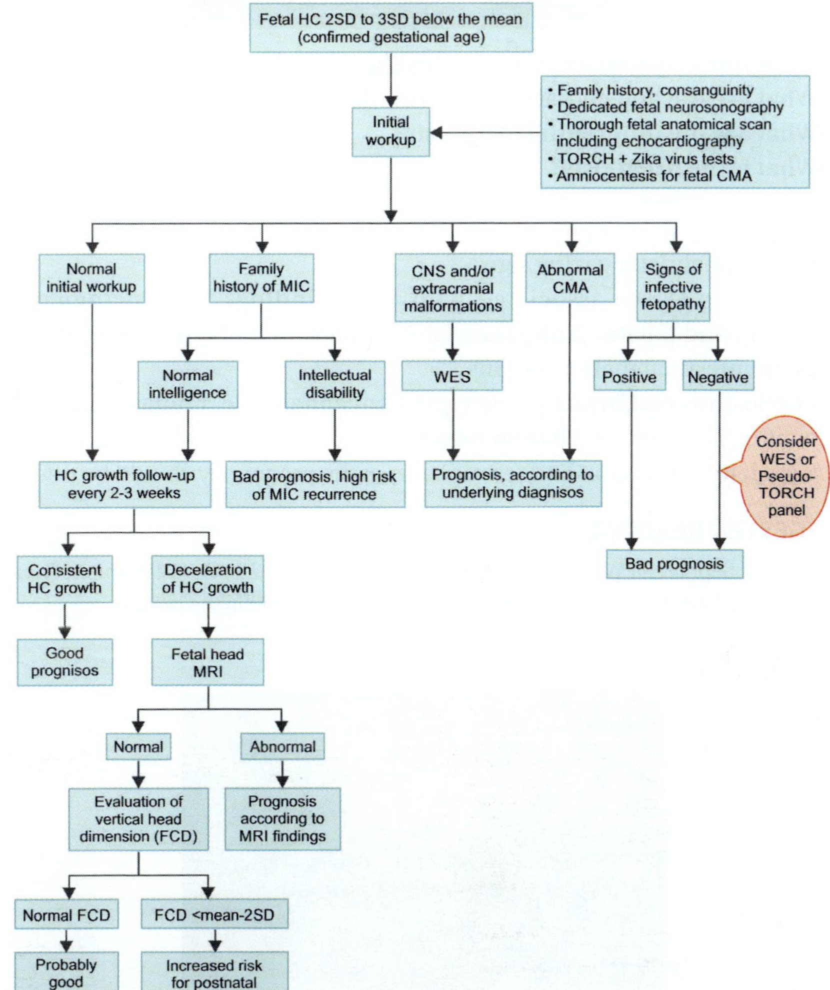

SUGGESTED READING

1. Leibovitz Z, Lerman-Sagie T. Diagnostic approach to fetal microcephaly. Eur J Paediatr Neurol. 2018;22(6):935-43.

STATION 15.

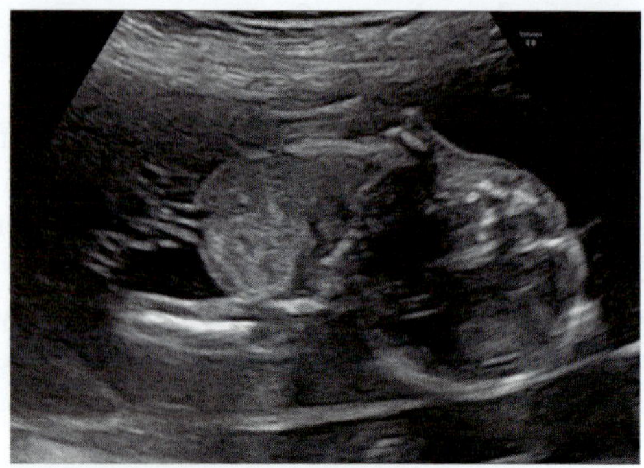

1. **What is the diagnosis? What is this sign called?**
2. **What are the defects associated with this condition?**
3. **What are the differential diagnosis?**
4. **What is the prognosis?**

Ans.

1. Iniencephaly/star gazing sign
2. It is often (80%) associated with other findings like micrognathia, cleft lip and palate, cardiovascular disorders, diaphragmatic hernia, and gastrointestinal malformations.
3. Cervical rib malformation, occipital encephalocele, craniorachischisis, teratomas, goiter, and lymphangioma
4. It is a lethal condition and termination of the pregnancy should be offered.

SUGGESTED READING

1. Sahid S, Sepulveda W, Dezerega V, Gutierrez J, Rodriguez L, Corral E. Iniencephaly: prenatal diagnosis and management. Prenat Diagn. 2000;20(3):202-5.

STATION 16.

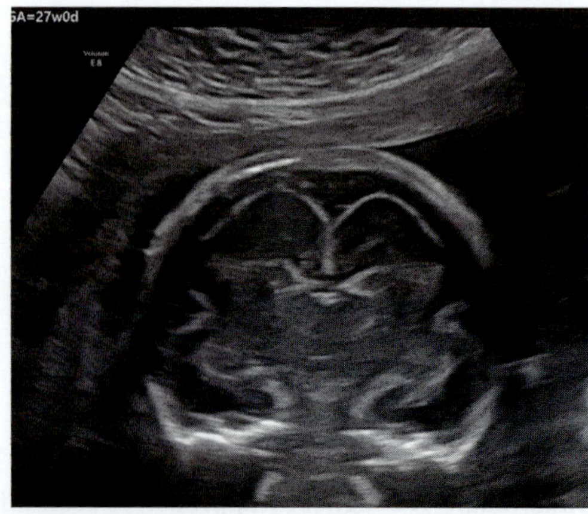

1. **This is a fetus at 26 weeks, describe the abnormalities seen in this coronal view.**
2. **What is the diagnosis?**
3. **How will you approach this case?**
4. **How will you counsel regarding the neurodevelopmental outcome?**

Ans.

1. The sylvian sulcus appears delayed, cingulate sulcus has not appeared yet, and increased subarachnoid space.
2. Malformation of cortical development
3. Work-up algorithm

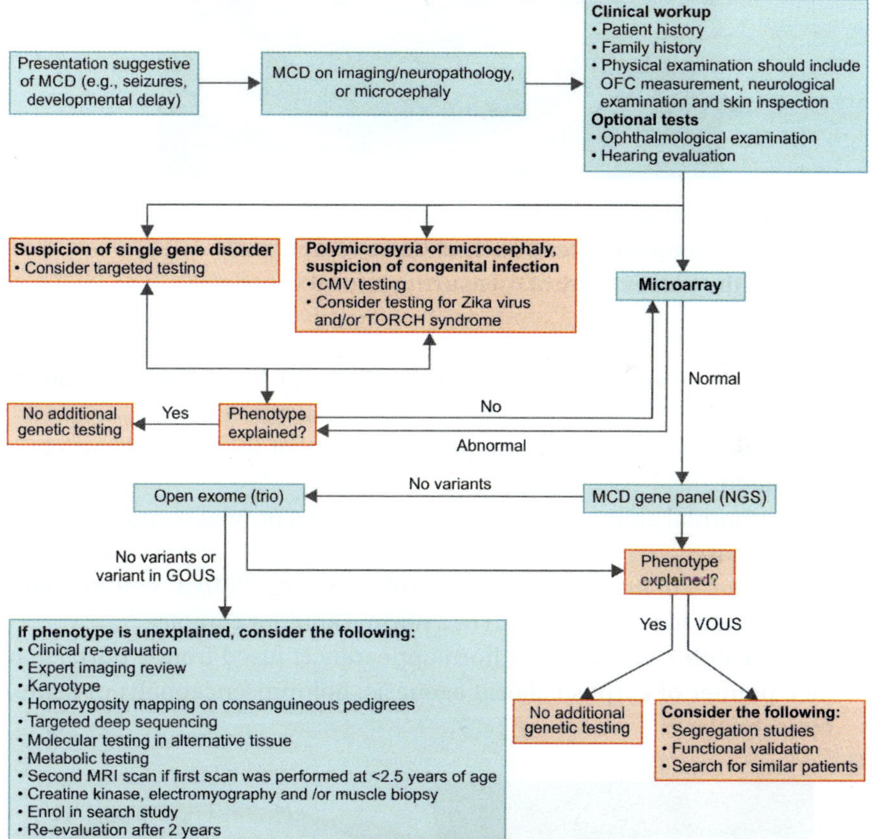

4. The prognosis is variable and can range from mild to severe intellectual disability and developmental delay depending on the cause.

SUGGESTED READING

1. Oegema R, Barakat TS, Wilke M, Stouffs K, Amrom D, Aronica E, et al. International consensus recommendations on the diagnostic work-up for malformations of cortical development. Nat Rev Neurol. 2020;16(11):618-35.

2. Pistorius LR, Stoutenbeek P, Groenendaal F, de Vries L, Manten G, Mulder E, et al. Grade and symmetry of normal fetal cortical development: a longitudinal two- and three-dimensional ultrasound study. Ultrasound Obstet Gynecol. 2010;36(6):700-8.

STATION 17.

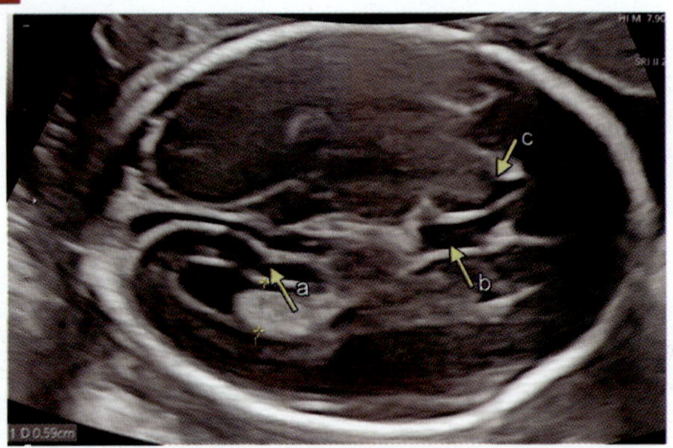

1. **Identify the structures labeled "a", "b", "c".**
2. **What is the importance of each of these structures?**
3. **What is the correct way of measuring lateral ventricle?**

Ans.

1. (a) Parieto-occipital (PO) sulcus, (b) CSP, (c) frontal horn of lateral ventricle
2. *PO sulcus:* Level at which the posterior horn of the lateral ventricle is measured.

   CSP: A normal appearing CSP is suggestive of a normal corpus callosum in most cases.

   Frontal horn of lateral ventricle: Its relation with CSP/CC and its shape is important to note as the part of a normal anterior complex.

   Abnormalities such as steer horn appearance, fused frontal horns may be a pointer of corpus callosal agenesis, holoprosencephaly, or septo-optic dysplasia
3.

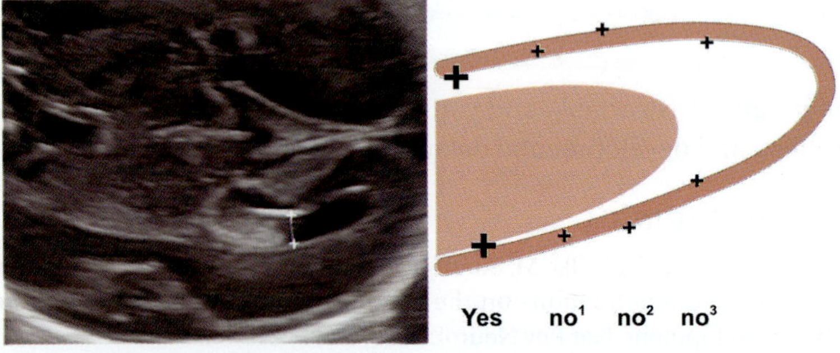

Callipers are placed correctly when touching inner edge of ventricular wall at its widest part and aligned perpendicular to long axis of ventricle.

SUGGESTED READING

1. Malinger G, Paladini D, Haratz KK, Monteagudo A, Pilu GL, Timor-Tritsch IE. ISUOG Practice Guidelines (updated): sonographic examination of the fetal central nervous system. Part 1: performance of screening examination and indications for targeted neurosonography. Ultrasound Obstet Gynecol. 2020; 56(3):476-84. Erratum in: Ultrasound Obstet Gynecol. 2022;60(4):591.

STATION 18.

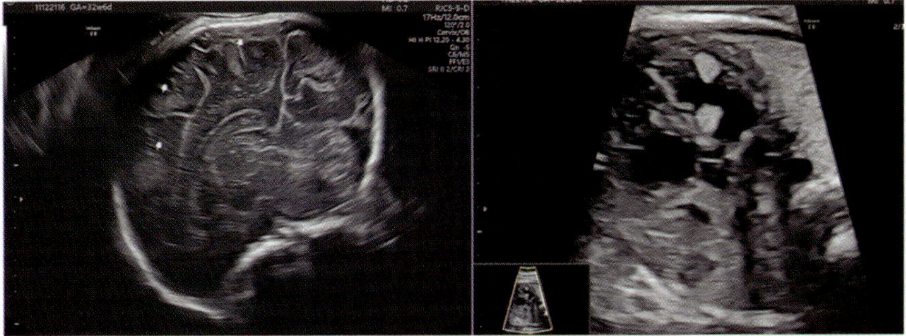

1. **What are the arrow hands pointing toward in the fetal brain?**
2. **What is this genetic syndrome called and what are the genes responsible for these?**
3. **How will you counsel?**
4. **What is the inheritance pattern?**

Ans.

1. Brain tubers
2. Tuberous sclerosis (TSC1 and SC2)
3. Rhabdomyomas usually regress postnatally. Brain tubers can cause postnatal seizures. There is a risk of neurodevelopmental delays along with other manifestations of the syndrome (renal involvement, dermatological manifestations, lung involvement, etc.). Sirolimus available as potential therapy-multidisciplinary care plan to be made with geneticist/pediatric neurologist.
4. Autosomal dominant

SUGGESTED READING

1. Malinger G, Prabhu A, Maroto González A, Brusilov M, Kidron D, Amster R, et al. Fetal neurosonography as accurate tool for diagnosis of brain involvement in tuberous sclerosis. Ultrasound Obstet Gynecol. 2023;62(3):391-7.

STATION 19.

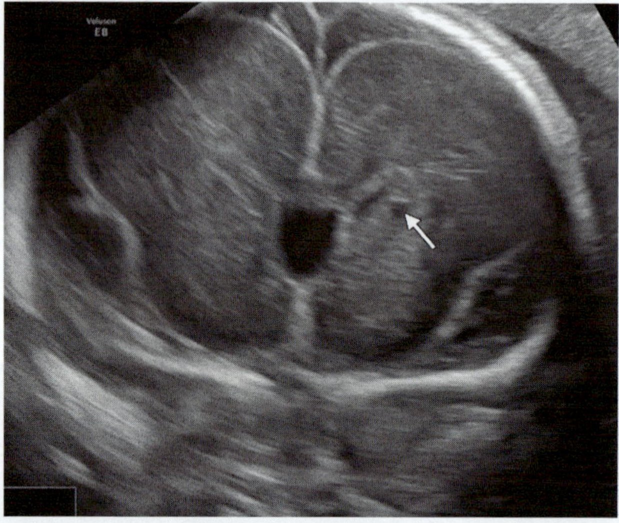

1. **Describe the location of this cyst.**
2. **What is the probable diagnosis? What are the other cysts around this area called and how will you differentiate between these?**
3. **How will you manage this case?**

Ans.

1. Anterior, inferior lateral to the angle of the frontal horn
2. Periventricular pseudocysts/connatal cysts (at the angle of the frontal horn)/periventricular leukomalacia (superior to the angle of the frontal horn)
3. Maternal TORCH immunoglobulin G/immunoglobulin M (IgG/IgM), discuss amniocentesis. Usually, benign outcomes if genetics and infections are ruled out.

SUGGESTED READING

1. Malinger G, Lev D, Ben Sira L, Kidron D, Tamarkin M, Lerman-Sagie T. Congenital periventricular pseudocysts: prenatal sonographic appearance and clinical implications. Ultrasound Obstet Gynecol. 2002;20(5):447-51.

STATION 20.

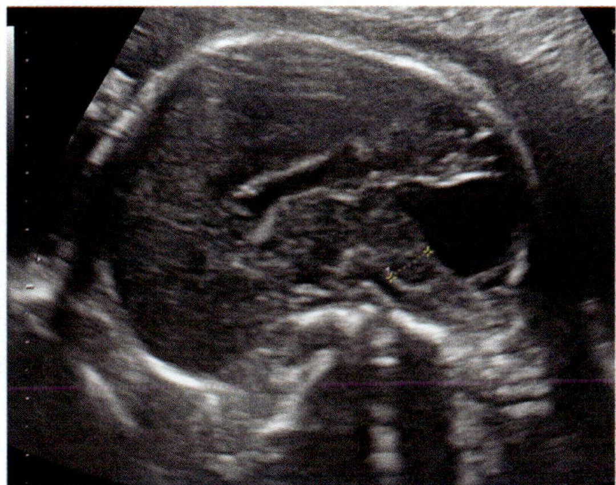

1. **Comment on the posterior fossa.**
2. **What is your diagnosis?**
3. **What are the different angles that will help to differentiate between various posterior fossa malformations?**
4. **What is the approach to such cases?**

Ans.

1. Open fourth ventricle and hypoplastic rotated vermis
2. Dandy–Walker malformation

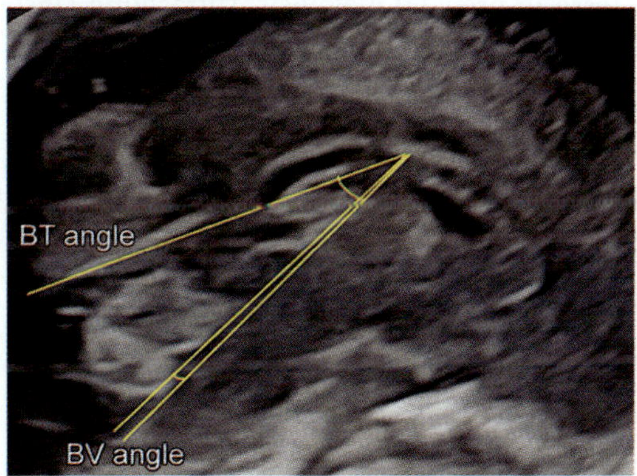

3. Measurement of the brainstem-vermis (BV) and brainstem-tentorium (BT) angles; (a) a median view of the fetal brain is obtained (in this case after the acquisition of an ultrasound volume starting from an axial view) and the main anatomic landmarks are identified; (b) a line is drawn tangentially to the dorsal aspect of the brainstem and a second line is drawn tangentially to the ventral contour of the cerebellar vermis; the interposed angle (1) is the BV angle; angle (2) the BT angle is measured between the former line and a third line tangential to the lower edge of the tentorium. Normally, the BV angle is <18° and BT angle is <45°.

   The BV angle and BT angle in fetuses with Blake's pouch cyst, cerebellar vermis hypoplasia, and Dandy-Walker malformation are 26°, 39°, and 73° respectively and 45°, 50°, and 66° respectively.
4. Amniocentesis (microarray /WES) to r/o genetic syndromes. Fetal MRI after 32 weeks. Patient and family need to be counseling about guarded prognosis. When they are isolated, there is a high possibility of spontaneous regression and normal developmental outcome. Dandy-Walker malformation and vermian hypoplasia have a guarded prognosis and are frequently associated with other abnormalities and neurologic impairment such as cognitive and psychomotor developmental delay.

SUGGESTED READING

1. Guibaud L, des Portes V. Plea for an anatomical approach to abnormalities of the posterior fossa in prenatal diagnosis. Ultrasound Obstet Gynecol. 2006; 27(5):477-8.
2. Praveen TLN, Surekha P. Demystifying Posterior Cranial Fossa Lesions in the Fetus. J Fetal Med. 2016;3:63-69.
3. Volpe P, Contro E, De Musso F, Ghi T, Farina A, Tempesta A, et al. Brainstem-vermis and brainstem-tentorium angles allow accurate categorization of fetal upward rotation of cerebellar vermis. Ultrasound Obstet Gynecol. 2012;39(6):632-5.

Skeletal Dysplasias

Manisha Kumar, Apoorva Kulshreshtha

STATION 1.

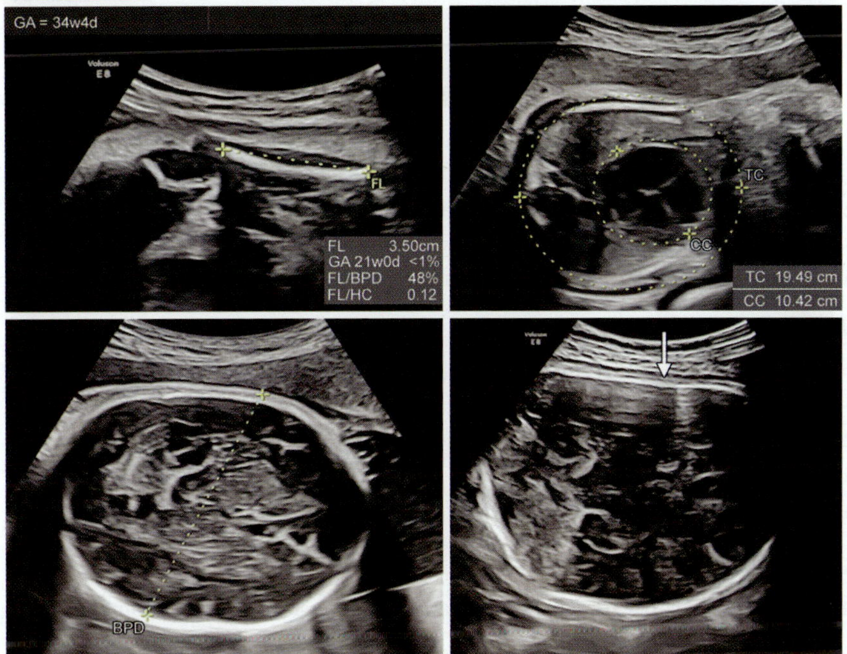

1. **What should be the standard deviation cut-off for the diagnosis of skeletal dysplasia?**
2. **What is the condition called when there is severe shortening of only femur and humerus?**
3. **What does distortion of the shape of the vault on ultrasound probe pressure suggest?**
4. **When do we say antenatally that the condition is lethal?**

Ans.

1. Below-2 SD
2. Rhizomelia
3. Poor mineralization
4. Thoracic circumference/abdominal circumference <0.7 *OR* femur length/abdominal circumference <0.16

SUGGESTED READING

1. Krakow D, Lachman RS, Rimoin DL. Guidelines for the prenatal diagnosis of fetal skeletal dysplasias. Genet Med. 2009;11(2):127-33.

STATION 2.

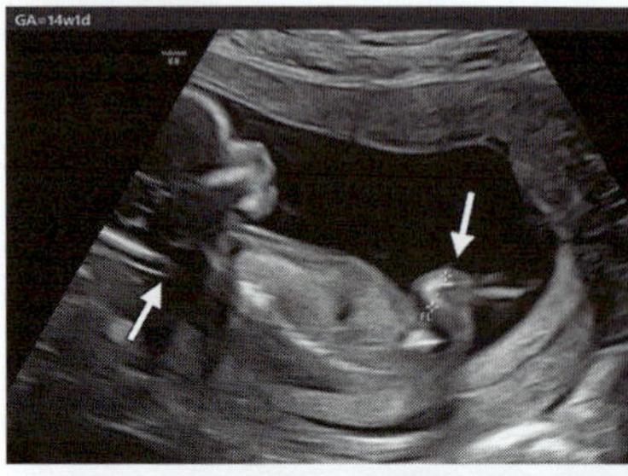

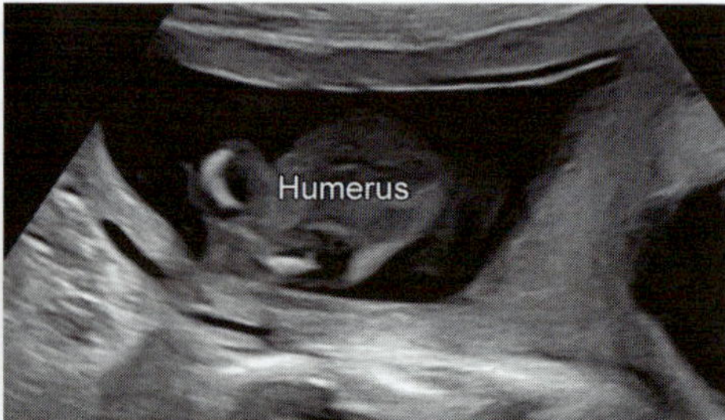

1. **What are the features suggestive of possibility of skeletal dysplasia in the first trimester?**
2. **What is the most common lethal skeletal dysplasia?**
3. **What is the eye finding typically seen with osteogenesis imperfecta?**
4. **What is the common mode of inheritance of the disorder?**

Ans.

1. Increased nuchal translucency (NT), short limbs, bending, and polydactyly
2. Osteogenesis imperfecta type 2
3. Blue sclera
4. Autosomal dominant

SUGGESTED READING

1. Khalil A, Pajkrt E, Chitty LS. Early prenatal diagnosis of skeletal anomalies. Prenat Diagn. 2011;31:115-24.

STATION 3.

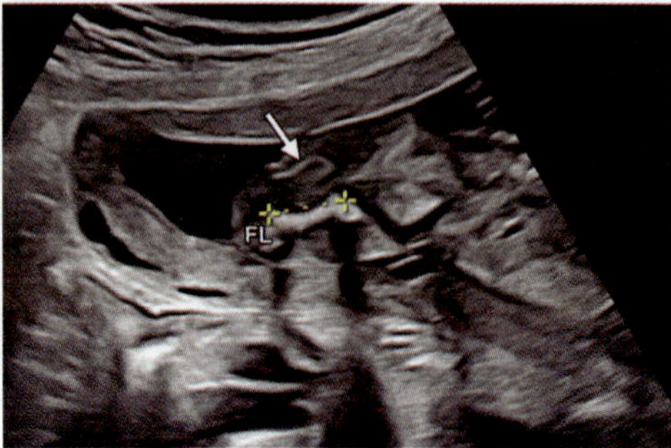

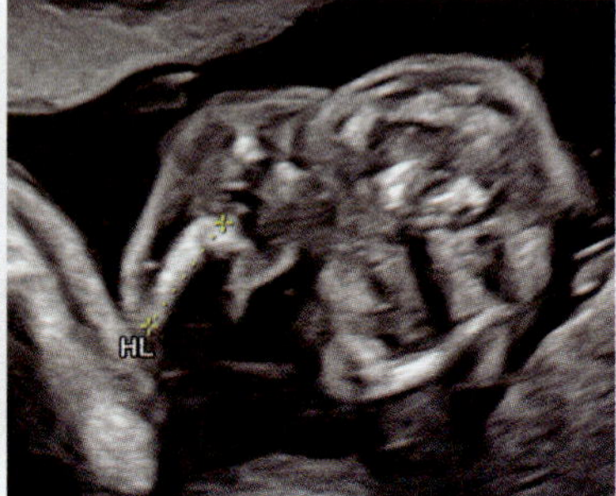

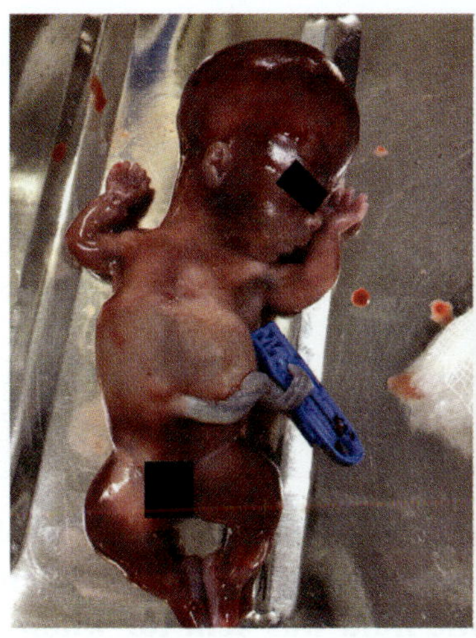
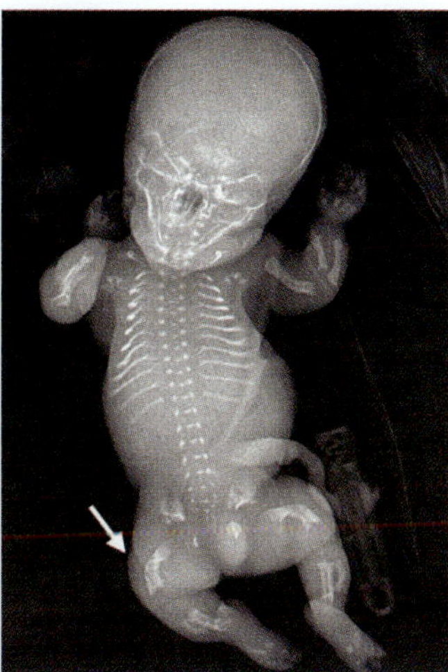

1. **What does the shape of femur in infantogram show?**
2. **What is the probable diagnosis based on ultrasound?**
3. **What is the typical skull shape in this condition?**
4. **What is the severe shortening of whole limb called?**

Ans.

1. Telephone receiver and bowing of femur
2. Thanatophoric dysplasia type 1
3. Cloverleaf skull
4. Micromelia

SUGGESTED READING

1. Omim.org. 166210 - OSTEOGENESIS IMPERFECTA, TYPE II; OI2. [online] Available from https://omim.org/entry/166210. [Last accessed June, 2025].

STATION 4.

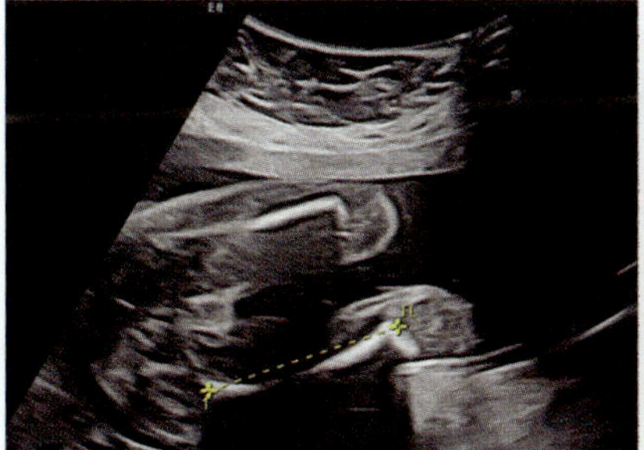
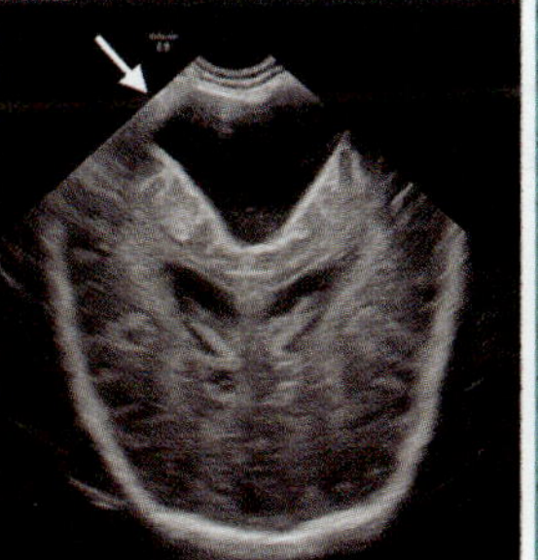

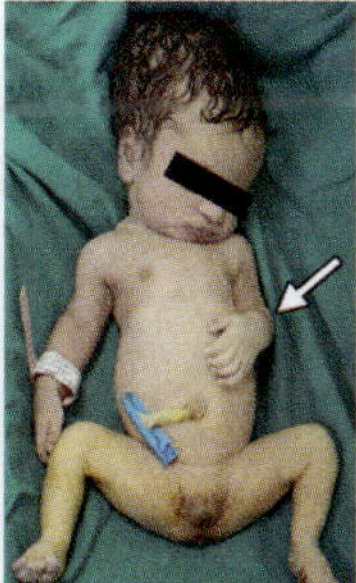

Contd...

Contd...

Gene and transcript	*Exon/ intron number*	*Variant nomenclature [variant depth/ total depth]*	*Zygosity*	*Classification*	*OMIM phenotype*	*Inheritance*
EVC2 (NM_147127.5)	Exon 17	c.2856_2857del p.Arg952SerfsTer51 [37x/67x]	Heterozygous	Pathogenic	Ellis-van Creveld syndrome	Autosomal recessive
EVC2 (NM_147127.5)	Exon 11	c.1633A>G p.Ile545Val [60x/136x]	Heterozygous	Uncertain significance	Ellis-van Creveld syndrome	Autosomal recessive

A G2 P1L0 with non-consanguineous marriage came at 30 weeks with short long bones, polydactyly, and Dandy-Walker malformation. Amniocentesis was done. Amniotic fluid was sent for whole exome sequencing, the report is shown above.

1. **What is a common visceral abnormality associated with this condition?**
2. **What is the mode of inheritance?**
3. **When can we earliest do the testing in the next pregnancy?**
4. **Can karyotyping help in diagnosis of the condition?**

Ans.

1. Heart defect
2. Autosomal recessive
3. At 11–12 weeks of gestation
4. No, molecular test is needed.

SUGGESTED READING

1. Omim.org. Entry - #225500 - ELLIS-VAN CREVELD SYNDROME; EVC. [online] Available from https://omim.org/entry/225500 [Last accessed June, 2025].

STATION 5.

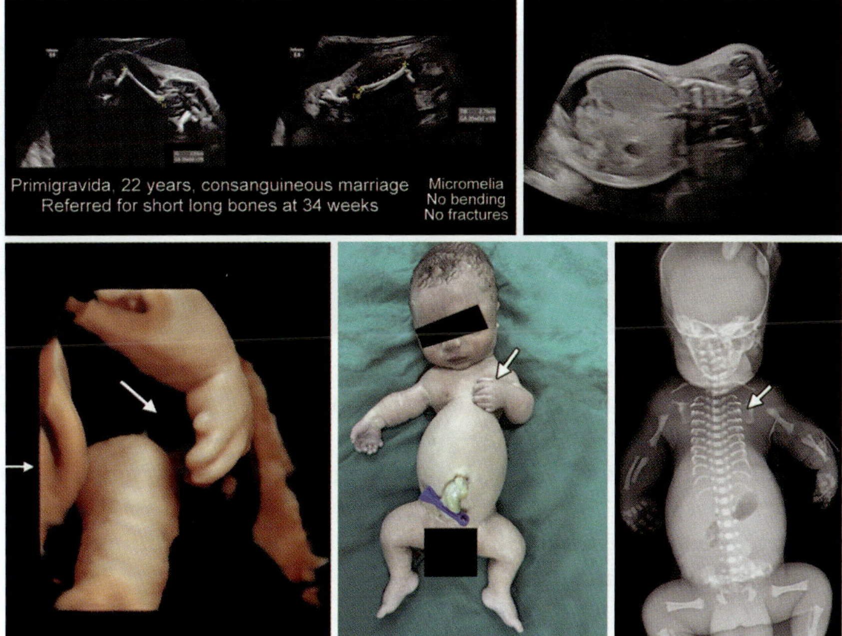

A primigravida, 22 years with consanguineous marriage, was referred at 34 weeks with short long bones.

1. **What additional feature is seen in thorax of fetus?**
2. **Fetus was found to have polydactyly on ultrasound and after delivery also, what is the probable diagnosis?**
3. **What additional visceral abnormality may be present in this group of disorders?**
4. **What is the chance of recurrence in next pregnancy?**

Ans.

1. Thorax is narrow with short ribs.
2. Short rib polydactyly syndrome
3. Heart defects, genitourinary defects, and brain malformations
4. Up to 25%

SUGGESTED READING

1. Badiner N, Taylor SP, Forlenza K, Lachman RS; University of Washington Center for Mendelian Genomics; Bamshad M, et al. Mutations in DYNC2H1, the cytoplasmic dynein 2, heavy chain 1 motor protein gene, cause short-rib polydactyly type I, Saldino-Noonan type. Clin Genet. 2017;92(2):158-65.

STATION 6. **A G2P1L1, 34 weeks period of gestation, presented with polyhydramnios, macrocrania, and short femur.**

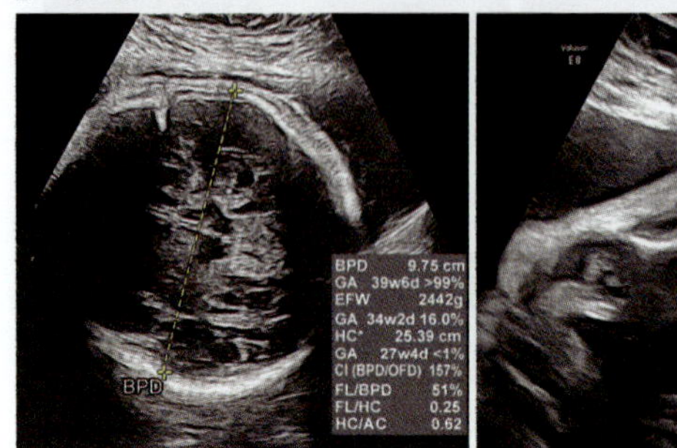

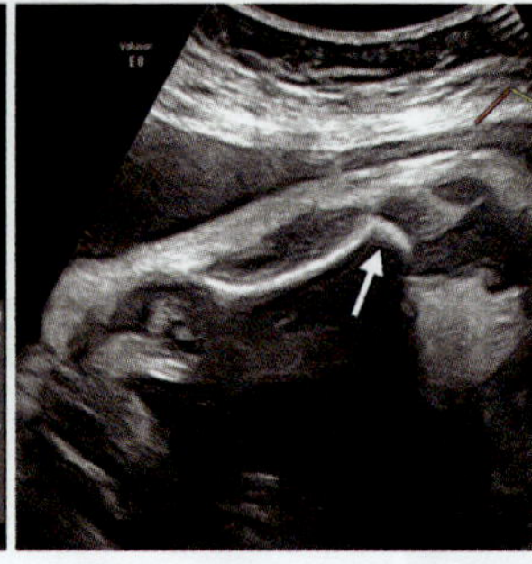
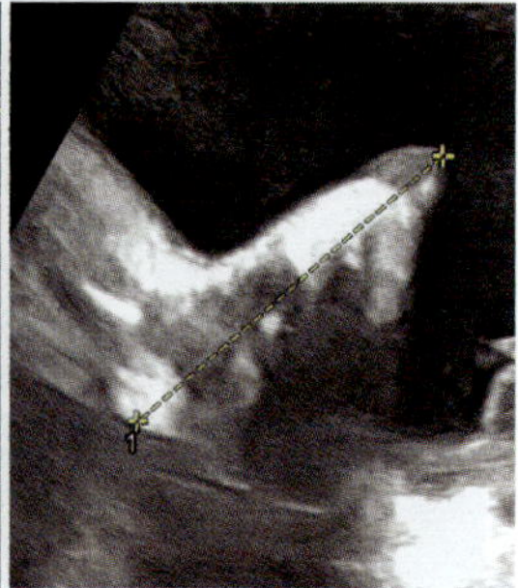

1. **Short limbs, short hands and fingers, large head with frontal bossing and depressed nasal bridge, and lumbar scoliosis are suggestive of which syndrome?**
2. **What cut-off of femur length/foot length is taken as suggestive of skeletal dysplasia?**
3. **What is the typical finding in the femur neck in this condition?**
4. **What is the gene involved?**

Ans.

1. Achondroplasia
2. 0.8
3. A wider than normal angle between the proximal diaphysis and metaphysis
4. *FGFR3* gene mutation

SUGGESTED READING

1. Vajo Z, Francomano CA, Wilkin DJ. The molecular and genetic basis of fibroblast growth factor receptor 3 disorders: the achondroplasia family of skeletal dysplasias, Muenke craniosynostosis, and Crouzon syndrome with acanthosis nigricans. Endocr Rev. 2000;21(1):23-39.

STATION 7.

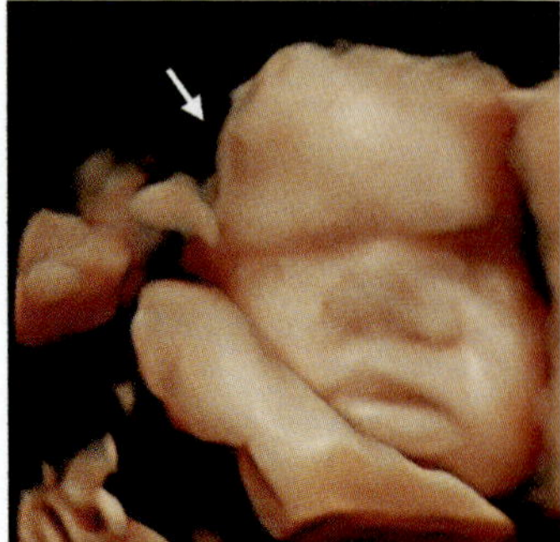
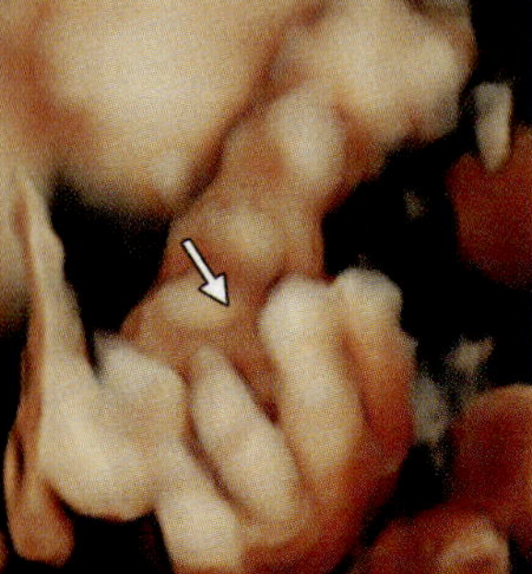
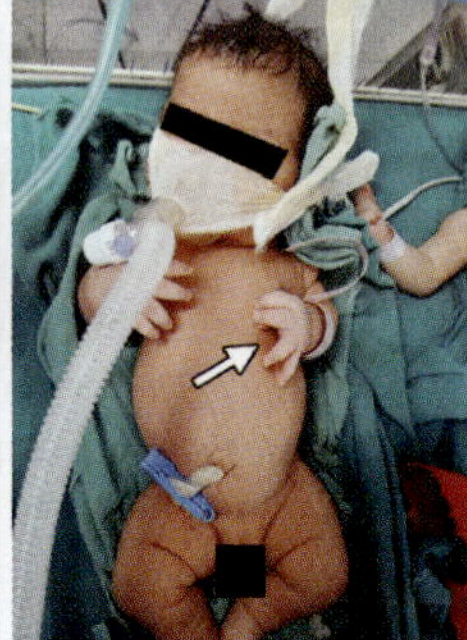

1. **Limb shortening and facial features become apparent after which gestation in achondroplasia?**
2. **What is the typical hand abnormality seen in this condition?**
3. **What is the mode of inheritance?**
4. **What will be the recurrence risk if parents are normal?**

Ans.

1. 20–22 weeks
2. Tri radiant hand
3. Autosomal dominant
4. Almost negligible

SUGGESTED READING

1. Vajo Z, Francomano CA, Wilkin DJ. The molecular and genetic basis of fibroblast growth factor receptor 3 disorders: the achondroplasia family of skeletal dysplasias, Muenke craniosynostosis, and Crouzon syndrome with acanthosis nigricans. Endocr Rev. 2000;21(1):23-39.

STATION 8. **G2P1L0, previous history of oligohydramnios and intrauterine death, presented at 23 weeks with oligohydramnios and bilateral echogenic kidneys. On ultrasound, along with enlarged hyperechogenic kidneys, echogenic liver, skeletal abnormality was also seen. Amniocentesis was done; sample was sent for genetic testing.**

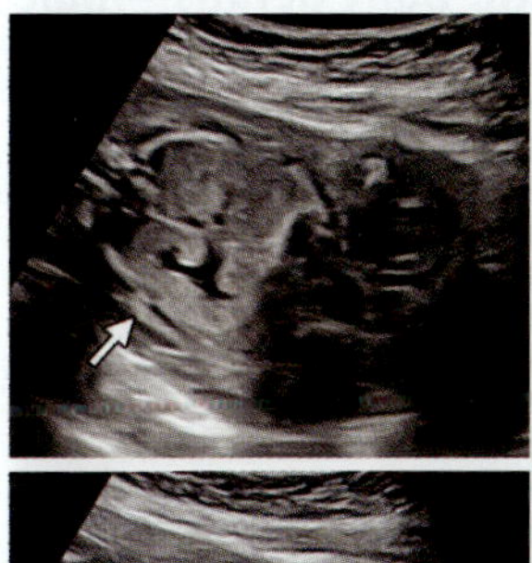

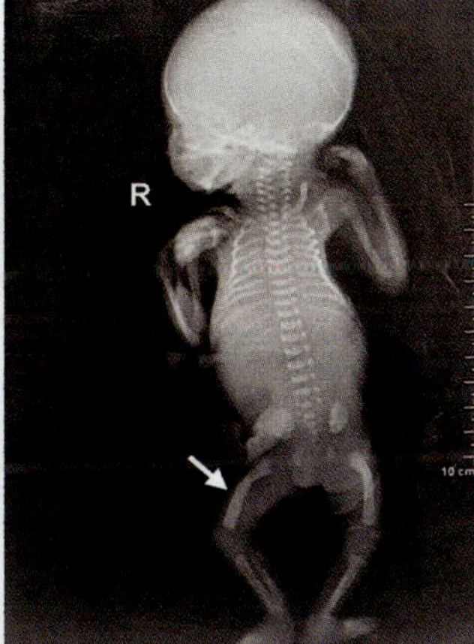

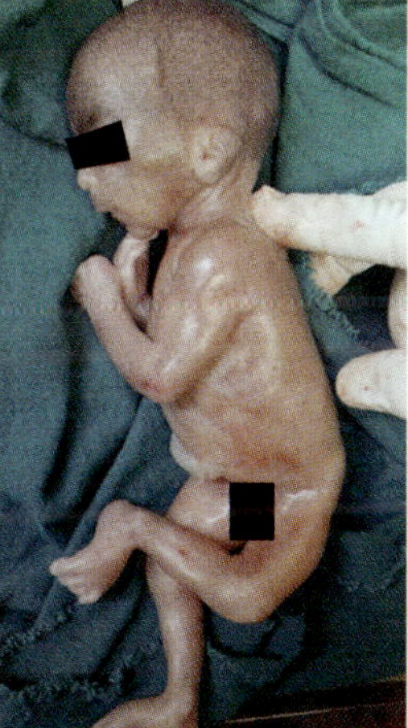

Gene[#] (Transcript)	*Location*	*Variant*	*Zygosity*	*Disease (OMIM)*	*Inheritance*	*Classifications*
NEK8 (+) (ENST00000268766.11)	Intron 8	c.1223-1G>T **(3′ Splice site)**	Compound Heterozygous	Renal-hepatic-pancreatic dysplasia 2 (OMIM#615415)	Autosomal recessive	Likely Pathogenic **(PVS1, PM2)**
	Exon 14	c.2022C>A **(p.Cys674Ter)**				Likely Pathogenic **(PVS1, PM2)**

1. **What is the skeletal abnormality on infantogram?**
2. **Is the defect genetic or sporadic?**
3. **What test will you perform from amniotic fluid?**
4. **When can we diagnose the condition at the earliest in the next pregnancy and by what test?**

Ans.

1. Bowing of femur
2. Genetic
3. Whole exome sequencing
4. 12 weeks by chorionic villous sampling (CVS) and mutation analysis by molecular test

SUGGESTED READING

1. Omim.org. RENAL-HEPATIC-PANCREATIC DYSPLASIA 2; RHPD2. [online] Available from https://omim.org/entry/615415. [Last accessed June, 2025].

STATION 9. A 35-year-old primigravida with diabetes, chronic hypertension with superimposed preeclampsia, with severe fetal growth restriction (FGR), was referred for unilateral short femur. Ultrasound examination showed a markedly asymmetrical shortening of the left femur. Fetus subsequently had intrauterine death. Baby details—male baby 400 g and placenta 180 g.

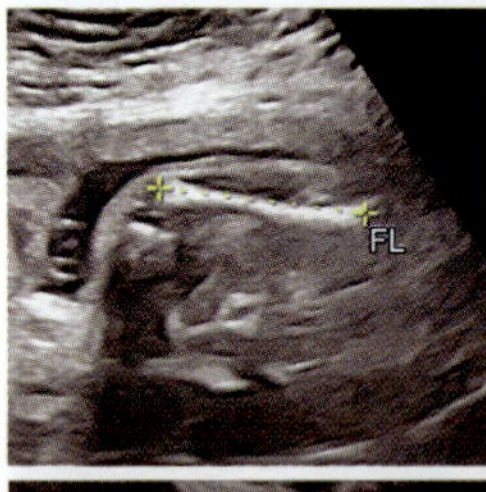

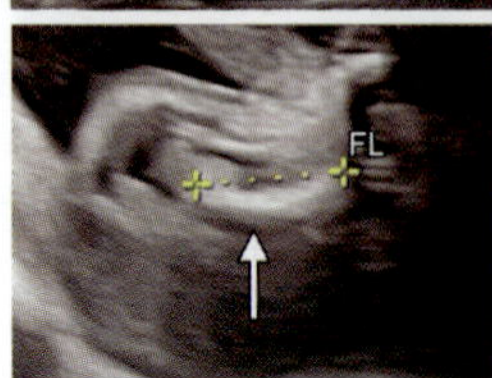

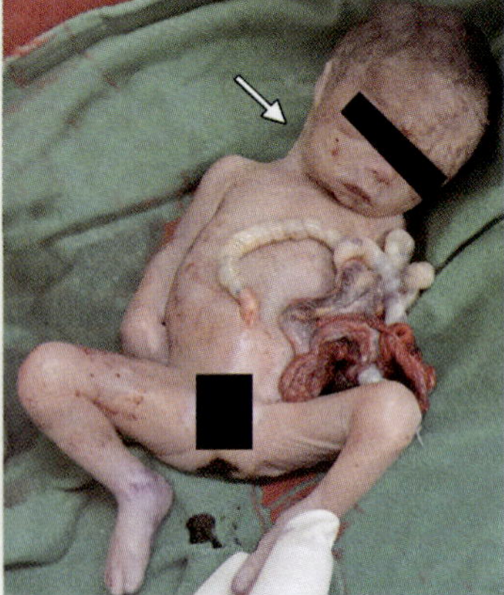

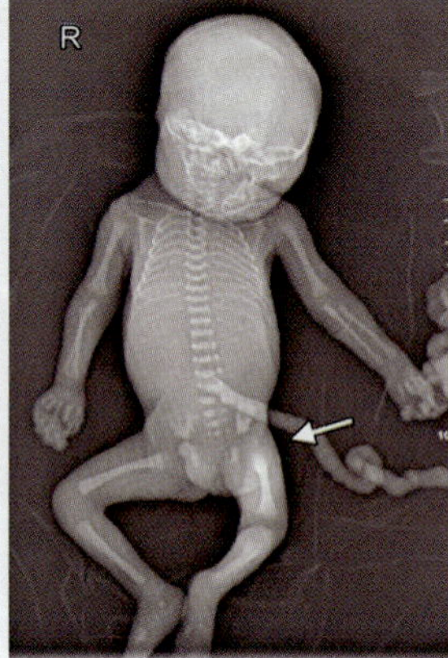

1. **What is the condition?**
2. **What are the typical facial features associated with it?**
3. **Is the condition multifactorial or genetic?**
4. **What maternal medical condition it is associated with?**

Ans.

1. Proximal femoral focal deficiency (PFFD)
2. Micrognathia and long philtrum thin upper lip
3. Multifactorial
4. Diabetes

SUGGESTED READING

1. Mailath-Pokorny M, Timor-Tritsch IE, Monteagudo A, Mittal K, Konno F, Santos R. Prenatal diagnosis of unilateral proximal femoral at 19 weeks' gestation: case report and review of the literature. Ultrasound Obstet Gynecol. 2011;38:594-59.

STATION 10. **Patient was referred at 17 weeks with skeletal abnormality in the upper limb. The lower limb was normal. Amniocentesis was done; sample sent for karyotyping. Medical termination of pregnancy (MTP) was done.**

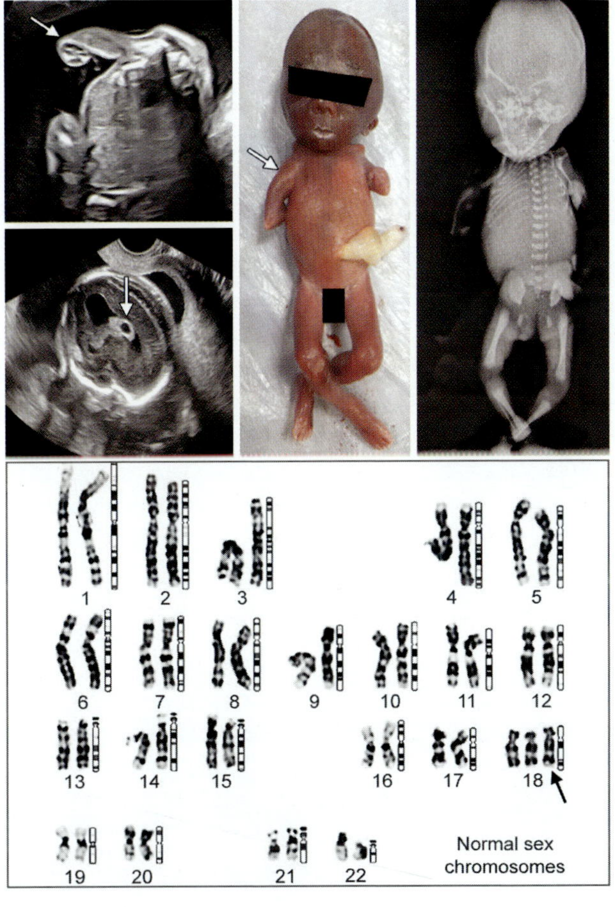

1. **What is the soft marker seen in the above case?**
2. **What is the skeletal defect associated with Down syndrome?**
3. **What is the chromosomal abnormality in this case?**
4. **What is the risk of recurrence in future pregnancy?**

Ans.

1. Choroid plexus cyst
2. Short humerus or femur
3. Trisomy 18
4. Less than 1:100

SUGGESTED READING

1. Baty BJ, Blackburn BL, Carey JC. Natural history of trisomy 18 and trisomy 13: I. Growth, physical assessment, medical histories, survival, and recurrence risk. Am J Med Genet. 1994;49(2):175-88.

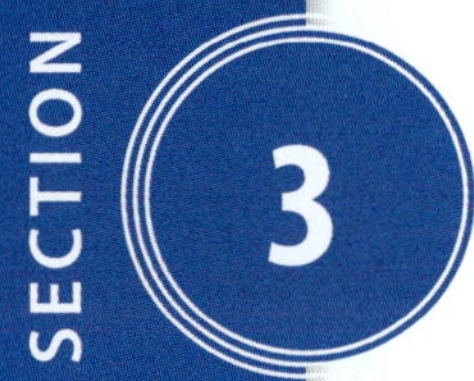

Soft Markers

13. **Soft Markers**
Sangeeta Yadav

CHAPTER 13

Soft Markers

Sangeeta Yadav

STATION 1.

Marker	*Present/Absent (choose from drop-down)*	*LR*
Intracardiac echogenic focus	Absent	0.80
Mild hydronephrosis	Absent	0.92
Short femur	Absent	0.80
Echogenic bowel	Absent	0.90
Increased nuchal fold	Absent	0.80
Aberrant right subclavian artery	Present	21.48
Absent or hypoplastic nasal bone	Normal size	0.46
Ventriculomegaly	Absent	0.94
LR for combination		**3.94**

1. **What are soft markers?**
2. **What is a priori risk?**
3. **What is likelihood ratio (LR)?**
4. **Which soft marker is associated with highest risk of aneuploidy?**
5. **What would be the approach if aberrant right subclavian artery is present as an isolated marker?**

Ans.

1. Soft markers are minor ultrasound (USG) findings identified in the midtrimester of pregnancy that most commonly do not represent a structural abnormality and may be normal variants but are noteworthy because of their association with an increased aneuploidy risk.
2. The baseline risk of aneuploidy for a pregnancy based on maternal age and period of gestation.
3. The LR is a measure of the sensitivity to false-positive rate. Higher the positive LR stronger the association of the soft marker with the aneuploidy.
4. Hypoplastic nasal bone carries the highest risk and increases the risk by six-to-sevenfold.
5. The a priori risk would be multiplied by the LR of the combination to arrive at the final risk.

SUGGESTED READING

1. Agathokleous M, Chaveeva P, Poon LC, Kosinski P, Nicolaides KH. Meta-analysis of second-trimester markers for trisomy 21. Ultrasound Obstet Gynecol. 2013;41(3):247-61.
2. Society for Maternal-Fetal Medicine. SMFM Consult Series #57: Evaluation and management of isolated soft ultrasound markers for aneuploidy in the second trimester. Am J Obstet Gynecol. 2021;225(4):B2-B15.

STATION 2.

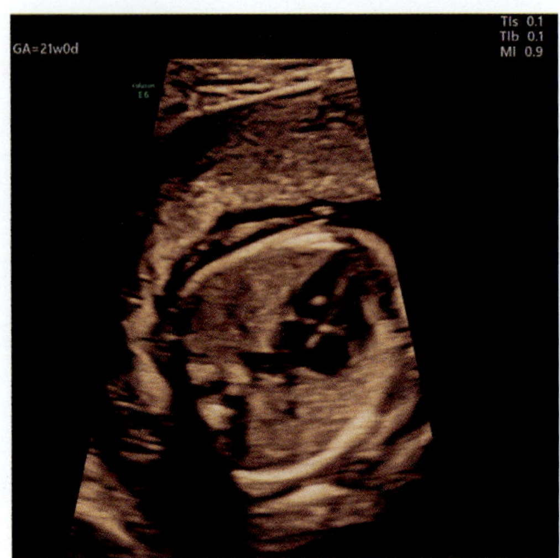

1. **Identify the marker and how is this formed?**
2. **What is the criterion for diagnosis?**
3. **What is the most common association and most common site?**
4. **What can be the adverse effect of echogenic intracardiac focus (EICF)?**
5. **How will you manage this condition?**

Ans.

1. This is EICF caused by microcalcification of the papillary muscles.
2. It should be as bright as the surrounding bone and visualized in at least two separate planes.
3. It is seen in 16% of fetuses with trisomy 21 and 5% of euploid fetuses and is usually located within the left ventricle.
4. EICF does not represent a structural or functional cardiac abnormality and is not associated with cardiac malformations in the fetus or newborn.
5. In isolated EICF with negative aneuploidy screening, no further evaluation is required.

SUGGESTED READING

1. O'Brien B, Choi W. Chromosomal abnormality. In: Rumack CM, Levine D (Eds). Diagnostic Ultrasound, 6th edition. Philadelphia: Elsevier; 2023.

2. Society for Maternal-Fetal Medicine. SMFM Consult Series #57: Evaluation and management of isolated soft ultrasound markers for aneuploidy in the second trimester. Am J Obstet Gynecol. 2021;225(4):B2-B15.

STATION 3.

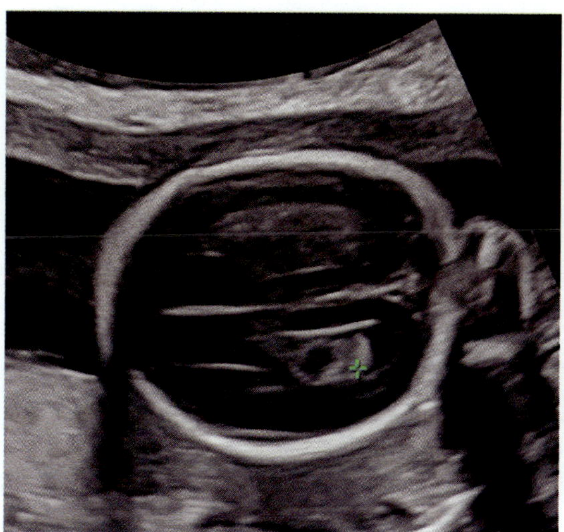

1. **What is the finding in USG image?**
2. **How are the dimensions of this marker measured on USG?**
3. **What is the significance of this condition?**
4. **What details should be specified in a report containing choroid plexus cyst (CPC)?**

Ans.

1. There is echolucent cyst within the echogenic choroid of the lateral ventricles of the fetal brain.
2. Outer-to-outer diameter.
3. A CPC is not considered a structural or functional brain abnormality, and nearly all CPCs resolve by 28 weeks. CPCs are associated with trisomy 18, as they are present in 30–50% of fetuses with this disorder. When a fetus is affected by trisomy 18, multiple structural anomalies are almost always evident. The presence of a CPC does not alter the risk of trisomy 21.
4. The size, number, unilaterality, or bilaterality should be mentioned in the report. If the size is >10 mm, it is associated with a higher risk of aneuploidy even as an isolated marker. The number of cysts and the cysts' distribution do not alter the risk of aneuploidy.

SUGGESTED READING

1. Sharma A, Dadhwal V, Rana A, Chawla J. Isolated large bilateral choroid plexus cysts associated with trisomy 18. BMJ Case Rep. 2019;12(3):e229216.

2. Society for Maternal-Fetal Medicine. SMFM Consult Series #57: Evaluation and management of isolated soft ultrasound markers for aneuploidy in the second trimester. Am J Obstet Gynecol. 2021;225(4):B2-B15.

STATION 4.

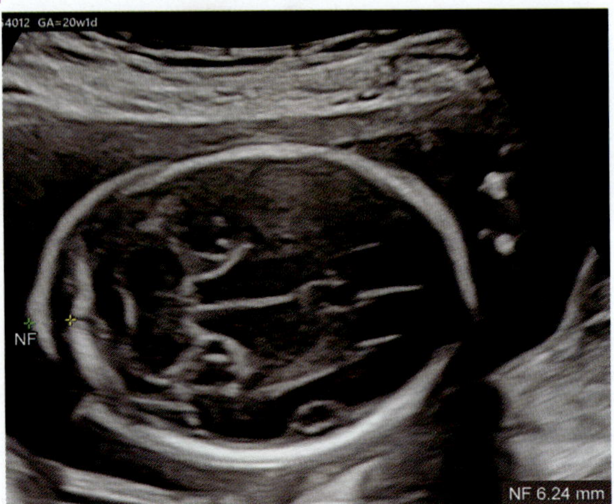

1. **What marker is shown in this image?**
2. **What is the significance?**
3. **What is the LR of this isolated marker?**
4. **What would be the next step if this marker is found on second trimester scan in the absence of a combined first trimester screen?**

Ans.

1. The image shows a thickened nuchal fold which is defined as the distance of >6 mm from the surface of the occipital bone to the surface of the skin edge in the axial view through trans cerebellar plane.
2. It is a soft marker for trisomy 21.
3. In isolation, it has the LR of 3.79.
4. Amniocentesis followed by fluorescence in situ hybridization (FISH) and chromosomal microarray (CMA) if the former is normal. Fetal echocardiography is also indicated.

SUGGESTED READING

1. Agathokleous M, Chaveeva P, Poon LC, Kosinski P, Nicolaides KH. Meta-analysis of second-trimester markers for trisomy 21. Ultrasound Obstet Gynecol. 2013;41(3):247-61.
2. Society for Maternal-Fetal Medicine. SMFM Consult Series #57: Evaluation and management of isolated soft ultrasound markers for aneuploidy in the second trimester. Am J Obstet Gynecol. 2021;225(4):B2-B15.

STATION 5.

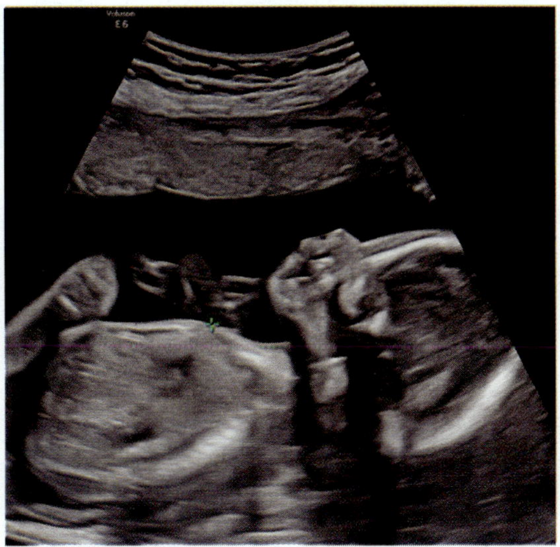

1. **What is the finding in this ultrasound image?**
2. **How should you proceed if this marker is found at 12 weeks?**
3. **What is the risk?**
4. **In addition to aneuploidies, what other genetic abnormalities are associated with this marker and how should they be ruled out?**

Ans.

1. This is midsagittal plane of the fetal face showing absent nasal bone.
2. The scan should be repeated at 16–17 weeks to look for ossification of the nasal bone.
3. Likelihood ratio of isolated absent or hypoplastic nasal bone for trisomy 21 is high (6.58).
4. If associated abnormalities seen, genetic conditions like Cri-du-chat, Pallister-Killian syndrome and rare pathogenic CNVs need to be ruled out. Amniocentesis followed by FISH followed by CMA/whole exome sequencing (WES).

SUGGESTED READING

1. Agathokleous M, Chaveeva P, Poon LC, Kosinski P, Nicolaides KH. Meta-analysis of second-trimester markers for trisomy 21. Ultrasound Obstet Gynecol. 2013;41(3):247-61.
2. Society for Maternal-Fetal Medicine. SMFM Consult Series #57: Evaluation and management of isolated soft ultrasound markers for aneuploidy in the second trimester. Am J Obstet Gynecol. 2021;225(4):B2-B15.

STATION 6.

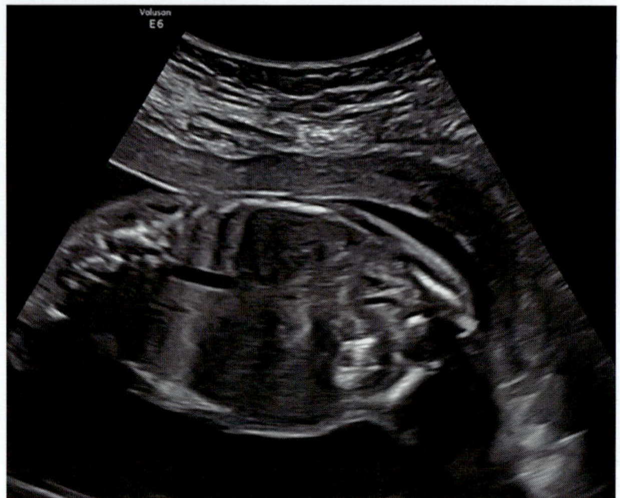

1. **What is this condition?**
2. **What precautions should be taken while reporting this marker?**
3. **What are the possible causes?**
4. **What test to be ordered when doing amniocentesis?**

Ans.

1. This is echogenic bowel
2. It should not be reported in the first trimester. In the second trimester, the gain should be reduced and it should only be reported if the echogenicity of the bowel is equivalent to the surrounding bone.
3. Possible causes are aneuploidy (LR 1.65), cystic fibrosis, congenital viral infection, primary gastrointestinal pathology, intra-amniotic bleeding, and fetal growth restriction.
4. Consider amniocentesis for karyotype, microarray, viral polymerase chain reaction (PCR), and mutation analysis for cystic fibrosis.

SUGGESTED READING

1. ISUOG. (2018). Echogenic bowel of the fetus, Visual encyclopedia of Ultrasound in Obstetrics and Gynecology. [online] Available from https://icc.gig.cymru/gwasanaethau-a-thimau/sgrinio/sgrinio-cyn-geni-cymru/gwybodaeth-i-weithwyr-proffesiynol1/dogfennau-uwchsain/v4-ultrasound-observations-pathways-jan-2022/ [Last accessed May, 2025].
2. Society for Maternal-Fetal Medicine. SMFM Consult Series #57: Evaluation and management of isolated soft ultrasound markers for aneuploidy in the second trimester. Am J Obstet Gynecol. 2021;225(4):B2-B15.

STATION 7.

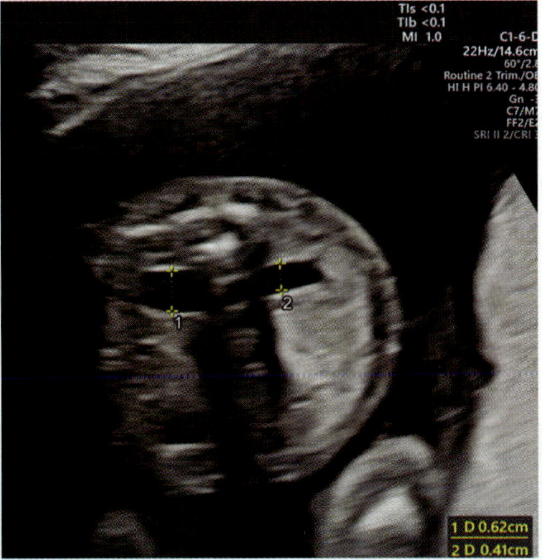

A 22-year-old G2P1L1 woman presents with the above marker on a 20-week anomaly scan.

1. **What is this condition?**
2. **How should the marker shown above be measured?**
3. **What are the pathological causes of fetal pyelectasis?**
4. **What are the other ultrasound features to be looked for if this marker is found?**
5. **What is the follow-up strategy?**

Ans.

1. This is bilateral fetal pyelectasis.
2. The maximum anteroposterior renal pelvis diameter in the transverse plane ideally with the fetal spine at 12 or 6 o'clock should be measured. Mild fetal pyelectasis (>4 mm in second trimester and >7 mm in third trimester) has been reported as a soft marker for trisomy 21.
3. The pathologic causes include vesicoureteral reflux (the most common etiology), ureteropelvic junction obstruction, ureterovesical junction obstruction, multicystic dysplastic kidneys, and posterior urethral valves.
4. Pelvi-calyceal system should be evaluated for the presence of central or peripheral calyceal dilatation, parenchymal appearance and thickness, status of ureter, bladder, and liquor should be evaluated.
5. Follow-up scans at 28 and 32 weeks depending upon severity of pyelectasis with planned postnatal follow-up.

SUGGESTED READING

1. Kolitsidakis A. (2020). Fetal hydronephrosis, Visual Encyclopedia of Ultrasound in Obstetrics and Gynecology. [online] Available from https://gynaecologia.com/2020/04/01/fetal-hydronephrosis/ [Last accessed May, 2025].
2. Nguyen HT, Benson CB, Bromley B, Campbell JB, Chow J, Coleman B, et al. Multidisciplinary consensus on the classification of prenatal and postnatal urinary tract dilation (UTD classification system). J Pediatr Urol. 2014;10(6):982-98.
3. Society for Maternal-Fetal Medicine. SMFM Consult Series #57: Evaluation and management of isolated soft ultrasound markers for aneuploidy in the second trimester. Am J Obstet Gynecol. 2021;225(4):B2-B15.

STATION 8.

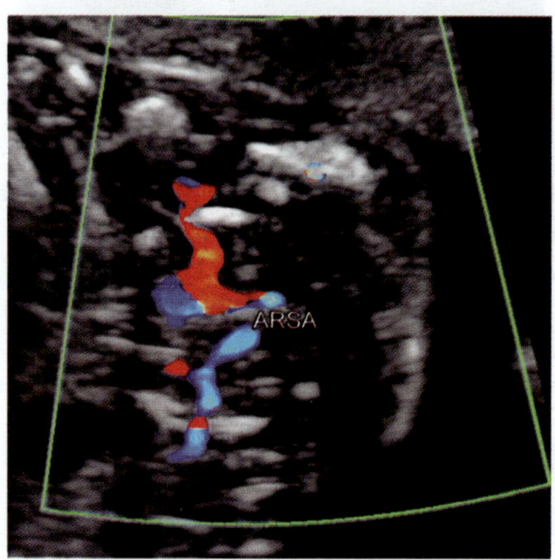

1. **What does the USG image depict?**
2. **What is the risk of aneuploidy?**
3. **What should be the next step if it is an isolated marker in the presence of low-risk noninvasive prenatal screening (NIPS)?**

Ans.

1. The USG image depicts the aberrant origin of the right subclavian artery (ARSA). This artery usually arises above the level of the aortic arch, as the first branch from the innominate (or brachiocephalic) artery. The aberrant vessel arises from the first portion of the descending aorta and passes behind the trachea and cranially as well as rightward.
2. There is risk of trisomy 21 (LR of isolated marker is 3.94).
3. There is insufficient evidence to recommend invasive testing in this case scenario.

SUGGESTED READING

1. Agathokleous M, Chaveeva P, Poon LC, Kosinski P, Nicolaides KH. Meta-analysis of second-trimester markers for trisomy 21. Ultrasound Obstet Gynecol. 2013;41(3):247-61.
2. Borenstein M, Minekawa R, Zidere V, Nicolaides KH, Allan LD. Aberrant right subclavian artery at 16 to 23 + 6 weeks of gestation: a marker for chromosomal abnormality. Ultrasound Obstet Gynecol. 2010;36(5):548-52.
3. Society for Maternal-Fetal Medicine. SMFM Consult Series #57: Evaluation and management of isolated soft ultrasound markers for aneuploidy in the second trimester. Am J Obstet Gynecol. 2021;225(4):B2-B15.

STATION 9.

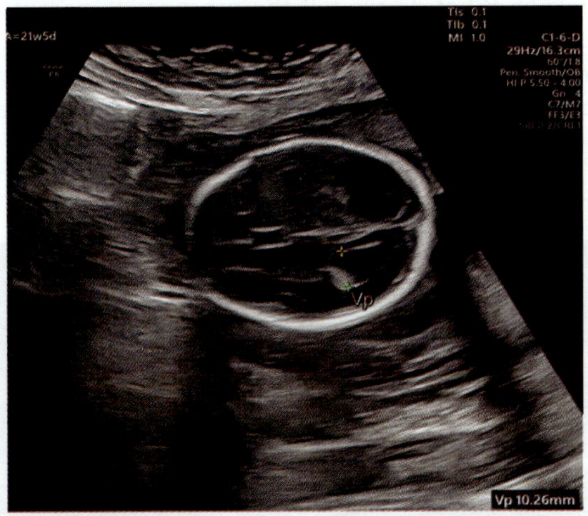

1. **What is the condition?**
2. **How do you measure this marker on a genetic sonogram?**
3. **What is the classification of severity?**
4. **What is the approach to a case with this marker?**
5. **How should the parents be counseled regarding neurodevelopmental outcome in this case?**

Ans.

1. It is mild ventriculomegaly (measurement of the atrial width of cerebral lateral ventricles of >10 mm).
2. The transventricular axial plane of fetal skull is focused and measurement of the lateral ventricle taken inner to inner at the level of the parieto-occipital sulcus.
3. Mild ≥10 mm and severe is ≥15 mm.
4. Mild ventriculomegaly is a soft marker for trisomy 21. Isolated mild ventriculomegaly has LR of 3.81 for trisomy 21.

Neurosonography ± MRI to look for associated central nervous system (CNS) and extracranial malformations and intracerebral hemorrhage, detailed anatomical survey, karyotype and CMA/WES, and maternal infection screen.

5. With mild ventriculomegaly, normal neurodevelopmental outcome can be expected in nearly 90% cases. With severe ventriculomegaly, survival is 88% albeit with neurologic, motor, and cognitive impairment in around 60% of these children.

SUGGESTED READING

1. Giorgione V, Haratz KK, Constantini S, Birnbaum R, Malinger G. Fetal cerebral ventriculomegaly: What do we tell the prospective parents? Prenat Diagn. 2022;42(13):1674-81.
2. ISUOG. Sonographic examination of the fetal central nervous system: guidelines for performing the 'basic examination' and the 'fetal neurosonogram'. Ultrasound Obstet Gynecol 2007;29:109-16.

STATION 10.

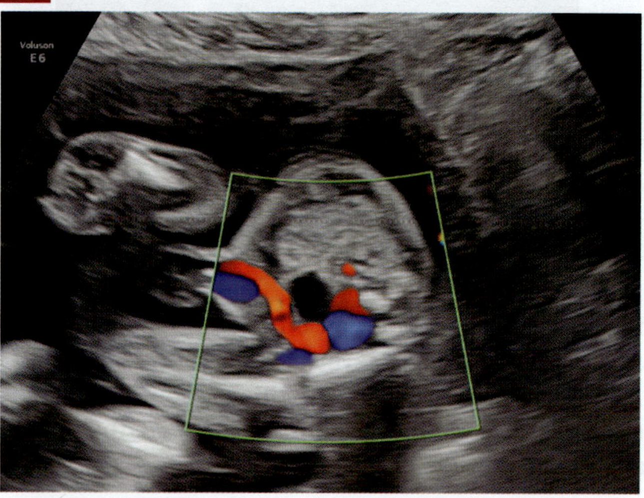

1. **What is this condition?**
2. **Which structural anomaly is most common with this condition?**
3. **What is the risk if it is isolated?**
4. **What is the follow-up in case of isolated marker?**

Ans.

1. Single umbilical artery (SUA)
2. It is isolated in most cases, however, a detailed anatomical survey to look for abnormalities in the cardiovascular, gastrointestinal tract (GIT), genitourinary, and skeletal systems should be offered.

3. Isolated SUA is not associated with aneuploidy; however, there is increased risk of fetal growth restriction (10%) and perinatal morbidity and mortality.
4. Serial growth scans to identify fetal growth restriction.

SUGGESTED READING

1. Society for Maternal-Fetal Medicine. SMFM Consult Series #57: Evaluation and management of isolated soft ultrasound markers for aneuploidy in the second trimester. Am J Obstet Gynecol. 2021;225(4):B2-B15.

STATION 11.

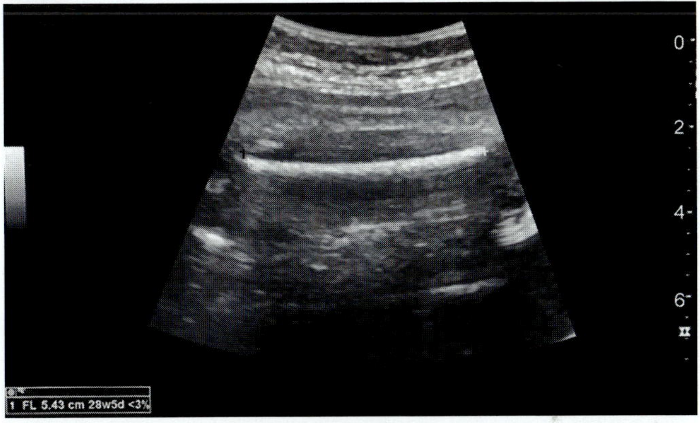

Courtesy: Dr Jaya Chawla.

1. **Identify the marker in the above image.**
2. **What are the criteria for the above marker to be clinically significant?**
3. **When the ratio of femur length to foot is <0.9 SD, one should evaluate for skeletal dysplasia. What are the common causes for this presentation?**
4. **What should be the follow-up?**
5. **How should parents be counseled in the presence of an isolated marker?**

Ans.

1. Short femur/short long bones
2. Ideally, –2/–3 standard deviations for the specified gestational age. Less than the third centile should be evaluated further.
3. Foot length
4. Aneuploidies, genetic syndromes, skeletal dysplasia in addition to maternal diabetes, are known associations. Therefore, when associated with major malformations or other soft markers, one should offer prenatal testing for FISH and microarray. Also, serial monitoring of

growth and appendicular long bones for evolving skeletal dysplasia in third trimester.

5. Prenatal fetal isolated short femur picked up during the late second and third trimester is associated with short stature. No neurodevelopmental impact has been observed.

SUGGESTED READING

1. Mohr-Sasson A, Toussia-Cohen S, Shapira M, Perlman S, Achiron R, Gilboa Y. Long-term follow-up on fetuses with isolated sonographic finding of short long bones: a cohort study. Arch Gynecol Obstet. 2020;301(2):459-63.

SECTION 4

Mixed Bag

14. **Fetal Infections**
Vandana Bansal, Nishigandha Mali

15. **Fetal Growth Restriction**
Madhusudan Dey, Seetha Ramamurthy Pal

16. **Red Cell Isoimmunization**
Mandakini Pradhan

17. **Hematological Disorders**
Saswati Mukhopadhyay

18. **Nonimmune Hydrops Fetalis**
Jaya Chawla, K Aparna Sharma

CHAPTER 14

Fetal Infections

Vandana Bansal, Nishigandha Mali

STATION 1.

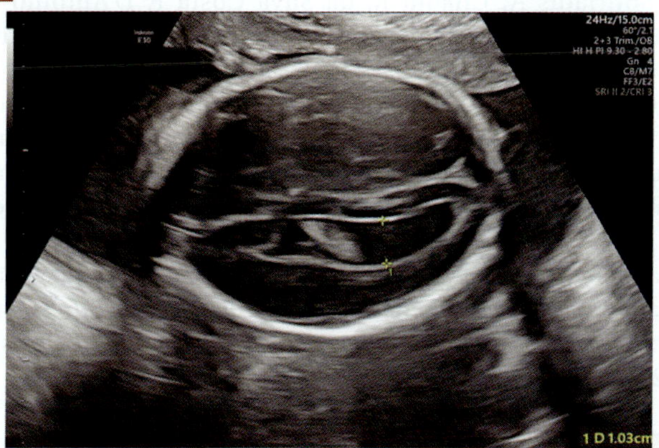

1. **Identify the above ultrasound findings. Write three possible etiologies for the same.**
2. **Name two causes of congenital infections which may cause this finding antenatally.**
3. **Enumerate at least four intracranial ultrasound findings of fetal intrauterine infection.**
4. **Enumerate at least four extracranial ultrasound findings of fetal intrauterine infection.**

Ans.

1. Mild ventriculomegaly. It may be isolated or associated with other anomalies.

   Possible etiology can be:
   a. Genetic or chromosomal (10–15%)
   b. Congenital infections [TORCH (toxoplasmosis, other infections, rubella, cytomegalovirus, herpes simplex) group] (8%)
   c. Structural brain anomalies (11%), e.g., neural tube defects
   d. Intracranial hemorrhage (2–4%)
   e. Normal variant
2. Cytomegalovirus and toxoplasmosis

3. Periventricular cysts, intracranial calcifications, lissencephaly, intraventricular adhesions, subependymal cysts, intracranial hemorrhage, corpus callosal agenesis, and mega cisterna magna.
4. Splenomegaly, hepatomegaly, cardiomegaly, pericardial effusion, echogenic bowel, placentomegaly, placental calcifications, oligohydramnios or polyhydramnios, fetal growth restriction (FGR), and ascites.

SUGGESTED READING

1. Khalil A, Sotiriadis A, Chaoui R, da Silva Costa F, D'Antonio F, Heath PT, et al. ISUOG Practice Guidelines: role of ultrasound in congenital infection. Ultrasound Obstet Gynecol. 2020;56(1):128-51.
2. Malinger G, Paladini D, Haratz KK, Monteagudo A, Pilu G, Timor-Tritsch IE. ISUOG Practice Guidelines (updated): sonographic examination of the fetal central nervous system. Part 1: performance of screening examination and indications for targeted neurosonography. Ultrasound Obstet Gynecol. 2020;56: 476-84.
3. Scala C, Familiari A, Pinas A, Papageorghiou AT, Bhide A, Thilaganathan B, et al. Perinatal and long-term outcomes in fetuses diagnosed with isolated unilateral ventriculomegaly: systematic review and meta-analysis. Ultrasound Obstet Gynecol. 2017;49(4):450-9.

STATION 2.

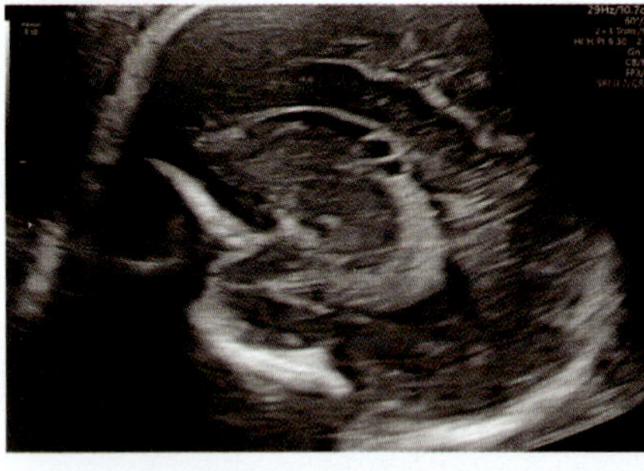

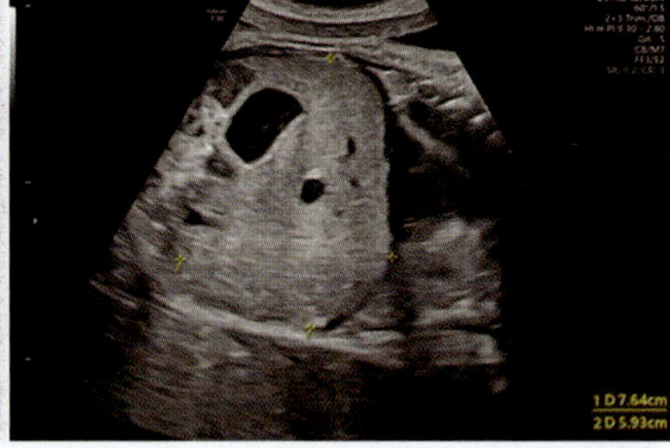

1. **Identify the above ultrasound findings of possible infectious etiology in the fetus.**
2. **What are the indications for maternal testing for TORCH infection in pregnancy? Write any three.**
3. **What are the ultrasound signs of suspected *Cytomegalovirus* (CMV) infections? Write two cranial, two extracranial, and two placental features.**
4. **How is maternal CMV infection confirmed?**

Ans.

1. Intraventricular synechia and hepatomegaly
2. Indications for maternal testing for TORCH infection in pregnancy include:
   a. Exposure to an infectious pathogen/travel to countries with Zika virus
   b. Sonographic markers of fetal infection with/without FGR such as ventriculomegaly, microcephaly, calcifications, intraventricular synechiae, intracranial hemorrhage, periventricular cysts, cerebellar hypoplasia, cortical abnormalities, hyperechogenic bowel, FGR, pericardial effusion, ascites, or fetal hydrops.
   c. Symptomatic maternal infections (nonvesicular rash, slapped cheek facial rash, and flu-like symptoms)
   d. Sudden intrauterine fetal death
   e. Human immunodeficiency virus (HIV)
3. Ultrasound findings can be categorized as fetal cranial, fetal extracranial, and placental/amniotic fluid abnormality.
   a. Ultrasonographic and MRI cranial features typical of CMV infection include mega cisterna magna, intracranial calcifications, ventriculomegaly, germinolytic cysts, agenesis of corpus callosum, intraventricular adhesions, periventricular cystic changes, lissencephaly, cerebral calcifications, and periventricular cysts and subependymal cysts.
   b. Ultrasonographic extracranial features typical of CMV infection include splenomegaly, cardiomegaly and pericardial effusion, and echogenic bowel and hepatomegaly.
   c. Ultrasonographic placental/amniotic fluid abnormalities typical of CMV infection include placentomegaly, placental calcifications, oligohydramnios, and/or polyhydramnios.
4. The diagnosis of primary CMV infection in pregnancy can be made following either: (i) Maternal appearance of CMV-specific immunoglobulin G (IgG) in a woman who was previously seronegative; or (ii) Maternal detection of CMV immunoglobulin M (IgM) antibody and low IgG avidity

SUGGESTED READING

1. Khalil A, Sotiriadis A, Chaoui R, da Silva Costa F, D'Antonio F, Heath PT, et al. ISUOG Practice Guidelines: role of ultrasound in congenital infection. Ultrasound Obstet Gynecol. 2020;56(1):128-51.

STATION 3.

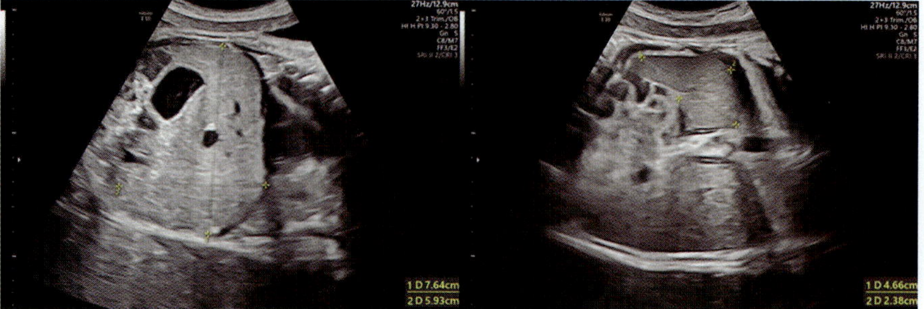

1. **How is fetal infection confirmed in a case of suspected CMV infection?**
2. **What is the ideal time for performing the confirmatory test for fetal affliction?**
3. **Name some neonatal features of congenital CMV infection. Name one late presenting complication of congenital CMV infection.**
4. **How is neonatal CMV infection confirmed? What is the best timing for the same?**

Ans.

1. Amniotic fluid polymerase chain reaction (PCR) for CMV DNA.
2. Amniocentesis should be performed at least 8 weeks after maternal infection and after 20 weeks of gestation to allow transplacental migration of the virus and subsequent shedding in the urine.
3. Small for gestational age, microcephaly, petechial rash, jaundice, hepatosplenomegaly, blueberry muffin rash, indicating extramedullary hematopoiesis; neurodevelopmental sequelae, sensorineural hearing loss. Sensorineural hearing loss can present late in neonates affected with congenital CMV.
4. Neonatal urine or saliva should be test for CMV-PCR as early as possible within 3 weeks of birth.

SUGGESTED READING

1. Khalil A, Sotiriadis A, Chaoui R, da Silva Costa F, D'Antonio F, Heath PT, et al. ISUOG Practice Guidelines: role of ultrasound in congenital infection. Ultrasound Obstet Gynecol. 2020;56(1):128-511.

STATION 4.

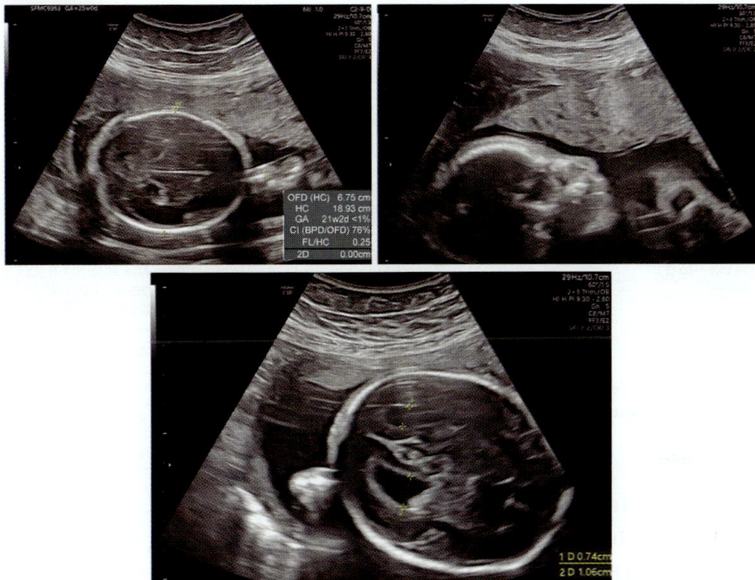

1. **Identify the above ultrasound findings.**
2. **Name two congenital infections which may cause the above ultrasound findings.**
3. **What is the causative organism of toxoplasmosis? How is toxoplasmosis transmitted?**
4. **What precautions must pregnant women take to avoid *Toxoplasma* infection?**

Ans.

1. Microcephaly and ventriculomegaly
2. Toxoplasmosis, CMV, and Zika virus (microcephaly)
3. *Toxoplasma gondii,* a parasite is the causative organism for toxoplasmosis. It is transmitted by the ingestion of infected tissues cysts found in undercooked meat or excreted by cats.
4. The precautions include:
    - Avoid uncooked/undercooked and processed meats in pregnancy!
    - Avoid contact with cats as they may be a reference of *Toxoplasma* cysts!
    - Uncooked salads/vegetables should be thoroughly washed before consumption as they may be contaminated by soil and water.

SUGGESTED READING

1. Khalil A, Sotiriadis A, Chaoui R, da Silva Costa F, D'Antonio F, Heath PT, et al. ISUOG Practice Guidelines: role of ultrasound in congenital infection. Ultrasound Obstet Gynecol. 2020;56(1):128-51.

STATION 5.

Summary report

Investigation outside reference range (Abnormal)			
Investigation	**Observed Value**	**Unit**	**Biological Reference Interval**
***Toxoplasma*—IgG** (Serum, CMIA)	**Reactive (>200.0)**	IU/mL	Non reactive: <1.6 Grayzone: 1.6–3.0 Reactive: >= 3.0
***Toxoplasma*—IgM** (Serum, CMIA)	**Reactive (1.71)**	S/CO	Non reactive: <0.50 Grayzone: 0.50–0.60 Reactive: >= 0.60
Medical Remarks: Rechecked by ELFA method			
***Toxoplasma* Avidity Test** (Serum, EIA)	**High Avidity (71.97)**	%	High avidity: Above 35% Grayzone avidity: 30–35% Low avidity: Below 30%

1. **How do you interpret the above report?**
2. **What would be further management in the following cases?**
   a. **IgM positive/equivocal and IgG negative**
   b. **IgM equivocal and IgG positive**
3. **What is the risk of congenital affliction following maternal infection without treatment?**
4. **What confirmatory test would you advise to detect fetal infection and when would you perform it?**

Ans.

1. Old *Toxoplasma* infection
2. Repeat testing after 2 weeks and do avidity testing!
3. The overall risk of congenital toxoplasmosis following maternal infection ranges from 20 to 50% without treatment. As with most viral infections in pregnancy, the risk of fetal infection increases with gestational age at maternal infection (being <1% before 4 weeks, 4–15% at 13 weeks, and >60% at 36 weeks). However, the earlier the gestational age at infection, the greater the risk that the fetus will be affected. Even though most infected infants do not have clinical signs of infection at birth, up to 90% will develop sequelae later in life.
4. Amniocentesis with amniotic fluid PCR for *Toxoplasma* DNA. It should be performed 4 weeks after maternal infection and after 18 weeks of gestation.

Interpretation of serological test results for *Toxoplasma* infection performed at clinical (nonreference) laboratories.

IgM test result	*IgG test result*	*Clinical relevance*
Negative	Negative	No evidence of maternal infection during pregnancy
Negative	Positive	During first or second trimester, likely indicated prepregnancy infection. If in third trimester, this result is more difficult to interpret. Although it is most consistent with an infection acquired prepregnancy, in some patients, this result may reflect an infection that was acquired early in gestation and that was accompanied by an increase in IgM titer and a decrease to nondetectable levels within a relatively short period of time
Positive or equivocal	Negative	Positive (or equivocal) IgM test result should be followed by confirmatory testing at *Toxoplasma* reference laboratory. IgM antibodies are detected early in acute infection and may persist for years
Positive or equivocal	Positive	Positive (or equivocal) IgM test result should be followed by confirmatory testing at *Toxoplasma* reference laboratory. IgM antibodies are detected early in acute infection and may persist for years

SUGGESTED READING

1. Khalil A, Sotiriadis A, Chaoui R, da Silva Costa F, D'Antonio F, Heath PT, et al. ISUOG Practice Guidelines: role of ultrasound in congenital infection. Ultrasound Obstet Gynecol. 2020;56(1):128-51.

STATION 6.

Summary report

Investigation outside reference range (Abnormal)			
Investigation	**Observed Value**	**Unit**	**Biological Reference Interval**
***Toxoplasma*—IgG** (Serum, CMIA)	**Reactive (>200.0)**	IU/mL	Non reactive: <1.6 Grayzone: 1.6–3.0 Reactive: >= 3.0
***Toxoplasma*—IgM** (Serum, CMIA)	**Reactive (1.71)**	S/CO	Non reactive: <0.50 Grayzone: 0.50–0.60 Reactive: >= 0.60
Medical remarks: Rechecked by ELFA method			
***Toxoplasma* Avidity Test** (Serum, EIA)	**High Avidity (71.97)**	%	High avidity: Above 35% Grayzone avidity: 30–35% Low avidity: Below 30%

1. **What treatment would you commence for the above patient? What can be the effect of this drug on the blood test?**
2. **What is the treatment regimen for the patient if amniotic fluid PCR is positive for *Toxoplasma* DNA?**
3. **How is the pregnancy followed up?**
4. **What are the neonatal sequelae of congenital toxoplasmosis?**

Ans.

1. The patient should be initiated on spiramycin 1 g thrice a day within 3 weeks of detecting maternal infection. It should be continued till amniotic fluid PCR reports are available. If amniotic fluid PCR is negative for *Toxoplasma* DNA, spiramycin should be continued till delivery. Spiramycin can delay the maturation of IgG antibodies and show prolonged low avidity.
2. Continue spiramycin for 1 week followed by pyrimethamine 50 mg orally once a day, sulfadiazine 1 g orally thrice a day and folinic acid 50 mg weekly till delivery, after testing for glucose-6-phosphate dehydrogenase (G6PD) deficiency. The infant treated for 1 further year.
3. Ultrasound examination every 4 weeks to assess brain, ocular features, and fetal growth.
4. *Central nervous system (CNS):* Microcephaly, hydrocephalus, ventriculomegaly, developmental delay, and epilepsy
   Other systems: Chorioretinitis with possibility of vision loss, pneumonitis, jaundice, hepatosplenomegaly, and rash.

SUGGESTED READING

1. Khalil A, Sotiriadis A, Chaoui R, da Silva Costa F, D'Antonio F, Heath PT, et al. ISUOG Practice Guidelines: role of ultrasound in congenital infection. Ultrasound Obstet Gynecol. 2020;56(1):128-51.

STATION 7.

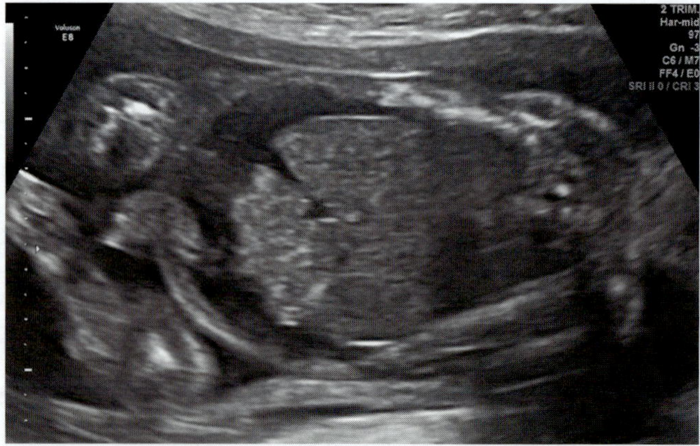

Questions below pertain to a specific viral infection in pregnancy that gives rise to the above image.

1. **Which intrauterine viral infection is most likely to result in this condition?**
2. **Identify the above condition and define it.**
3. **Enumerate the causes of the above condition.**

4. If the above condition was caused by an intrauterine viral infection, what is another name for this viral infection? What is the term for the characteristic rash due to this infection?

5. How does this virus cause the above condition?

Ans.

1. Parvovirus
2. The above image shows hydrops fetalis. It is defined as fluid collection in two or more body compartments which could be subcutaneous edema, pleural effusion, pericardial effusion, or ascites. Polyhydramnios and placentomegaly usually coexist.
3. Following can be the etiology of fetal hydrops:
   - *Immune hydrops:* As a result of Rh incompatibility in an isoimmunized mother, rarely with other blood group incompatibility, e.g., Kell blood group. Immune hydrops fetalis caused by presence of maternal circulating antibodies against red blood cells and is responsible for 10% of cases of hydrops.
   - *Nonimmune hydrops:* Nonimmune hydrops fetalis (NIHF) is caused by etiologies other than immune with absence of hemolytic antibodies and is responsible for 76–87% of cases.
     - Chromosomal or genetic disorders
     - Infections like parvovirus B19
     - Complications of monochorionic twins such as twin-to-twin transfusion syndrome (TTTS) or twin anemia polycythemia sequence (TAPS).
     - Due to cardiac overload in hyperdynamic circulation, e.g., sacrococcygeal teratoma and placental chorioangioma
     - As a result of space-occupying lesions in the fetal thorax, e.g., congenital pulmonary airway malformation (CPAM) and cardiac teratoma
4. Human parvovirus B19 infection is also known as "fifth disease". Clinical features include fever with characteristic rash known as "slapped-cheek appearance".

   Parvovirus B19 is a single-stranded DNA, nonenveloped virus from the family Parvoviridae and the only member of the family that can cause human disease. Also known as fifth disease, it is such a common childhood viral infection that approximately 60–75% of pregnant women are immune. Infected children exhibit a characteristic facial rash and fever, which is known as slapped-cheek syndrome.
5. Parvovirus B19 is vertically transmitted to the fetus from infected mother and targets fetal erythroid precursor cells, myocardium, and first trimester placenta.

It causes transient bone marrow suppression. It then inhibits red cell production leading to aplastic crisis, fetal anemia which eventually causes hydrops fetalis if not corrected.

SUGGESTED READING

1. Bellini C, Hennekam RC, Fulcheri E, Rutigliani M, Morcaldi G, Boccardo F, et al. Etiology of nonimmune hydrops fetalis: a systematic review. Am J Med Genet A. 2009;149A(5):844-51.
2. Khalil A, Sotiriadis A, Chaoui R, da Silva Costa F, D'Antonio F, Heath PT, et al. ISUOG Practice Guidelines: role of ultrasound in congenital infection. Ultrasound Obstet Gynecol. 2020;56(1):128-51.

STATION 8.

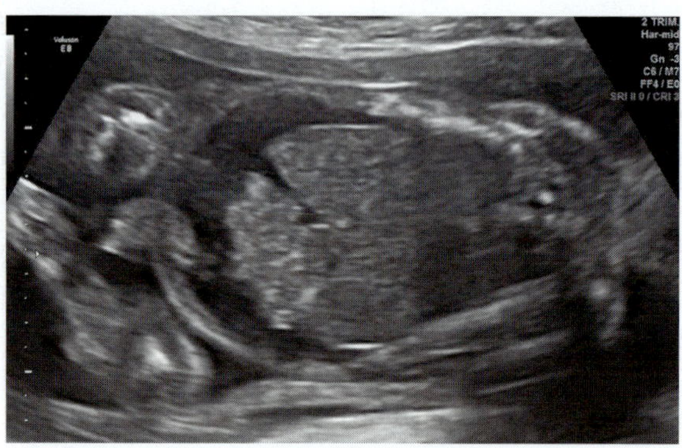

1. **What are the ultrasound features of fetal affliction with this virus?**
2. **How is the pregnancy monitored in a suspected/confirmed case of maternal infection?**
3. **When is fetal intrauterine transfusion indicated in this infection?**
4. **What is the risk of vertical transmission following maternal infection?**
5. **Why does this infection have serious implications for the fetus but not adults?**

Ans.

1. Ultrasound abnormalities in fetuses infected by parvovirus B19

	Abnormality
Cardiac system	• Increased cardiac biventricular outer diameter • Myocarditis
Nonimmune hydrops fetalis	• Pleural effusion • Pericardial effusion • Ascites • Abdominal wall edema • Bilateral hydroceles • Amniotic fluid disorder

Contd...

Contd...

	Abnormality
Brain abnormalities following brain hemorrhage	• Hydrocephalus • Microcephaly • Intracranial calcification
Gastrointestinal system	• Fetal liver calcification • Meconium peritonitis
Other findings	• Sporadic cases of contracture • Increased nuchal translucency thickness • Intrauterine growth restriction

2. Serial ultrasound monitoring should be started 4 weeks after maternal infection or seroconversion and repeated every 1–2 weeks till 12 weeks after infection. Ultrasound parameters evaluated are evidence of ascites, cardiomegaly, hydrops, and raised middle cerebral artery-peak systolic velocity (MCA-PSV) suggestive of fetal anemia. Fetal blood sampling, with preparation for intrauterine blood transfusion, is indicated when MCA-PSV >1.5 MoM, or when there is fetal ascites or hydrops.
3. Fetal intrauterine blood transfusion is indicated when MCA-PSV is >1.5 multiples or median or when there is evidence of fetal hydrops.
4. When a mother contracts infection, the risk of vertical transmission to the fetus ranges from 25 to 32%.
5. The main receptor for parvovirus B19 is globoside, a blood group P antigen, which is found primarily in erythroid precursors, but also in myocardium and the first trimester placenta. Parvovirus B19 causes fetal anemia by inhibiting erythropoiesis, thus leading to aplastic crisis. In healthy adults, this crisis is well-tolerated, with minimal anemia. However, the fetus has a greater relative demand for red blood cells and a larger red cell mass, with associated rapid cell turnover. This renders the fetus particularly vulnerable to any insult to erythropoiesis, and profound anemia may result from infection with parvovirus B19. In the fetus, the virus affects mainly the bone marrow, but it can also affect areas of extramedullary hematopoiesis, such as the liver or spleen. The fetal anemia, as well as the associated hepatitis, hypoalbuminemia and myocarditis, can lead to cardiac failure and subsequent hydrops fetalis.

SUGGESTED READING

1. Bellini C, Hennekam RC, Fulcheri E, Rutigliani M, Morcaldi G, Boccardo F, et al. Etiology of nonimmune hydrops fetalis: a systematic review. Am J Med Genet A. 2009;149A(5):844-51.
2. Khalil A, Sotiriadis A, Chaoui R, da Silva Costa F, D'Antonio F, Heath PT, et al. ISUOG Practice Guidelines: role of ultrasound in congenital infection. Ultrasound Obstet Gynecol. 2020;56(1):128-51.

STATION 9.

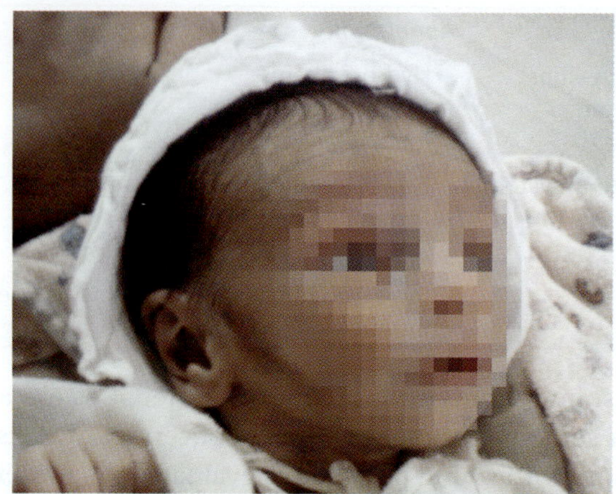

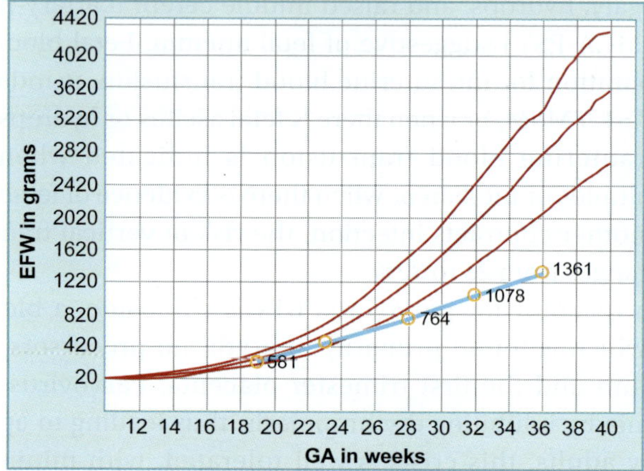

The questions below pertain to an intrauterine infection characterized by the images above.

1. **What infection do the above images refer to?**
2. **What is the classical triad of this infection? Identify one of the triad in the given newborn.**
3. **Is this congenital infection preventable? If yes, how?**
4. **What is the relationship between gestational age at maternal infection with vertical transmission (fetal infection) and severity of fetal affection in this case?**
    - **<12 weeks**
    - **>16 weeks**

Ans.

1. Rubella
2. Congenital rubella triad comprises sensorineural deafness and ocular abnormalities (cataract, retinopathy, glaucoma, and microphthalmia)

and congenital heart disease [pulmonary artery stenosis and patent ductus arteriosus (PDA)]. This child has congenital cataract.

3. Rubella is a preventable congenital infection as vaccination is available and is a part of the immunization schedule.
4. Risk of fetal infection decreases with increasing gestational age in rubella infections. Severity of fetal disease is greatest in the first trimester and minimal after 16 weeks.

   Risk of fetal infection is around 90% before 12 weeks' gestation, 55% from 12 to 16 weeks, and 45% after 16 weeks.

   Risk of an infected fetus being affected (i.e., risk of developing congenital defects) is greatest when infection occurs earlier in gestation: it is 97% when infection is before 12 weeks (termination of pregnancy can be considered, even without invasive testing); 20% when it is from 12 to 16 weeks, while infection from 16 to 20 weeks is associated with a minimal risk of deafness only.

SUGGESTED READING

1. Khalil A, Sotiriadis A, Chaoui R, da Silva Costa F, D'Antonio F, Heath PT, et al. ISUOG Practice Guidelines: role of ultrasound in congenital infection. Ultrasound Obstet Gynecol. 2020;56(1):128-51.

STATION 10.

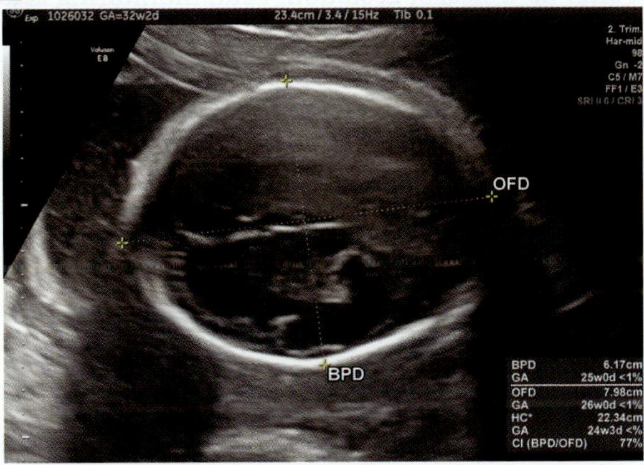

The above ultrasound findings pertain to a virus that is acquired by travel to endemic areas. Please answer questions that follow about this viral infection.

1. **Identify the above ultrasound finding. Name the virus described above.**
2. **How is the abnormality shown above defined? At what cut-off is the risk for brain abnormalities highest?**
3. **How is this virus transmitted? How do we identify high-risk pregnant woman at risk of this viral infection?**

4. **How is maternal infection with the above virus diagnosed?**
5. **In a confirmed case of maternal infection, how is fetal infection confirmed?**
6. **What are the ultrasound features of fetal infection?**

Ans.

1. The image shows microcephaly. Zika virus
2. Microcephaly is defined as head circumference <2 standard deviations below the mean for gestational age. However, brain abnormalities are associated with head circumference <3 standard deviations below the mean for gestational age.
3. Zika virus is a *Flavivirus* transmitted by the *Aedes* mosquito and also by sexual contact. Pregnant women with symptoms suggestive of Zika virus infection such as fever, skin rash, conjunctivitis, muscle and joint pain, malaise, and headache and (a) history of recent travel to area of Zika virus risk or (b) sexual contact with person returning from affected area.
4. The primary diagnostic test for Zika virus infection is real-time reverse transcriptase PCR (rt-PCR) of maternal serum and urine.
5. Amniocentesis for fetal Zika virus infection detection should be performed after 20 weeks of gestation. Fetal monitoring is done by serial ultrasound examination in a fetal medicine unit.
6. Following are the fetal ultrasound abnormalities that have been reported in pregnancies with congenital Zika syndrome (CZS):
   - *Microcephaly:* Head circumference <2 standard deviations below mean for gestational age.
   - Cerebral calcifications
   - Cerebral atrophy
   - Cerebellar atrophy
   - Ventriculomegaly
   - Cortical and white matter abnormalities, e.g., agyria, pachygyria, and lissencephaly
   - Periventricular cysts
   - Choroid plexus cysts
   - Mega cisterna magna
   - Vermian agenesis/dysgenesis
   - Corpus callosum abnormalities

SUGGESTED READING

1. CDC. (2024). Travelers' Health: Zika Travel Information. [online] Available from https://wwwnc.cdc.gov/travel/page/zika-travel-information [Last accessed May, 2025].

2. Khalil A, Sotiriadis A, Chaoui R, da Silva Costa F, D'Antonio F, Heath PT, et al. ISUOG Practice Guidelines: role of ultrasound in congenital infection. Ultrasound Obstet Gynecol. 2020;56(1):128-51.

STATION 11.

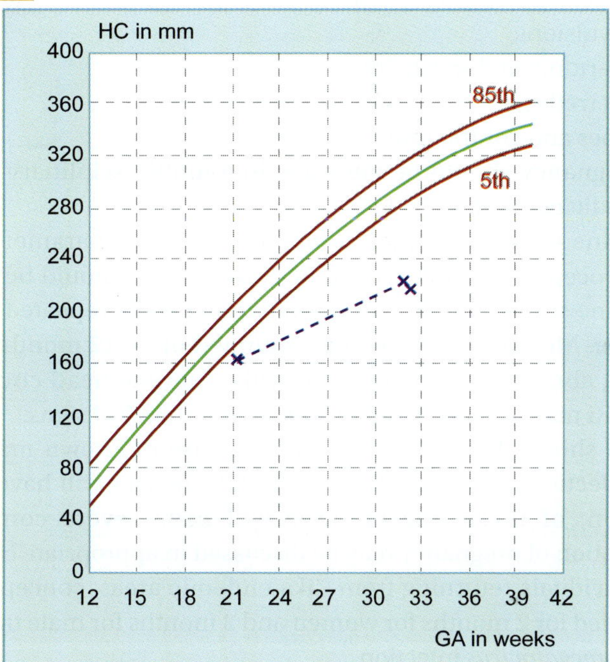

The above ultrasound findings pertain to a virus that is acquired by travel to endemic areas. Please answer questions that follow about this viral infection.

1. **Write three antenatal and three postnatal complications you will counsel parents about?**
2. **How would you monitor a pregnancy with maternal exposure/infection?**
3. **How will you counsel a woman who is contemplating termination of pregnancy after confirmed fetal infection?**
4. **For how long should sexual contact be avoided after visit to an endemic area?**
5. **Name two more viruses that can cause the abnormality shown in the images above.**

Ans.

1. Antenatal complications:
   a. Preterm birth
   b. Fetal growth restriction

c. Intrauterine fetal demise
d. Stillbirth

Postnatal/neonatal complications:

a. Microcephaly
b. Craniofacial disproportion
c. Convulsions
d. Hypertonia and spasticity
e. Hyperreflexia
f. Talipes and contractures

The pregnancy should be managed in a multidisciplinary setting in a fetal medicine unit.

2. A baseline fetal ultrasound to look for biometry parameters (to look for microcephaly and FGR) and neurosonogram should be performed. If baseline scan is normal, an examination can be repeated in the third trimester. Monitoring should be continued up to 12 months after birth as brain abnormalities may occur with a normal head circumference. Fetal MRI may be considered to look for neurological signs.
3. Women should be counseled that in a case of known maternal Zika virus infection, approximation one in four fetuses will have congenital infection, of these one in three will have severe complications. Termination of pregnancy may be discussed in appropriate cases.
4. For individuals returning from Zika endemic areas, conception should be avoided for 2 months for women and 3 months for male travelers.
5. a. *Cytomegalovirus* infection
   b. Rubella
   c. Toxoplasmosis

SUGGESTED READING

1. CDC. (2024). Travelers' Health: Zika Travel Information. [online] Available from https://wwwnc.cdc.gov/travel/page/zika-travel-information [Last accessed May, 2025].
2. Khalil A, Sotiriadis A, Chaoui R, da Silva Costa F, D'Antonio F, Heath PT, et al. ISUOG Practice Guidelines: role of ultrasound in congenital infection. Ultrasound Obstet Gynecol. 2020;56(1):128-51.

CHAPTER 15

Fetal Growth Restriction

Madhusudan Dey, Seetha Ramamurthy Pal

STATION 1.

1. **What is the first step before diagnosing small for gestational age (SGA)/fetal growth restriction (FGR)?**
2. **How should growth be assessed?**
3. **Which assessment tool should be used to monitor growth velocity?**
4. **What is appropriate for gestational age (AGA)?**

Ans.

1. The first step before diagnosing SGA/FGR is to ensure correct gestational age with accurate dating scan done between 7 and 14 weeks of pregnancy.
2. Growth should always be assessed on charts which show centiles.
3. Standard charts such as Hadlock charts can be used to monitor the growth velocity.
4. Appropriate for gestational age is when estimated fetal weight (EFW) is between the 10th and 90th centile for that gestational age.

SUGGESTED READING

1. Morris RK, Johnstone E, Lees C, Morton V, Smith G, the Royal College of Obstetricians and Gynaecologists. Investigation and Care of a Small-for-Gestational-Age Fetus and a Growth Restricted Fetus (Green-top Guideline No. 31). 2024.

STATION 2.

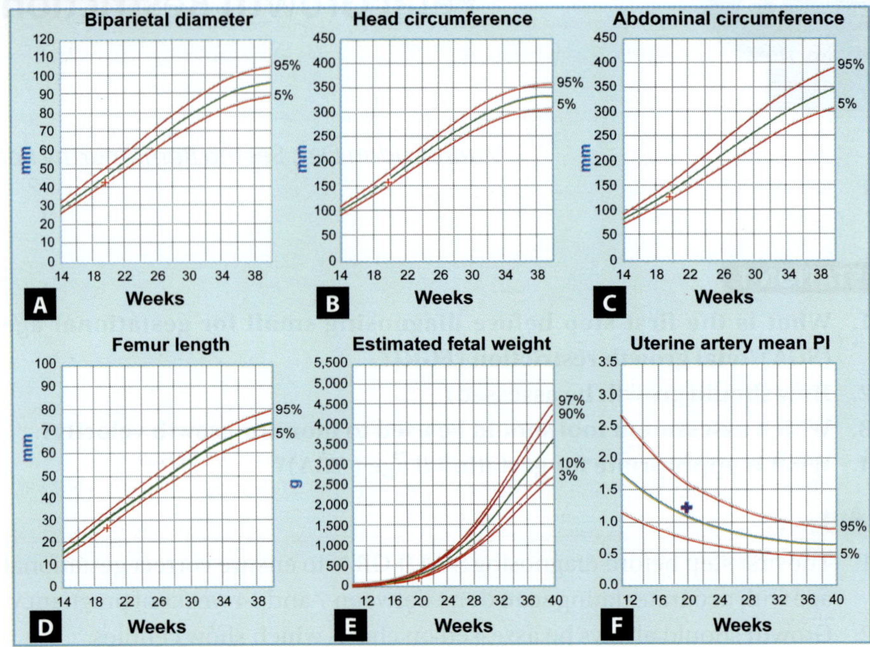

Source: (A to D) Snijders RJ, Nicolaides KH. Fetal biometry at 14–40 weeks' gestation. Ultrasound Obstet Gynecol. 1994;4(1):34-48. (E) Hadlock FP, Harrist RB, Martinez-Poyer J. In utero analysis of fetal growth: a sonographic weight standard. Radiology. 1991;181(1):129-33. (F) Gómez, O et al. Reference ranges for uterine artery mean pulsatility index at 11–41 weeks of gestation. Ultrasound Obstet Gynecol. 2008;32(2):128-32.

1. **How is SGA defined?**
2. **How is FGR defined?**
3. **What constitutes dropping centiles?**
4. **What are the tools used to differentiate between FGR and SGA?**

Ans.

1. A fetus with an EFW below the 10th percentile but with normal uterine and umbilical artery Doppler.
2. A fetus with an EFW or abdominal circumference (AC) below 3rd centile or below the 10th percentile for gestational age with signs of placental insufficiency, such as abnormal umbilical artery Doppler studies.
3. When there is a drop in fetal growth centiles by 50%. For example, a fetus with drop in EFW from 70th centile to <20th centile
4. Doppler of uterine artery and umbilical artery

SUGGESTED READING

1. Morris RK, Johnstone E, Lees C, Morton V, Smith G, the Royal College of Obstetricians and Gynaecologists. Investigation and Care of a Small-for-Gestational-Age Fetus and a Growth Restricted Fetus (Green-top Guideline No. 31). 2024.

STATION 3.

1. **Which measurement is the ONLY routine screening for FGR that is endorsed by the ACOG and Society for Maternal-Fetal Medicine (2021)?**
2. **If this parameter differs by more than or equal to ____________ cm in the absence of an obvious explanation, sonography is indicated.**
3. **Is routine third trimester sonography to assess fetal growth recommended?**
4. **What period of gestation is taken as cutoff for differentiation between early versus late fetal growth restriction?**

Ans.

1. Symphysio fundal height
2. 3
3. Though studies have shown that compared to clinically indicated ultrasonography in the third trimester, universal screening triples the detection rate of late smallness for gestational age and as opposed to early third-trimester ultrasound, scanning late in pregnancy (around 37 weeks) increases the detection rate for birthweight <3rd centile.
4. 32 weeks

SUGGESTED READING

1. Fetal Growth Restriction: ACOG Practice Bulletin, Number 227. Obstet Gynecol. 2021;137(2):e16-e28.
2. Figueras F, Caradeux J, Crispi F, Eixarch E, Peguero A, Gratacos E. Diagnosis and surveillance of late-onset fetal growth restriction. Am J Obstet Gynecol. 2018;218(2S):S790-S802.e1.

STATION 4.

1. **When should high risk women be called for growth assessment?**
2. **Enumerate the diagnostic criteria for early FGR in absence of congenital anomalies.**
3. **Enumerate the diagnostic criteria for late FGR in absence of congenital anomalies.**
4. **What is meant by static growth?**

Ans.

1. High risk should have serial growth scans at 28, 32, 34, and 36 weeks for growth and Doppler assessment.
2. *<32 weeks:*

   AC/EFW <3rd centile or umbilical artery absent end-diastolic flow (UmbA-AEDF)

   Or AC/EFW <10th centiles combined with:

   a. Uterine artery pulsatility index (UtA-PI) >95th centiles and/or
   b. UmbA-PI >95th centiles

3. *>32 weeks:*
   AC/EFW <3rd centile
   Or at least two out of three of the following:
   a. AC/EFW, 10th centiles
   b. AC/EFW crossing centiles >2 quartiles on growth centiles
   c. Cerebroplacental ratio (CPR) <5th centiles or UmbA PI >95th centile
4. No forward growth velocity in EFW, or AC measured at least 14 days apart

SUGGESTED READING

1. Morris RK, Johnstone E, Lees C, Morton V, Smith G, the Royal College of Obstetricians and Gynaecologists. Investigation and Care of a Small-for-Gestational-Age Fetus and a Growth Restricted Fetus (Green-top Guideline No. 31). 2024.

STATION 5.

1. **What is the Doppler index used to assess waveforms?**
2. **What does increased PI in the uterine artery signify?**
3. **What does increased PI or absent EDF in the umbilical artery signify?**
4. **What does reduced PI in middle cerebral artery (MCA) signify?**

Ans.

1. Pulsatility index
2. Reflect inadequate trophoblastic invasion of spiral artery
3. Increased fetal afterload resistance and reduction in the placental surface area available for exchange
4. Brain sparing effect in response to fetal hypoxemia

SUGGESTED READING

1. Morris RK, Johnstone E, Lees C, Morton V, Smith G, the Royal College of Obstetricians and Gynaecologists. Investigation and Care of a Small-for-Gestational-Age Fetus and a Growth Restricted Fetus (Green-top Guideline No. 31). 2024.

STATION 6.

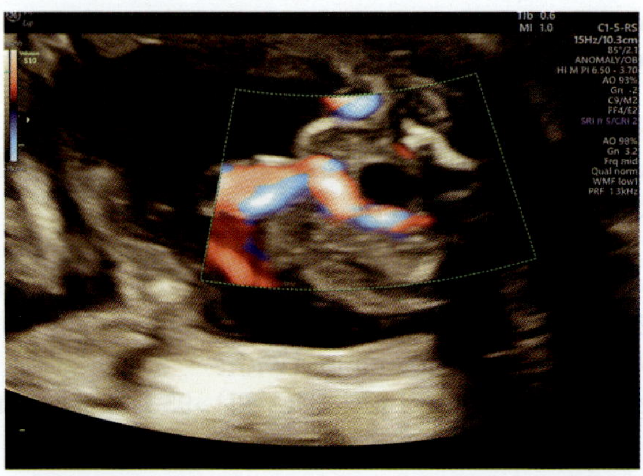

1. **Spot the diagnosis**
2. **Name any two biochemical markers which are used for aneuploidy screening, and which can be used as a risk factor for SGA and FGR.**
3. **Presence of single umbilical artery (SUA) raises risk of SGA by almost ________________ fold.**
4. **Women at risk of preeclampsia and/or placental dysfunction should take aspirin ______________ mg once daily at night from 12 to 36 weeks to reduce their chances of SGA and FGR.**
5. **According to guideline minimum time interval between two ultrasound examination for diagnosing FGR and interval growth.**

Ans.

1. Single umbilical artery
2. Low pregnancy-associated plasma protein-A (PAPP-A), raised alpha-fetoprotein (AFP), raised inhibin
3. 03
4. 150
5. 2 weeks

SUGGESTED READING

1. Morris RK, Johnstone E, Lees C, Morton V, Smith G, the Royal College of Obstetricians and Gynaecologists. Investigation and Care of a Small-for-Gestational-Age Fetus and a Growth Restricted Fetus (Green-top Guideline No. 31). 2024.

STATION 7.

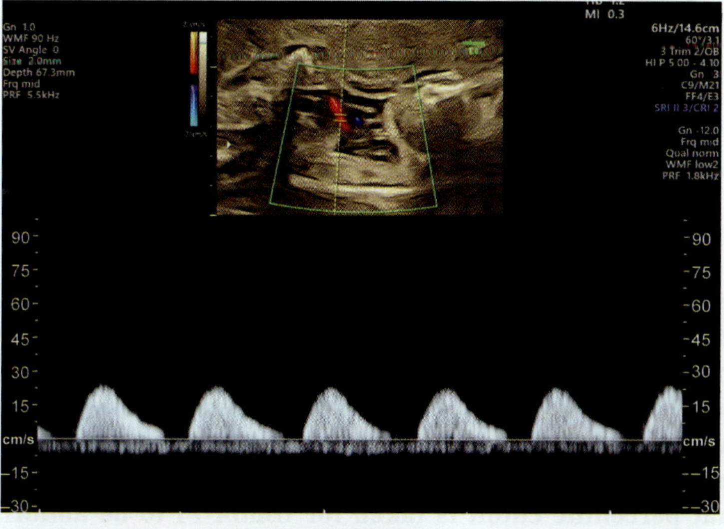

1. **What is the diagnosis of above trace?**
2. **What is the value of end-diastolic flow in above trace?**

3. **What is the management of a primigravida at 31 weeks period of gestation (POG) with early onset FGR with above trace already received steroid induction 5 days back?**
4. **Which part of umbilical cord is taken for above measurement as a reference?**

Ans.

1. Absent end-diastolic flow in umbilical artery
2. Zero
3. Measurement of ductus venosus (DV) and computed cardiotocography (cCTG)
4. Free loop of cord

SUGGESTED READING

1. Lees CC, Stampalija T, Baschat A, da Silva Costa F, Ferrazzi E, Figueras F, et al. ISUOG Practice Guidelines: diagnosis and management of small for gestational age fetus and fetal growth restriction. Ultrasound Obstet Gynecol. 2020;56(2): 298-312.

STATION 8.

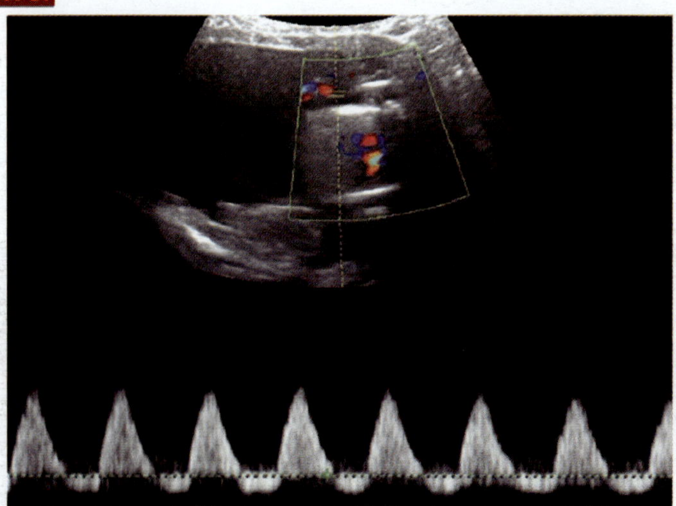

1. **Identify the above trace.**
2. **A 23-year-old primigravida presents at 34 weeks gestation (dating confirmed) with an EFW <3rd percentile for gestational age. Doppler velocimetry of the umbilical artery reveals the waveform shown above. What is your next course of action?**
3. **Absolute immediate indication of delivery in late FGR?**
4. **What percentile cutoff is taken for UmbA-PI to be abnormal in monitoring of FGR fetuses?**

Ans.

1. Reverse end-diastolic flow (REDF).
2. Proceed with primary cesarean delivery.
3. Spontaneous repeated persistent unprovoked fetal heart rate deceleration, altered biophysical profile (BPP) (<4), reversed UA EDF and cCTG <3.5 ms at 32 + 0 to 33 + 6 weeks and <4.5 ms >34 weeks.
4. 95%

SUGGESTED READING

1. Morris RK, Johnstone E, Lees C, Morton V, Smith G, the Royal College of Obstetricians and Gynaecologists. Investigation and Care of a Small-for-Gestational-Age Fetus and a Growth Restricted Fetus (Green-top Guideline No. 31). 2024.

STATION 9. **A 22-year-old Primi at routine 32 weeks USG was found to have fetus with an EFW on 9th centile suggestive of GA**

1. **Surveillance tool in the SGA fetus?**
2. **When umbilical artery flow indices are normal it is reasonable to repeat surveillance every ____________ days.**
3. **For SGA fetuses, interpretation of amniotic fluid volume should be based on four quadrant technique, or single deepest vertical pocket.**
4. **Biophysical profile should not be used for fetal surveillance in preterm SGA fetuses. Is this statement true or false?**

Ans.

1. Uterine and umbilical artery Doppler
2. 14
3. Single deepest pocket (SDP)
4. True

SUGGESTED READING

1. Morris RK, Johnstone E, Lees C, Morton V, Smith G, the Royal College of Obstetricians and Gynaecologists. Investigation and Care of a Small-for-Gestational-Age Fetus and a Growth Restricted Fetus (Green-top Guideline No. 31). 2024.

STATION 10.

1. **What is sildenafil and what is its mechanism of action?**
2. **What is the dose used in the trial?**
3. **Effects of sildenafil in fetal growth restriction treatment.**

Ans.

1. A phosphodiesterase type 5 inhibitor—potential vasodilatory effect

2. 25 mg three times a day
3. Maternal use of sildenafil has no effect on fetal growth velocity.

SUGGESTED READING

1. Morris RK, Johnstone E, Lees C, Morton V, Smith G, the Royal College of Obstetricians and Gynaecologists. Investigation and Care of a Small-for-Gestational-Age Fetus and a Growth Restricted Fetus (Green-top Guideline No. 31). 2024.

STATION 11.

1. **What is the full form of cCTG?**
2. **Name the criteria used to interpret a cCTG.**
3. **Of all variables of cCTG which dataset is used in pregnancy to make clinical decision?**
4. **Based on TRUFFLE study, between 26 + 0 and 28 + 6 weeks, delivery indicated if STV is less than ________ ms.**

Ans.

1. Computerised CTG
2. Dawes and Redman
3. Short-term variation (STV)
4. 2.6

SUGGESTED READING

1. Lees CC, Stampalija T, Baschat A, da Silva Costa F, Ferrazzi E, Figueras F, et al. ISUOG Practice Guidelines: diagnosis and management of small for gestational age fetus and fetal growth restriction. Ultrasound Obstet Gynecol. 2020;56(2):298-312.

STATION 12.

1. **What are the biochemical markers that can predict FGR?**
2. **What are the ultrasound markers that can predict FGR?**
3. **What is the sensitivity of these markers?**
4. **What does abnormal UtA-PI in the third trimester signify?**

Ans.

1. Pregnancy-associated plasma protein-A-0.4 multiples of the median (MoM) or less, low placental growth factor (PlGF), high AFP >2 MoM
2. Uterine artery PI >95th centile, marginal, or velamentous cord insertion, single umbilical artery or short femur
3. Sensitivity of the above markers is 86% for preterm SGA and 66% for term SGA for an FPR of 10%.
4. FGR with Abn-UtA Doppler in 3rd trimester have a two-fold increased risk of abnormal brain Doppler at term, poor perinatal outcome, and increased risk of late maternal preeclampsia.

SUGGESTED READING

1. Crovetto F, Triunfo S, Crispi F, Rodriguez-Sureda V, Dominguez C, Figueras F, et al. Differential performance of first trimester screening in predicting small-for-gestational-age neonate or fetal growth restriction. Ultrasound Obstet Gynecol. 2017;49(3):349-56.
2. Martinez-Portilla RJ, Caradeux J, Meler E, Lip-Sosa DL, Sotiriadis A, Figueras F. Third-trimester uterine artery Doppler for prediction of adverse outcome in late small-for-gestational-age fetuses: systematic review and meta-analysis. Ultrasound Obstet Gynecol. 2020;55(5):575-85.

STATION 13.

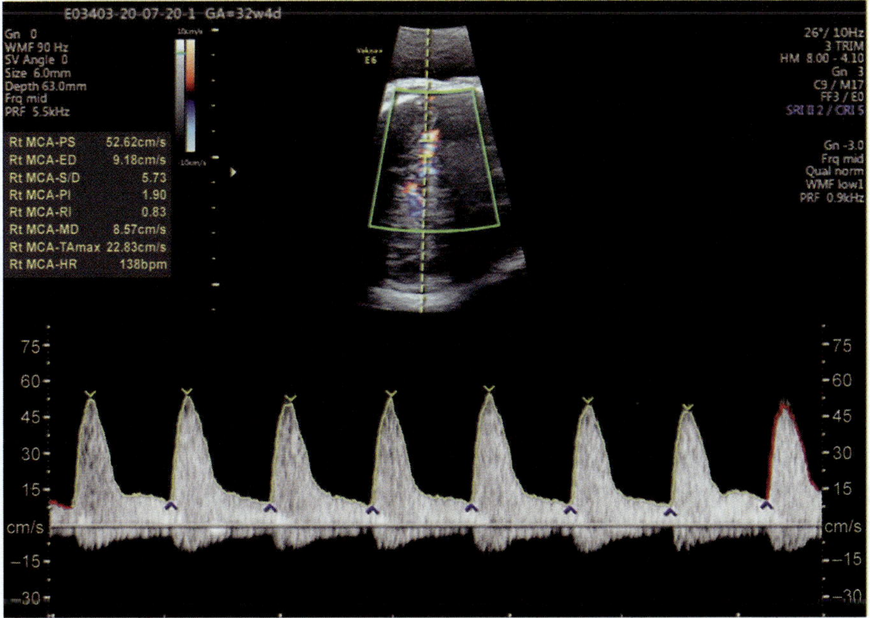

1. **Which arterial flow pattern is shown in the above image?**
2. **What is CPR?**
3. **What does CPR reflect?**
4. **What is unique about late FGR?**

Ans.

1. Middle cerebral artery waveform
2. CPR stands for cerebroplacental ratio—ratio of MCA PI and UmbA PI
3. May reflect fetal hypoxia and become abnormal before MCA, but should not be used to determine delivery before 37 weeks
4. Late FGR fetuses are more susceptible to hypoxia and hence sudden stillbirth and abnormalities in growth and Dopplers are seen late (34–36 weeks) or UA Dopplers can remain normal, but CPR may be abnormal.

SUGGESTED READING

1. Morris RK, Johnstone E, Lees C, Morton V, Smith G, the Royal College of Obstetricians and Gynaecologists. Investigation and Care of a Small-for-Gestational-Age Fetus and a Growth Restricted Fetus (Green-top Guideline No. 31). 2024.

STATION 14.

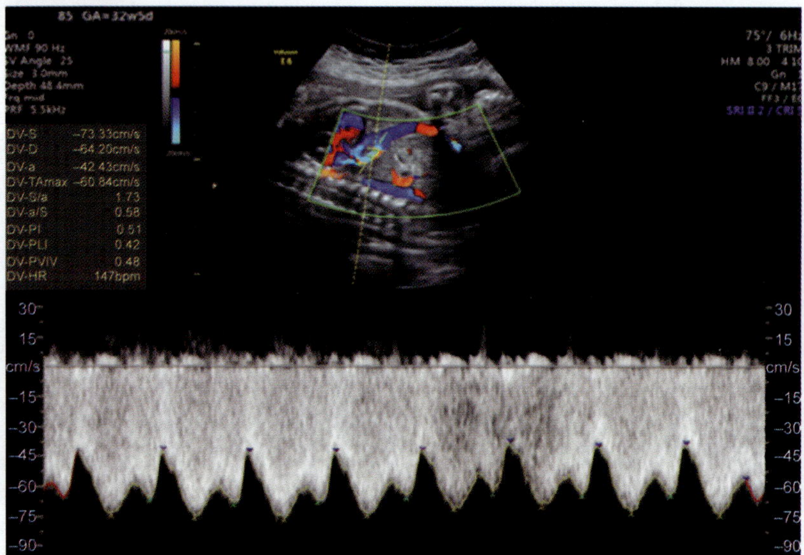

1. **What does the above image depict?**
2. **Which organ function does the above vessel corelate to?**
3. **What is the clinical utility of the above vessel in FGR?**
4. **What are the findings of the TRUFFLE study?**

Ans.

1. Ductus venosus Doppler
2. Fetal cardiovascular status
3. In early FGR, DV Doppler abnormalities are the best predictors of adverse perinatal outcome and trigger for delivery.
4. TRUFFLE study showed that timing of delivery based on ductus venosus Doppler measurement in conjunction with cCTG safety-net criteria improves long-term (2-year) neurodevelopmental outcome in surviving infants.

SUGGESTED READING

1. Morris RK, Johnstone E, Lees C, Morton V, Smith G, the Royal College of Obstetricians and Gynaecologists. Investigation and Care of a Small-for-Gestational-Age Fetus and a Growth Restricted Fetus (Green-top Guideline No. 31). 2024.

STATION 15.

Regarding delivery in small for gestational age (SGA)

1. **What do SGA babies need monitoring?**
2. **When can SGA fetuses be delivered?**
3. **What should be the mode of delivery in SGA babies?**
4. **What additional precautions should be taken intrapartum?**

Ans.

1. Small for gestational age with normal fetoplacental Doppler can be associated with accelerated placental aging, signs of placental under perfusion, lower umbilical vein blood flow volume, altered maternal hemodynamics, and greater incidence of cesarean section for fetal distress compared with AGA fetuses.
2. SGA fetuses can be delivered after 38 + 0 weeks of gestation, and the pregnancy should not exceed 39 + 0 weeks.
3. Induction of labor can be done depending on the clinical situation.
4. Continuous fetal heart rate monitoring in labor should be performed in these cases.

SUGGESTED READING

1. Morris RK, Johnstone E, Lees C, Morton V, Smith G, the Royal College of Obstetricians and Gynaecologists. Investigation and Care of a Small-for-Gestational-Age Fetus and a Growth Restricted Fetus (Green-top Guideline No. 31). 2024.

STATION 16.

According to the Barcelona staging

1. **What is stage I FGR and what is the frequency of monitoring in stage I FGR?**
2. **What is stage II FGR and what is the frequency of monitoring in stage II FGR?**
3. **What is stage III FGR and what is the frequency of monitoring in stage III FGR?**
4. **What is stage IV FGR and what is the frequency of monitoring in stage IV FGR?**

Ans.

1. Stage I FGR is mild placental insufficiency where EFW <3rd centile with UA PI >95th centile and UtA-PI >95th centile. They should be monitored weekly and delivery can be done at 37 weeks.
2. Stage II FGR indicates severe placental insufficiency where UA has absent EDF and DV PI >95th centile and they should be monitored twice weekly with delivery at 34 weeks.

3. Stage III FGR indicates low suspicion of fetal acidosis where the UA has reverse EDF. Here the Dopplers need to be repeated daily with delivery at 30 weeks.
4. Stage IV FGR indicates high suspicion of fetal acidosis where there is DV reversal and CTG changes and such fetuses should be monitored every 12 hours before delivery.

SUGGESTED READING

1. Figueras F, Gratacos E. An integrated approach to fetal growth restriction. Best Pract Res Clin Obstet Gynaecol. 2017;38:48-58.

STATION 17.

1. **What postnatal evaluation should be done in cases of FGR?**
2. **What are the long-term risks for FGR fetuses?**
3. **What is the recurrence risk?**
4. **What are the modifiable risk factors?**

Ans.

1. **Histological examination of the placenta and testing for thrombophilia in cases of severe early onset FGR**
2. **Prematurity-associated complications and worse neurodevelopmental outcome in early FGR and increased risk of non-communicable diseases in adulthood**
3. **Birth of a baby with FGR is a major risk factor for FGR in subsequent pregnancy with Odds ratio of 8.1**
4. **Lifestyle modification such as reduced exposure to smoking, decreasing body mass index (BMI), and optimizing medical conditions.**

SUGGESTED READING

1. Morris RK, Johnstone E, Lees C, Morton V, Smith G, the Royal College of Obstetricians and Gynaecologists. Investigation and Care of a Small-for-Gestational-Age Fetus and a Growth Restricted Fetus (Green-top Guideline No. 31). 2024.

CHAPTER 16

Red Cell Isoimmunization

Mandakini Pradhan

STATION 1. A primigravida with blood group is "A negative" with her partner is "B positive" presents to your antenatal OPD at 18 weeks of gestation.

1. **What specific test would you like to do as regards to her blood group?**
2. **If the above investigation report comes as positive, what would be your next step?**
3. **If the above investigation report is negative, when should it be repeated definitely?**
4. **When would you plan to deliver this patient if there are no other complications in pregnancy and the test remains negative?**

Ans.

1. ICT (indirect Coombs test)
2. Antibody titer
3. At 28 weeks of gestation
4. At 40 weeks, preferably not beyond 40 weeks

SUGGESTED READING

1. Practice bulletin no 181: prevention of Rh D alloimmunization. Obstet Gynecol. 2017;130(2):e57-e70.

STATION 2.

1. **What documentation is necessary while administering anti-D prophylaxis?**
2. **Why should anti-D be administered in the deltoid muscle?**
3. **How should anti-D be offered if intramuscular (IM) injections are contraindicated?**
4. **What are the common reasons for failure of anti-D?**

Ans.

1. It is necessary to document negative ICT and written informed consent should be taken.
2. Deltoid muscle is preferred to avoid slow absorption from subcutaneous tissue in case of gluteus muscle.

3. Anti-D can be administered intravenously in the same dose if IM injections are contraindicated.
4. Wrong site, wrong dose, wrong storage, and unawareness

SUGGESTED READING

1. FOGSI TOG 2021: Anti D immunoglobulin for rhesus prophylaxis: key practice points, 2021.
2. Royal College of Obstetricians and Gynaecologists (RCOG). Green-top Guideline No. 65: The Prevention of RhD Haemolytic Disease in the Newborn, 2014.

STATION 3. **A primigravida with Rh D antibody titers of one in 256 presents to you.**

1. **What could be the two possible causes for such a high antibody titer?**
2. **What will be the method of monitoring of fetus for development of complications related to this?**
3. **While monitoring if values are normal when will you ask the patient to come back?**
4. **If this fetus has not required any fetal therapy, when will you deliver this woman if there are no other indications for early delivery?**

Ans.

1. History of blood transfusion and grandmother phenomenon
2. By ultrasound for middle cerebral artery peak systolic velocity (MCA PSV)
3. 2 weekly
4. 36 weeks

SUGGESTED READING

1. Cunningham FG, Leveno KJ, Dashe JS, Hoffman BL, Spong CY, Casey BM. Williams obstetrics. Rh Disease and Hemolytic Disease of Fetus and Newborn, 26th edition. McGraw Hill; 2022. pp. 904-33.

STATION 4.

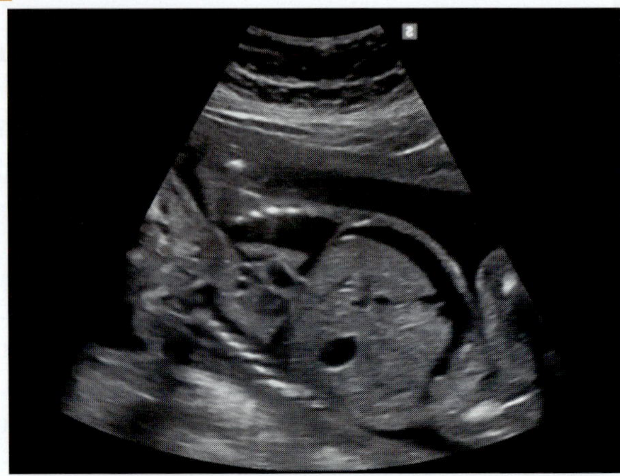

1. **What is the diagnosis?**
2. **What could be three most common possible causes for this fetal finding?**
3. **Name one most relevant additional USG finding you would look for?**
4. **What could be possible treatment if fetal heart rate (FHR) >200 bpm.**

Ans.

1. Fetal hydrops
2. Rh isoimmunized, infections, metabolic disorders, cardiac malformation, and cardiac rhythm abnormalities
3. MCA PSV
4. Treatment can be given through transplacental route, e.g., digoxin, amiodarone, and flecainide.

SUGGESTED READING

1. American College of Obstetrics and Gynecology. ACOG practice bulletin no 75: management of alloimmunization during pregnancy. Obstet Gynecol. 2006;108(2):457-64.
2. American Heart Association. Pharmacological management of cardiac arrhythmias in the fetal and neonatal periods: A scientific statement from the American Heart Association. Circulation. 2024;149(10):e937-52.

STATION 5.

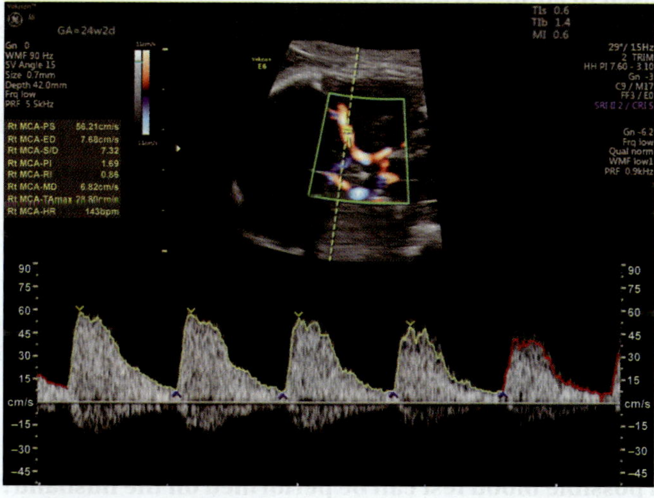

1. **What does the image depict?**
2. **Which parameter of the above image is used to predict fetal anemia?**
3. **Why is the velocity increased in the above vessel in cases of fetal anemia?**
4. **What is the cut off for diagnosing fetal anemia and what is the sensitivity?**

Ans.

1. The image depicts middle cerebral artery Doppler
2. Peak systolic velocity and the values are converted to multiples of the median (MoM)
3. Anemia causes less viscosity which causes hyperdynamic circulation and increased velocity
4. PSV >1.5 MoM for that gestational age or more than twice the gestational age

SUGGESTED READING

1. Mari G, Deter RL, Carpenter RL, Rahman F, Zimmerman R, Moise KJ, et al. Noninvasive Diagnosis by Doppler Ultrasonography of Fetal Anemia Due to Maternal Red-Cell Alloimmunization. N Engl J Med. 2000;342(1):9-14.
2. Martinez-Portilla RJ, Lopez-Felix J, Hawkins-Villareal A, Villafan-Bernal JR, Paz Y Miño F, Figueras F, et al. Performance of fetal middle cerebral artery peak systolic velocity for prediction of anemia in untransfused and transfused fetuses: systematic review and meta-analysis. Ultrasound Obstet Gynecol. 2019;54(6):722-31.

STATION 6. A G7P4111, Rh isoimmunized pregnancy with fetal anemia.

1. **What could be various sites for fetal blood transfusion?**
2. **What blood group blood is given to fetus?**
3. **Hematocrit (Hct) of blood transfused to fetus is equal to Hct of blood transfused to adult—True or False.**
4. **Volume of blood given to fetus will depend on which three factors?**

Ans.

1. **Intravascular (cord insertion or intrahepatic), intraperitoneal**
2. **Fresh O RhD-negative blood**
3. **False**
4. **Estimated fetal weight, bag Hct, and pretransfusion Hct**

SUGGESTED READING

1. Royal College of Obstetricians and Gynaecologists. The management of women with red cell antibodies during pregnancy. Green-top Guideline No. 65. London: RCOG; 2014.

STATION 7. If wife is RhD-negative and husband is RhD-positive.

1. **Which possible blood test can be performed on the husband?**
2. **Which blood test in the mother can identify the fetal blood group?**
3. **If this woman does not require any fetal therapy and delivers normally, which test should be sent from cord blood?**
4. **Can amniocentesis be done at 18 weeks to determine fetal RhD grouping.**

Ans.

1. Zygosity of husband
2. Noninvasive prenatal screening (NIPS) or cell free fetal DNA
3. Blood group, direct Coombs test (DCT), and reticulocyte count
4. Yes, it can be done.

SUGGESTED READING

1. Cunningham FG, Leveno KJ, Dashe JS, Hoffman BL, Spong CY, Casey BM. Williams obstetrics. Rh Disease and Hemolytic Disease of Fetus and Newborn, 26th edition. McGraw Hill; 2022. pp. 904-33.

STATION 8. Rh-negative pregnant woman who has received antenatal anti-D prophylaxis at 28 weeks presents to you.

1. **With spotting per vaginum at 34 weeks which stopped after one episode only, would you like to give injection anti-D?**
2. **If she delivers twins and both twins have RhD-positive blood group, then how much injection anti-D you will give?**
3. **Injection anti-D is best given at which site?**
4. **What is the dose of injection anti-D to be given in a patient with abruptio placentae with fetal intrauterine death?**

Ans.

1. Yes, after 6 weeks it needs to be repeated.
2. 300 µg (same dose as recommended in singleton delivery)
3. Intramuscular route at deltoid
4. Double the dose, i.e. 600 µg

SUGGESTED READING

1. American College of Obstetrics and Gynecology. ACOG practice bulletin no 75: management of alloimmunization during pregnancy. Obstet Gynecol. 2006;108(2):457-64.

STATION 9. A 36-year-old woman G7P3211 presented at 10 weeks with RhD-negative blood group with history of previous pregnancy having fetal death at 28 weeks following fetal hydrops.

1. **At what gestation, you would like to do an aneuploidy screening for her and what test you will do?**
2. **What is the likely D antibody titer in this woman?**
3. **At what gestation, you will give injection anti-D to this woman?**
4. **At what gestation would you like the patient to start monitoring with ultrasound?**

Ans.

1. At 10 weeks, NIPS or non-invasive prenatal testing (NIPT) or cell free fetal DNA test
2. More than critical titer for that laboratory
3. Never
4. From 18 weeks onwards

SUGGESTED READING

1. American College of Obstetrics and Gynecology. ACOG practice bulletin no 75: management of alloimmunization during pregnancy. Obstet Gynecol. 2006;108(2):457-64.

STATION 10. A 36-year-old woman, G7P3211 with Rh isoimmunized pregnancy with history of previous fetal death at 28 weeks following hydrops, is under your follow-up.

1. **When will you do or send the patient for intrauterine fetal blood transfusion [intrauterine transfusion (IUT)]?**
2. **If she has received one IUT, and the post transfusion Hb is reported to be 15 g/dL, when is she likely to have the next IUT?**
3. **What will you tell the couple about the success rate of IUT, if the fetus is non-hydropic?**
4. **When will you do the blood grouping of the fetus/newborn?**

Ans.

1. When MCA PSV is >1.5 MoM for the gestation.
2. After 15 days
3. More than 90%
4. Before the first IUT

SUGGESTED READING

1. Cunningham FG, Leveno KJ, Dashe JS, Hoffman BL, Spong CY, Casey BM. Williams obstetrics. Rh Disease and Hemolytic Disease of Fetus and Newborn, 26th edition. McGraw Hill; 2022. pp. 904-33.

STATION 11. A 30-year-old primigravida woman presented to your antenatal OPD at 18 weeks gestation with RhD-negative blood group without any antibody.

1. **Give two indications of giving injection anti-D to this patient at this gestation.**
2. **Dose of injection anti-D given to this woman at 28 weeks.**
3. **After she received injection anti-D, when will you order for the antibody titer?**

4. **She had a normal vaginal delivery at term and baby's blood group was found to be B RhD-positive. Your staff forgot to give injection anti-D that you have ordered after delivery that you noticed after 7 days when she came to show you the episiotomy stich line as she was having pain. Would you like to give the dose of injection anti-D and at what dose and which route?**

Ans.

1. Amniocentesis, bleeding P/V
2. 300 μg
3. Never
4. Yes, to be given at 300 μg, intramuscular

SUGGESTED READING

1. Cunningham FG, Leveno KJ, Dashe JS, Hoffman BL, Spong CY, Casey BM. Williams obstetrics. Rh Disease and Hemolytic Disease of Fetus and Newborn, 26th edition. McGraw Hill; 2022. pp. 904-33.

STATION 12.

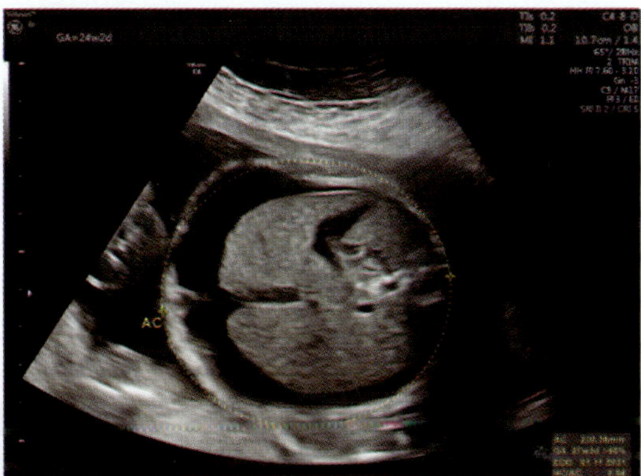

1. **Describe the above image.**
2. **What are the other ultrasound features in Rh isoimmunized fetuses?**
3. **Which cardiac function gets affected before the development of hydrops?**
4. **What is the success rate of IUT in cases of hydropic fetuses?**

Ans.

1. Fetal ascites
2. Hydrops, hepatomegaly, splenomegaly, pericardial effusion, placentomegaly, and hydramnios
3. Tricuspid regurgitation.
4. Even in the presence of hydrops, IUT has a success rate of 40%.

SUGGESTED READING

1. Abbasi N, Johnson JA, Ryan G. Fetal anemia. Ultrasound Obstet Gynecol. 2017; 50(2):145-53.

STATION 13. **A 28-year-old primigravida has been given intrauterine blood transfusion.**

1. **Mention three indications of fetal blood transfusion.**
2. **Mention the drugs used to paralyze the fetus for intrauterine transfusion.**
3. **Mention the best site which offers less complications of fetal transfusion.**
4. **Mention the special preparation of the blood used for fetal transfusion.**

Ans.

1. Rh isoimmunization, Parvovirus B19 infection, chorioangioma, and monochorionic twin pregnancy with anemia-polycythemia syndrome
2. Atracurium and vecuronium
3. Intrahepatic portion of the umbilical vein
4. Leuco-reduced, gamma-irradiated, crossmatched with mother's blood with hematocrit between 75 and 85%.

SUGGESTED READING

1. Cunningham FG, Leveno KJ, Dashe JS, Hoffman BL, Spong CY, Casey BM. Williams obstetrics. Rh Disease and Hemolytic Disease of Fetus and Newborn, 26th edition. McGraw Hill; 2022. pp. 904-33.

STATION 14.

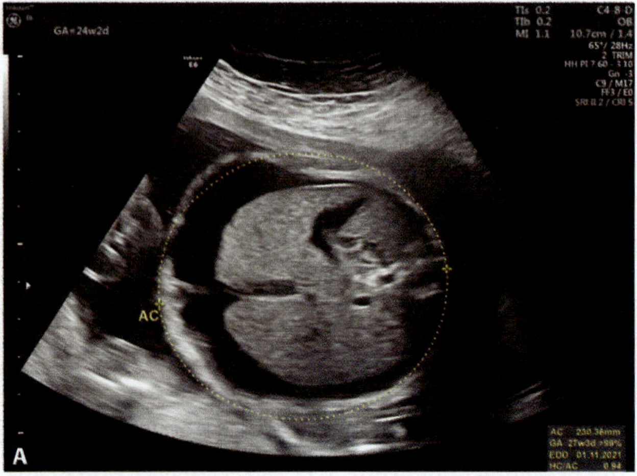

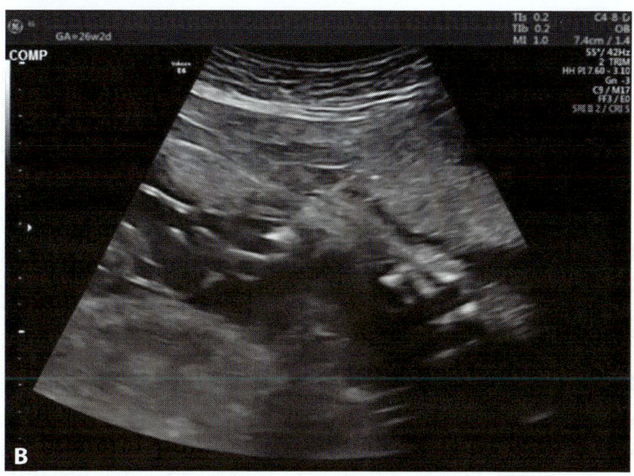

1. **Describe the above two images A and B.**
2. **From how many weeks can the procedure be done?**
3. **When is the last procedure usually timed and what precautions should be taken?**
4. **What are the possible complications?**

Ans.

1. Image A—fetal hydrops; image B—cordocentesis for IUT
2. IUT can be done from 18 weeks onwards till term
3. The last IUT is usually timed at around 35 weeks. The procedure should be done under steroid cover and OT back up in case of the patient needing emergency delivery
4. Transient bradycardia, preterm labor (PTL), prolonged bradycardia needing emergency cesarean section (CS), cord hematoma and rarely IUD

SUGGESTED READING

1. Van Kamp IL, Klumper FJCM, Meerman RH, Oepkes D, Scherjon SA, Kanhai HHH. Treatment of fetal anemia due to red-cell alloimmunization with intrauterine transfusions in the Netherlands, 1988-1999. Acta Obstet Gynecol Scand. 2004;83(8):731-7.

STATION 15.

1. **How is the fetus monitored post IUT?**
2. **What is the rate of fall of Hct in the anemic fetus?**
3. **What is the sensitivity of MCA PSV post-transfusion?**
4. **Why does the sensitivity of MCA PSV reduce post-transfusion?**

Ans.

1. Post-transfusion, the fetus is monitored with MCA PSV MoM and some use a higher cutoff of 1.69 MoM to diagnose fetal anemia
2. The rate of fall of Hct is 0.4 g/dL/day, 0.3 g/dL/day, and 0.2 g/dL/day.
3. The sensitivity of MCA PSV decreases to 85–90% post-transfusion.
4. MCA PSV performs less well for timing the second and subsequent IUTs as fetal MCA blood flow is different when replaced by adult RBCs and adult RBCs are smaller, less rigid, and have different oxygen carrying capacity and oxygen delivery characteristics.

SUGGESTED READING

1. Abdelshafi S, Okasha A, Elsirgany S, Khalil A, El-Dessouky S, AbdelHakim N, et al. Peak systolic velocity of fetal middle cerebral artery to predict anemia in Red Cell Alloimmunization in un-transfused and transfused fetuses. Eur J Obstet Gynecol Reprod Biol. 2021;258:437-42.
2. Moise KJ. The usefulness of middle cerebral artery Doppler assessment in the treatment of the fetus at risk for anemia. Am J Obstet Gynecol. 2008;198(2): 161.e1-161.e4.

Hematological Disorders

Saswati Mukhopadhyay

STATION 1.

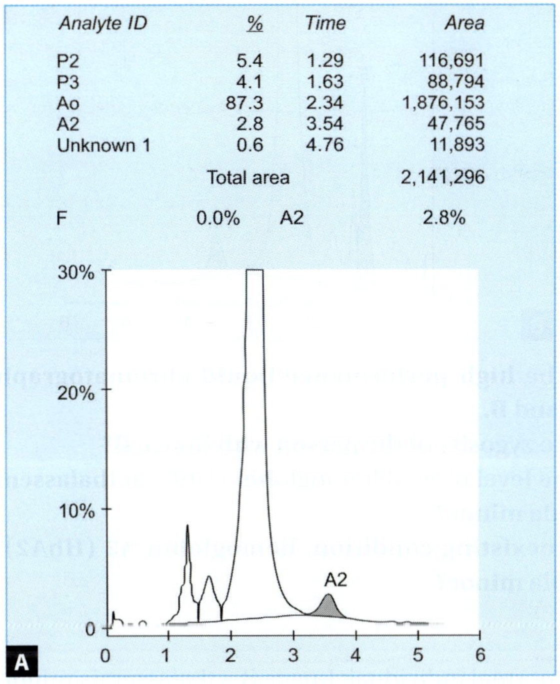

Analyte ID	%	Time	Area
P2	5.4	1.29	116,691
P3	4.1	1.63	88,794
Ao	87.3	2.34	1,876,153
A2	2.8	3.54	47,765
Unknown 1	0.6	4.76	11,893
	Total area		2,141,296
F	0.0%	A2	2.8%

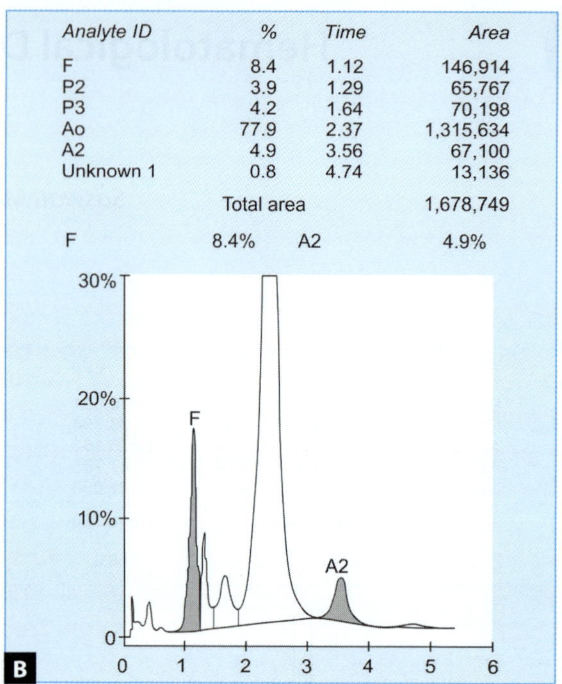

1. **Identify the high-performance liquid chromatography (HPLC) in images A and B.**
2. **What is the zygosity of the person with image B?**
3. **What is the level of fetal hemoglobin (HbF) in thalassemia major and thalassemia minor?**
4. **In what coexisting condition, hemoglobin A2 (HbA2) is normal in thalassemia minor?**

Ans.

1. Image A—normal individual; Image B—thalassemia minor
2. Image B—heterozygous for thalassemia mutation
3. Thalassemia minor—<5%, thalassemia major—up to 95%
4. Coinherited δ-thalassemia, coinherited α-thalassemia, and iron deficiency anemia

SUGGESTED READING

1. Jha R, Jha S. Beta thalassemia—a review. J Pathol Nepal. 2014;4:663-71.

STATION 2.

1. **What is the blood image of thalassemia?**
2. **Name another condition with similar blood image.**
3. **At which age in a thalassemia patient is this blood image found?**
4. **What is the treatment for correcting anemia in a thalassemia patient?**

Ans.

1. Microcytic hypochromic anemia, anisocytosis, basophilic stippling, Pappenheimer bodies, target cells, and circulating nucleated red cells.
2. Iron deficiency anemia
3. After 6 months of age
4. Blood transfusion at regular intervals, with iron chelators.

SUGGESTED READING

1. Lee YK, Kim HJ, Lee K, Park SH, Song SH, Seong MW, et al. Recent progress in laboratory diagnosis of thalassemia and hemoglobinopathy: a study by the Korean Red Blood Cell Disorder Working Party of the Korean Society of Hematology. Blood Res. 2019;54(1):17-22.

STATION 3.

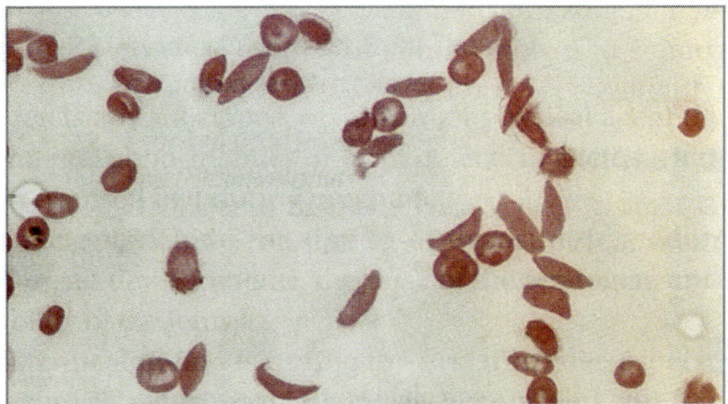

1. **Describe the peripheral smear.**
2. **What is the disease with this type of peripheral smear?**
3. **Which genetic mutation causes this disease?**
4. **What is the inheritance pattern?**

Ans.

1. Red blood cells (RBCs) are pale, some are nucleated, and some are distorted into sickle shape.
2. Sickle cell disease
3. A single base-pair point mutation (GAG to GTG) results in the substitution of the amino acid glutamic acid (hydrophilic) to valine (hydrophobic) in the 6th position of the β-chain of hemoglobin referred to as hemoglobin S, this mutation is in *HBB* gene.
4. Autosomal recessive pattern

SUGGESTED READING

1. Inusa BPD, Hsu LL, Kohli N, Patel A, Ominu-Evbota K, Anie KA, et al. Sickle Cell Disease-Genetics, Pathophysiology, Clinical Presentation and Treatment. Int J Neonatal Screen. 2019;5(2):20.

STATION 4. **A lady came for preconceptional counseling. Her previous child, a 6-year-old boy, with anemia, fever, and dehydration was admitted with sudden pain in the legs. The child frequently suffers from respiratory infections and complains of pain in the legs, upper abdomen, and chest. She sought advice about recurrence risk in her next pregnancy.**

1. **What was the diagnosis of her previous child?**
2. **What was the cause of pain in his legs?**
3. **Give two clinical features of this disease.**
4. **Name two disease modifiers of this disease.**

Ans.

1. Sickle cell disease
2. Vaso-occlusion of microcirculation by sickled RBC causes stimulation of nociceptive nerve fibers thus pain in the organ
3. Recurrent infection and anemia
4. Coinheritance of α-thalassemia (decreases severity) and level of HbF (greater HbF, lesser severity)

SUGGESTED READING

1. Inusa BPD, Hsu LL, Kohli N, Patel A, Ominu-Evbota K, Anie KA, et al. Sickle Cell Disease-Genetics, Pathophysiology, Clinical Presentation and Treatment. Int J Neonatal Screen. 2019;5(2):20.

STATION 5.

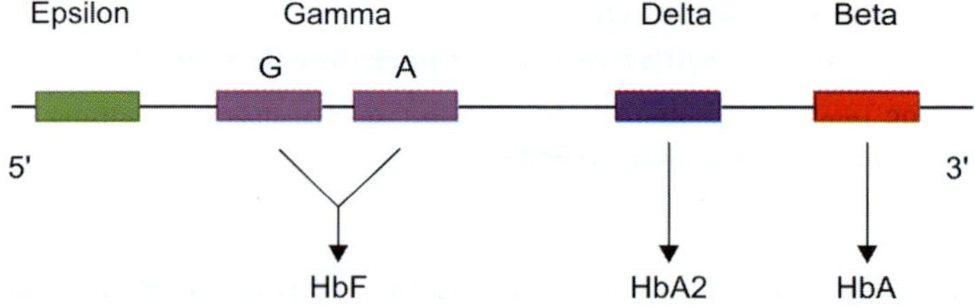

1. **Describe the above image.**
2. **What is hemoglobin E β-thalassemia?**
3. **What is the severity of anemia in hemoglobin E β-thalassemia?**
4. **In what concomitant conditions of the partner would prenatal testing be indicated?**
5. **Can prenatal testing of thalassemia be done, if so, when?**

Ans.

1. This is a schematic drawing of *HBB* gene, showing gene clusters—from 5 prime end to 3 prime end—*epsilon* gene, *gamma* gene, *delta* gene, and *beta* gene.

2. This is a type of compound heterozygous thalassemia, carrying both E mutation and β-mutation in two different alleles.
3. Ranges from severe (hemoglobin 4–5 g/dL) to mild and moderate (a hemoglobin 9–12 g/dL and 6–7 g/dL, respectively).
4. β-thalassemia, α-thalassemia, sickle cell, and Hb D-Punjab
5. Prenatal testing can be done if both parents mutation of *HBB* gene are known, by Sanger sequencing of *HBB* gene, using chorionic villus sampling or amniocentesis.

SUGGESTED READING

1. Keohane EM, Otto CN, Walenga JM. Rodak's Hematology: Clinical Principles and Applications, 6th edition. Philadelphia: Elsevier; 2020.

STATION 6. This consanguineous couple, with two previous daughters and ongoing pregnancy of 18 weeks, came to the outpatient department (OPD) with the following mutation analysis report, after undergoing amniocentesis.

Sample	*Mutations*
Father	HBB c.92G>C
Mother	HBB c.92 + 5G>C
Daughter 1[a]	HBB c.92G>C
	HBB c.92 + 5G>C
Daughter 2[a]	HBB c.92 + 5G>C
Amniotic fluid	HBB c.92G>C
	HBB c.92G>C

[a]Information given by the clinician.

1. **Will daughter one require blood transfusion?**
2. **Will daughter two have anemia?**
3. **What test was done to get the information from amniotic fluid?**
4. **What is the status of the fetus in present pregnancy?**

Ans.

1. Yes, she has thalassemia major.
2. Daughter two may/may not have anemia. If she has anemia, it will be very mild.
3. Sanger sequencing of *HBB* gene, using amniotic fluid.
4. Fetus is compound heterozygous thalassemia major.

SUGGESTED READING

1. Muncie HL Jr, Campbell J. Alpha and beta thalassemia. Am Fam Physician. 2009;80(4):339-44.

STATION 7. The parents of this child came for preconceptional counseling. Their child of 8 years had presented to pediatric OPD with chief complaints of easy fatigability, decreased appetite, and progressive abdominal distension for 6 months. She had severe pallor and massive hepatosplenomegaly. Peripheral blood smear (PBS) showed signs of microcytic hypoplastic anemia.

High-performance liquid chromatography of father, mother, and child had been done. Their HPLC reports are as shown below:

	HbA	*HbA2*	*HbF*	
Father	77.4%	12.0%	1.7%	
Mother	78.3%	11.9%	1.4%	
Child	0.3%	25%	74.4%	Two peaks noted, HbA2 and HbF

1. **What is the diagnosis of the child?**
2. **How will you offer prenatal testing in next pregnancy?**
3. **What sample and when should be sent for prenatal testing?**
4. **What could be an alternative explanation for the HPLC image of parents?**

Ans.

1. Homozygous Hb Lepore/HbE. Child has a rare type of hemoglobinopathy, with hemoglobin made of hybrid or fused globin chain comprising a δ-chain and a β-chain. This abnormal globin chain is formed by unequal crossing over between the δ- and β-*globin* genes resulting in a 7.4 kb deletion between the δ- and β-*globin* genes.
2. As this is a fusion type of thalassemia, mutation in the next fetus to be confirmed by Sanger sequencing and multiplex ligation-dependent probe amplification (MLPA) of the *HBB* gene.
3. Chorionic villus sampling at 13 weeks in a subsequent pregnancy
4. HbE if thought of, to be confirmed by sequencing *HBB* gene in the fetus and both parents.

SUGGESTED READING

1. Bhusal A, Bhandari S, Seth T, Sah RP. Homozygous Lepore Syndrome: A case report. Ann Med Surg (Lond). 2022;80:104168.

STATION 8.

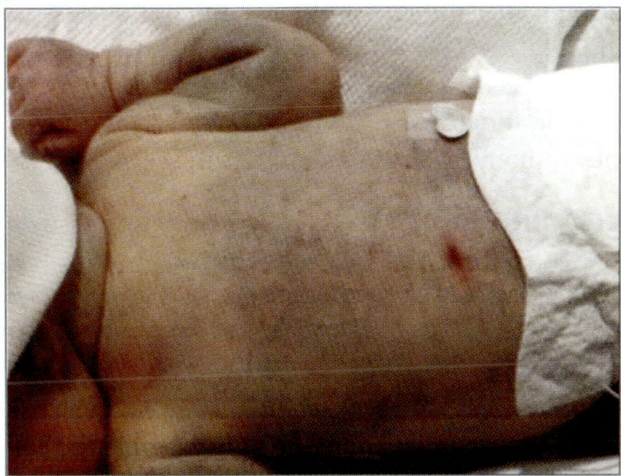

This neonate had petechiae (generalized) from the time of delivery, progressively increasing. Bluish discoloration in arms and back noticed, indicating hemorrhage under skin. Complete blood count (CBC) report shows thrombocytopenia (<50,000/mL), similar symptoms noted in previous two siblings in early infancy, self-corrected.

1. **What is the provisional diagnosis?**
2. **How can it be confirmed?**
3. **What are the complications of this disorder?**
4. **How to offer prenatal diagnosis?**

Ans.

1. Fetal and neonatal alloimmune thrombocytopenia (FNAIT)
2. Testing the mother's blood for anti-human platelet antigen (anti-HPA) antibodies and HPA genotyping of the mother, father, and newborn. Genotyping of HPAs is done to check for the presence or absence of *HPA* genes.
3. Severe case of FNAIT may have bleeding in major organs, such as the brain, gastrointestinal tract, lungs, or eyes. Severe symptoms can cause death or lead to lifelong disability.
4. The history of a previously affected child, especially if that child developed intracerebral hemorrhage (ICH), is the strongest predictor of recurrence and severity of FNAIT in a future pregnancy.

Fetal HPA group can be obtained by amniocentesis and analysis of cultured amniocytes and should be considered if there is a previously affected child with FNAIT and a heterozygous partner. However, fetal genotyping using cell-free fetal DNA is becoming a more popular choice in order to avoid the invasive procedure, which (at least in theory) may increase the antibody level and potentially the severity of the disease.

SUGGESTED READING

1. Espinoza JP, Caradeux J, Norwitz ER, Illanes SE. Fetal and neonatal alloimmune thrombocytopenia. Rev Obstet Gynecol. 2013;6(1):e15-21.
2. NORD. (2022). Fetal and Neonatal Alloimmune Thrombocytopenia. [online] Available from https://rarediseases.org/rare-diseases/fetal-and-neonatal-alloimmune-thrombocytopenia/ [Last accessed May, 2025].

STATION 9.

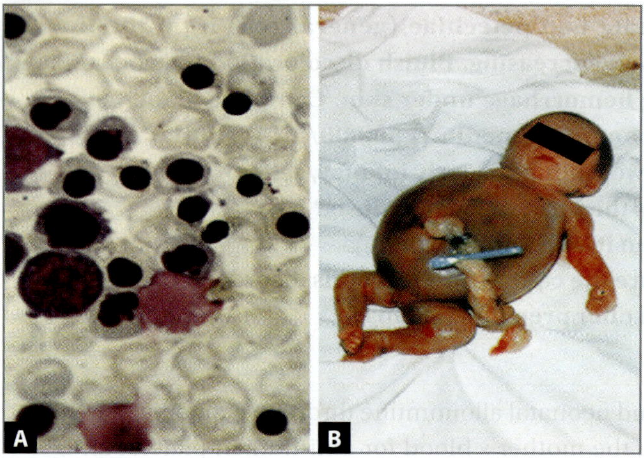

Image A: Peripheral blood film with immature red-cell precursors and hypochromic, microcytic, red cells showing anisocytosis and poikilocytosis

Image B: Stillborn hydropic infant

1. **Which hemoglobinopathy can give rise to the clinical image shown above?**
2. **What is the genetic test to confirm this hemoglobinopathy?**
3. **What is the genotype and hemoglobin present in this fetus?**
4. **How will you offer prenatal testing in a subsequent pregnancy?**

Ans.

1. Hemoglobin Bart (Hb Bart) syndrome
2. MLPA for the α-thalassemia genes
3. *Genotype*—homozygous deletion of both HbA1 and HbA2 on both chromosomes; --/--; *Hemoglobin* present—Hb Bart 85–90% and

hemoglobin Portland (Hb Portland) 10–15%. Hb Bart—four γ-globin chains (γ4) and Hb Portland. Two ζ-globin chains and two γ-globin chains (ζ2γ2).

4. Prenatal testing in next pregnancy, USG at 14 weeks, showing hydrops fetalis and chorionic villus biopsy and MLPA of HbA1 and HbA2 to see the homozygous deletions in the fetus

SUGGESTED READING

1. Tamary H, Dgany O. Alpha-Thalassemia. In: Adam MP, Feldman J, Mirzaa GM, et al., (Eds). GeneReviews® [Internet]. Seattle (WA): University of Washington, Seattle; 1993-2025.

STATION 10.

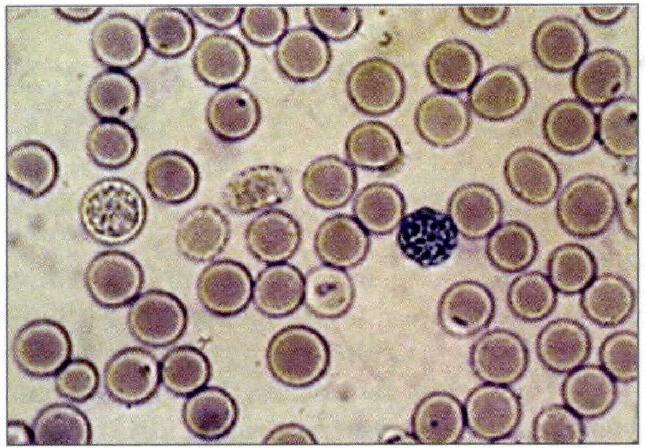

Red blood cell supravital stain following incubation of fresh blood smears with 1% brilliant cresyl blue for 1–3 hours.

1. **Describe the peripheral smear.**
2. **What is the disease?**
3. **What is the genotype of this patient?**
4. **What is the hemoglobin analysis of this disease?**

Ans.

1. Hemoglobin H (HbH) inclusions (β4 tetramers) deposit in RBCs
2. HbH disease (α-thalassemia phenotype)
3. Biallelic pathogenic variants in both *HbA1* and *HbA2* genes that result in deletion/inactivation of three α-globin genes (--/-α)
4. HbA 60–90%, HbH 0.8–40%, and Hb Bart 2–5%

SUGGESTED READING

1. Fucharoen G, Yooyen K, Chaibunruang A, Fucharoen S. A newly modified hemoglobin H inclusion test as a secondary screening for α(0)-thalassemia in Southeast Asian populations. Acta Haematol. 2014;132(1):10-4.

STATION 11. **A male neonate developed jaundice in the first 24 hours of life, with a history of a brother who also developed neonatal jaundice. Tandem mass spectrometry (TMS) report done by newborn screening indicated glucose-6-phosphate dehydrogenase (G6PD) deficiency.**

1. **What is the inheritance pattern of G6PD deficiency?**
2. **Name two drugs which can precipitate jaundice in these patients.**
3. **What is the neonatal complication of G6PD deficiency?**
4. **What is the treatment in neonatal period for jaundice due to G6PD deficiency?**

Ans.

1. X-linked recessive
2. Chloroquine and primaquine
3. Kernicterus
4. Phototherapy, in severe cases—exchange transfusion

SUGGESTED READING

1. Richardson SR, O'Malley GF. Glucose-6-Phosphate Dehydrogenase Deficiency. In: StatPearls [Internet]. Treasure Island (FL): StatPearls Publishing; 2025.

STATION 12. **A couple came for preconceptional counseling. They had previous baby with neonatal jaundice, failure to grow, anemia, and splenomegaly. Peripheral blood film showed pale round RBC. The husband also had complaints of easy fatigability, moderate anemia, and his peripheral blood image showed pale round RBCs. His Hb was 9 g/dL.**

1. **Identify the disease.**
2. **Describe the blood image.**
3. **What is the inheritance pattern?**
4. **What is the cause of anemia in this disorder?**

Ans.

1. Hereditary spherocytosis
2. The RBCs are spherical and pale.
3. Autosomal dominant (75%) and autosomal recessive (25%)
4. Deficiency of RBC membrane proteins—loss of RBC membrane stability and deformability—so decreased RBC lifespan and increased clearance in spleen.

SUGGESTED READING

1. Zamora EA, Schaefer CA. Hereditary Spherocytosis. In: StatPearls [Internet]. Treasure Island (FL): StatPearls Publishing; 2025.

STATION 13. **A 20-year-old primigravida patient with *20 weeks gestation* with known case of thalassemia major, receiving blood transfusion at**

monthly frequency developed cardiac problems such as heart failure, peripheral edema, and respiratory distress. ECG showed ventricular tachycardia.

1. **What is the cause of cardiomyopathy?**
2. **What can be done to prevent cardiomyopathy in this patient?**
3. **What complications can occur in other organs in this patient?**
4. **What is the diagnostic evaluation in this case?**

Ans.

1. Iron overload in the heart following repeated blood transfusions
2. Iron chelators to be given prior to transfusion—deferoxamine.
3. Hepatic fibrosis, hepatic carcinoma, endocrine—thyroid disorders, pancreatic insufficiency
4. Serum ferritin levels (>1,000 μg/L), cardiac, pancreatic and hepatic MRI, and ECG

SUGGESTED READING

1. Cianciulli P. Iron chelation therapy in thalassemia syndromes. Mediterr J Hematol Infect Dis. 2009;1(1):e2009034.
2. RCOG. (2014). Management of Beta Thalassaemia in Pregnancy (Green-top Guideline No. 66). [online] Available from https://www.rcog.org.uk/guidance/browse-all-guidance/green-top-guidelines/management-of-beta-thalassaemia-in-pregnancy-green-top-guideline-no-66/ [Last accessed May, 2025].

STATION 14. The recent therapeutic advances have been made for thalassemia and sickle cell anemia in the form of HSCT. This represents an alternative to RBC transfusions and iron chelation therapy.

1. **What is the full form of HSCT?**
2. **What type of cells are the ones described in the above question?**
3. **Who is the ideal donor for HSCT?**
4. **What are the complications of HSCT?**

Ans.

1. Hematopoietic stem cell therapy
2. Pluripotent cells, capable of differentiating to any type of cell
3. Human leukocyte antigen (HLA)-matched sibling. In its absence, haploidentical mother-to-child transplantation
4. Severe acute graft-versus-host disease (GVHD)

SUGGESTED READING

1. Sodani P, Isgrò A, Gaziev J, Paciaroni K, Marziali M, Simone MD et al. T cell-depleted hla-haploidentical stem cell transplantation in thalassemia young patients. Pediatr Rep. 2011;3:e13.

STATION 15.

1. **What gene editing technologies are now the Food and Drug Administration (FDA) approved for thalassemia major?**
2. **Which viral vector is used for gene addition?**
3. **How is the modified gene introduced in the patient?**
4. **What are the two FDA approved gene therapy used for thalassemia?**

Ans.

1. Gene addition using viral vectors introduce a functional β-globin chain and gene knockdown using CRISPR Cas 9 technology to silence *BCL11A* to induce γ-globin chain production.
2. Lentivirus
3. Autologous hematopoietic stem cells are collected from an affected individual, and gene-editing techniques are used to modify the stem cells ex vivo. Individuals undergo conditioning chemotherapy before infusion of genetically modified stem cells.
4. Betibeglogene autotemcel (beti-cel) and Exagamglogene autotemcel (exa-cel)

SUGGESTED READING

1. Locatelli F, Thompson AA, Kwiatkowski JL, Porter JB, Thrasher AJ, Hongeng S, et al. Betibeglogene Autotemcel Gene Therapy for Non-β0/β0 Genotype β-Thalassemia. N Engl J Med. 2022;386(5):415-27.

STATION 16. **A nonconsanguineous couple delivered a boy, who developed recurrent respiratory tract infection (RTI), anemia, and failed to gain weight from early infancy. The father carried a sickle cell trait and mother was a carrier of β-thalassemia.**

1. **What is the provisional diagnosis of this child?**
2. **What is the genotype of this child?**
3. **What prenatal testing should have been done in this pregnancy, and how?**
4. **How can the patient's diagnosis be confirmed?**

Ans.

1. Sickle cell disease
2. Hb S/β0-thalassemia
3. Mutation testing of *HBB* gene (by Sanger sequencing) of fetus by chorionic villus sampling or amniocentesis
4. Mutation testing of *HBB* gene (by Sanger sequencing)

SUGGESTED READING

1. Bender MA, Carlberg K. Sickle Cell Disease. In: Adam MP, Feldman J, Mirzaa GM, Pagon RA, Wallace SE, Amemiya A, editors. GeneReviews® [Internet]. Seattle (WA): University of Washington, Seattle; 1993–2025.

STATION 17. A consanguineous couple came for preconceptional counseling, as two brothers of the wife had died at 3 and 5 years of life, after having recurrent fever, RTI, and she recalls her mother saying that they had hugely distended abdomens. Her parents were also consanguineously married. They wanted to know whether her babies could have early deaths like her brothers.

1. **What counseling should be given to this couple?**
2. **What prenatal test should be advised and when?**
3. **What is an autosomal recessive disorder?**
4. **What is the risk of having an affected offspring in autosomal recessive disorder?**

Ans.

1. They should do couple carrier screening by whole exome sequencing prior to conception.
2. Targeted prenatal testing by Sanger sequencing of fetus, using chorionic villus sampling or amniocentesis
3. Both the genes should carry the mutation to manifest the relevant disease.
4. 25% risk of having the disease.

SUGGESTED READING

1. Aiello LB, Chiatti BD. Primer in Genetics and Genomics, Article 4-Inheritance Patterns. Biol Res Nurs. 2017;19(4):465-72.

STATION 18. A 4th gravida, para 3, came with 12 weeks pregnancy and history of previous two boys with neonatal jaundice. The girl child had no neonatal jaundice. The younger son, born at 34 weeks (preterm), was admitted in neonatal intensive care unit (NICU) and given exchange transfusion. There was one episode of jaundice following malaria in the elder son.

1. **What could be the cause of neonatal and post-malaria jaundice in the children?**
2. **How can it be confirmed?**
3. **What prenatal testing should be advised for this couple?**
4. **What is the likely inheritance pattern for the disease in this case?**

Ans.

1. G6PD deficiency
2. G6PD enzyme assay or mutation analysis of *G6PD* gene
3. In case of confirmed G6PD deficiency, the mother should have chorionic villus sampling at 13 weeks for targeted Sanger sequencing of *G6PD* gene.
4. X-liked recessive pattern

SUGGESTED READING

1. Ravikumar N, Greenfield G. Glucose-6-phosphate Dehydrogenase Deficiency: A Review. Int J Med Stud. 2020;8(3):281-7.

STATION 19. A consanguineous couple came for preconceptional counseling with history of one infant death at 10 months age. There was splenomegaly, jaundice, and severe pallor, requiring frequent blood transfusions. Peripheral blood smear indicated sickled RBC. Death was due to meningitis. No newborn screening (NBS) was done.

1. **What is the diagnosis?**
2. **What vaccine would have benefitted this child?**
3. **What could be the possible genotypes of this infant?**
4. **What should be the advice for this couple?**

Ans.

1. Sickle cell disease
2. Apart from routine vaccination, pneumococcal vaccination
3. HbSS (homozygous), Hb S/C, Hb S/β^+, and Hb S/β^0 (compound heterozygous)
4. Mutation analysis by Sanger sequencing of *HBB* gene for the couple. Prenatal testing of fetus by Sanger sequencing of *HBB* gene for the fetus.

SUGGESTED READING

1. Bender MA, Carlberg K. Sickle Cell Disease. In: Adam MP, Feldman J, Mirzaa GM, Pagon RA, Wallace SE, Amemiya A, editors. GeneReviews® [Internet]. Seattle (WA): University of Washington, Seattle; 1993–2025.

CHAPTER 18

Nonimmune Hydrops Fetalis

Jaya Chawla, K Aparna Sharma

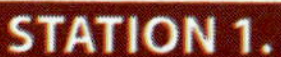

STATION 1.

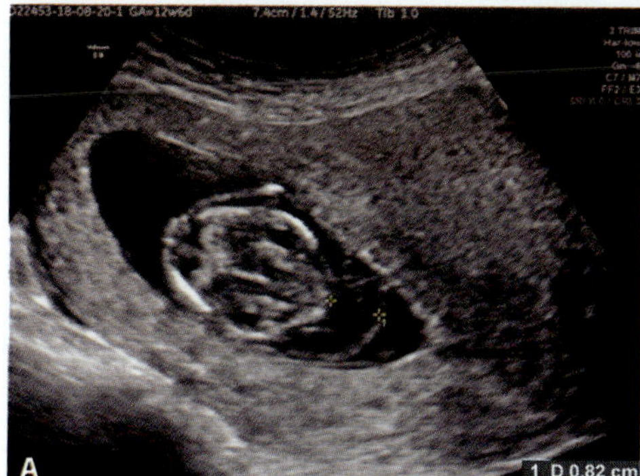

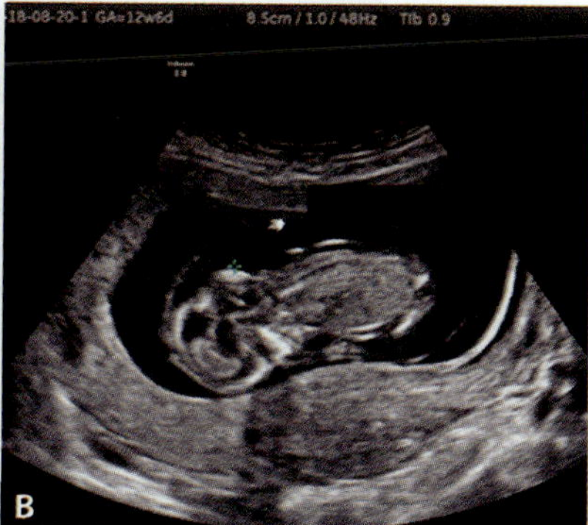

A 32-year-old lady, G2A1, presents with above fetal status at 12 weeks 6 days on nuchal translucency (NT) scan.

The following questions pertain to the images A and B above:

1. **Identify the condition.**
2. **What is the most common etiology of this condition in the first trimester?**
3. **What is the most appropriate prenatal test to be offered at this period of gestation?**
4. **What is the most appropriate genetic test to be offered on the test sample?**

Ans.

1. Cystic hygroma
2. Aneuploidy (70%), Turner's syndrome, and Down syndrome
3. Chorionic villous sampling
4. Fluorescence in situ hybridization (FISH) followed by 750 K resolution chromosomal microarray if FISH is normal.

SUGGESTED READING

1. Khairudin D, Alfirevic Z, Mone F, Navaratnam K. Non-immune hydrops fetalis: a practical guide for obstetricians. Obstet Gynecol. 2023;25:110-20.

STATION 2.

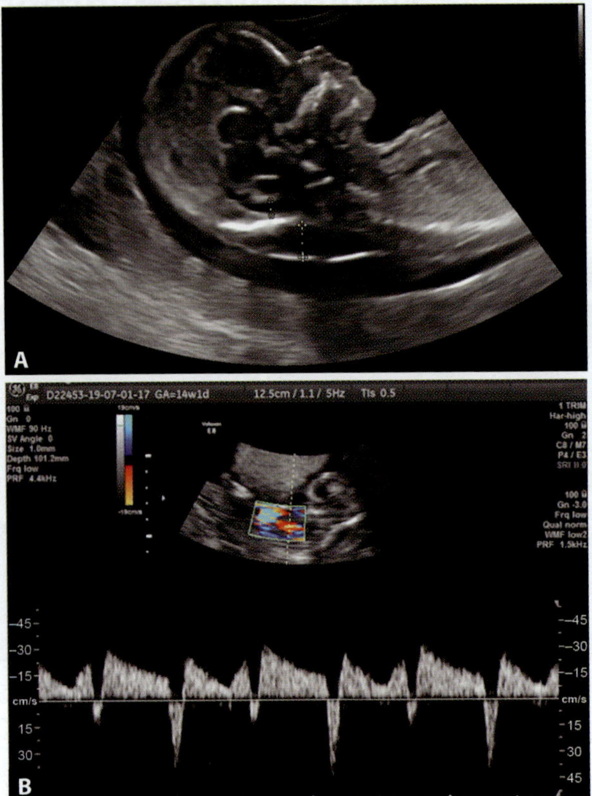

A 28-year-old primigravida with above NT scan findings has persistence of raised nuchal fold thickness in second trimester anomaly scan. Her FISH and chromosomal microarray analysis (CMA) are normal.

1. **Identify the abnormality in the images A and B above.**
2. **What could be the possible etiology? Name one genetic syndrome associated with this condition.**
3. **What genetic tests should now be offered to diagnose the underlying genetic disorder?**
4. **What is the incremental yield of the test offered in question 3 above in identifying the genetic abnormality after a normal karyotype and chromosomal microarray?**
5. **Is noninvasive prenatal screen (NIPS) a valid option in the workup of this case?**

Ans.

1. Raised NT and a wave reversal in ductus venosus (DV)
2. Single gene disorders, e.g., Noonan syndrome

3. Whole exome sequence
4. 29%
5. No

SUGGESTED READING

1. Khairudin D, Alfirevic Z, Mone F, Navaratnam K. Non-immune hydrops fetalis: a practical guide for obstetricians. Obstet Gynecol. 2023;25:110-20.

STATION 3.

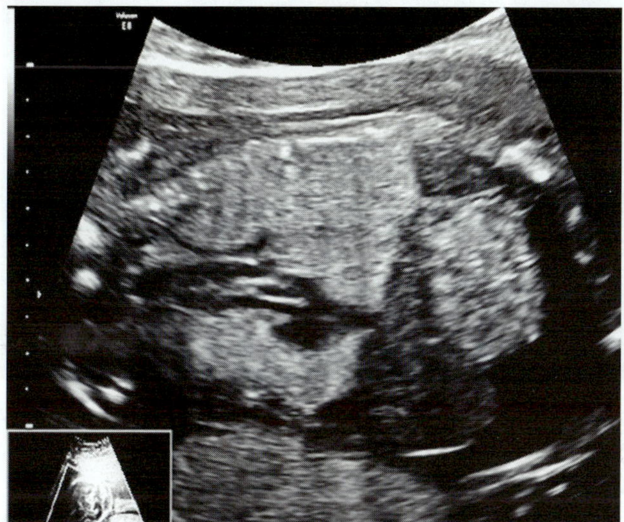

A 27-year-old G2P1L1 patient presents with 22 weeks pregnancy showing above ultrasound findings in addition to scalp edema measuring 5.3 mm.

1. **What are the ultrasound findings shown in the image above?**
2. **What is your provisional diagnosis based on these findings?**
3. **What possible etiologies could lead to this presentation?**
4. **Name three syndromes associated with this condition.**
5. **Name one intervention that can be used to salvage the fetus in the above case.**

Ans.

1. Hyperechoic uniformly bulging lungs everting the diaphragm and mesocardia.
2. Congenital high airway obstruction syndrome (CHAOS)
3. Laryngeal web, laryngeal atresia, tracheal atresia, and laryngeal cysts
4. Fraser syndrome, short-rib polydactyly syndrome, cri du chat syndrome, and velocardiofacial defect
5. Ex utero intrapartum treatment (EXIT)

SUGGESTED READING

1. Moussaoui KE, Slaoui A, Baidada A, Kharabch A. Syndrome congénital d´obstruction des voies aériennes supérieures (syndrome du CHAOS): à propos d'un cas [Congenital high airway obstruction syndrome (CHAOS): a case report]. Pan Afr Med J. 2021;38:1.

STATION 4.

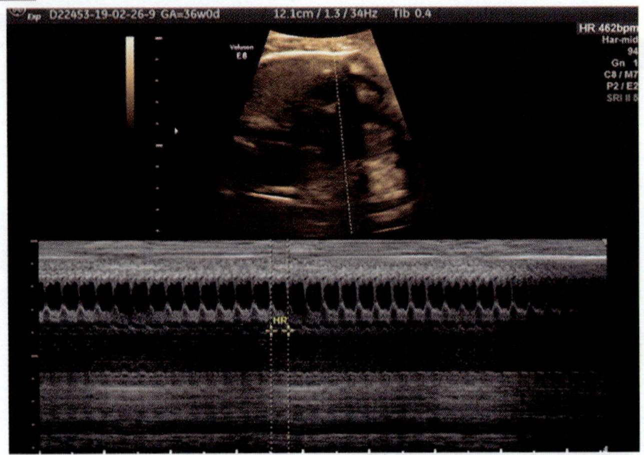

A primi 35 weeks 5 days gestation presents with nonimmune hydrops and the above heart rate pattern.

1. **Identify the disorder of cardiac rate and rhythm.**
2. **Name two drugs that can be used to manage this condition in utero along with their first-line routes of administration.**
3. **What prenatal intervention can be offered to refractory cases?**
4. **Name one modality of postnatal management.**

Ans.

1. Atrial flutter with varying conduction 1:1 to 1:2
2. Oral digoxin and oral β-blockers such as sotalol or flecainide or amiodarone
3. Intramuscular digoxin, intraperitoneal/intra-amniotic amiodarone
4. Cardioversion

SUGGESTED READING

1. Lin PH, Wu HH, Tsai HD, Hsieh CT. Successful treatment of atrial flutter by repeated intraperitoneal and intra-amniotic injections of amiodarone in a fetus with hydrops. Taiwan J Obstet Gynecol. 2016;55(3):434-6.

STATION 5.

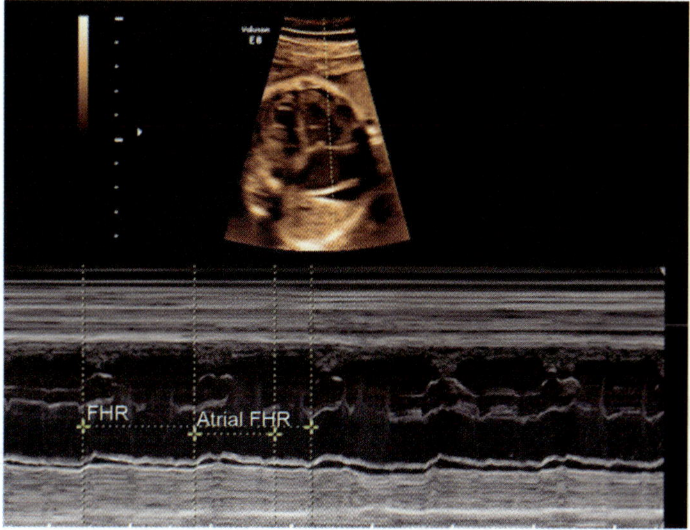

A primigravida woman 22 years of age presents with chronic hypertension, gestational diabetes, malar rash, and nonimmune fetal hydrops along with above ultrasound findings on prenatal scan at 23 weeks of gestation.

1. **Identify the fetal condition shown in the scan above.**
2. **Name the most common maternal medical disorder associated with this condition and the antibodies responsible.**
3. **What are the other possible associations of this condition in the fetus?**
4. **What maternal disease-modifying drug is an essential part of management of this condition.**
5. **What drugs can help ameliorate the fetal symptoms in this case?**
6. **Name one structural malformation of the heart and one syndrome associated with congenital heart block.**
7. **How can women with anti-Rho/anti-La antibodies be monitored for the development of heart block?**

Ans.

1. Congenital atrioventricular block
2. Systemic lupus erythematosus (SLE), maternal anti-Rho, and anti-La antibodies
3. Structural malformations of the heart are most commonly transposition of great vessels and endocardial fibroelastosis

4. Hydroxychloroquine (HCQ) 300 mg a day administered orally to the mother
5. Maternal salbutamol 40 mg/day and steroids (tablet Omnacortil 4 mg/day)
6. Endocardial cushion defects and heterotaxy syndrome
7. With mPR interval

SUGGESTED READING

1. Friedman DM, Kim MY, Copel JA, Llanos C, Davis C, Buyon JP. Prospective evaluation of fetuses with autoimmune-associated congenital heart block followed in the PR Interval and Dexamethasone Evaluation (PRIDE) Study. Am J Cardiol. 2009;103(8):1102-6.

STATION 6.

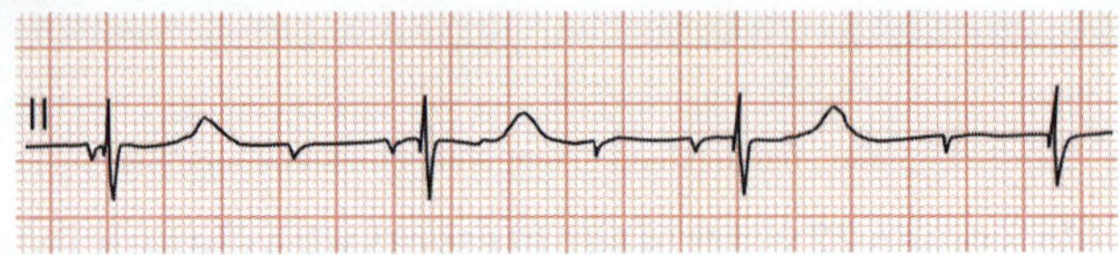

Say yes or no for the following (Questions 1–2):

1. **Congenital heart block of the fetus has four degrees.**
2. **There is orderly progression from first degree to second and so on.**
3. **Name three prognosticating factors for fetal atrioventricular (AV) block.**
4. **Name the postnatal intervention that can be offered to salvage babies with complete congenital heart block.**
5. **What is the risk of developing recurrence when a prior pregnancy has been affected by fetal autoimmune congenital heart block?**

Ans.

1. No, it has three
2. No
3. Heart rate below 55 beats/min, development of fetal hydrops and endocardial fibroelastosis, early gestational age at onset of heart block, and degree of tricuspid regurgitation
4. Permanent pacemaker
5. 17–22%

SUGGESTED READING

1. Melim C, Pimenta J, Areias JC. Congenital atrioventricular heart block: From diagnosis to treatment. Rev Port Cardiol. 2022;41(3):231-40.

STATION 7.

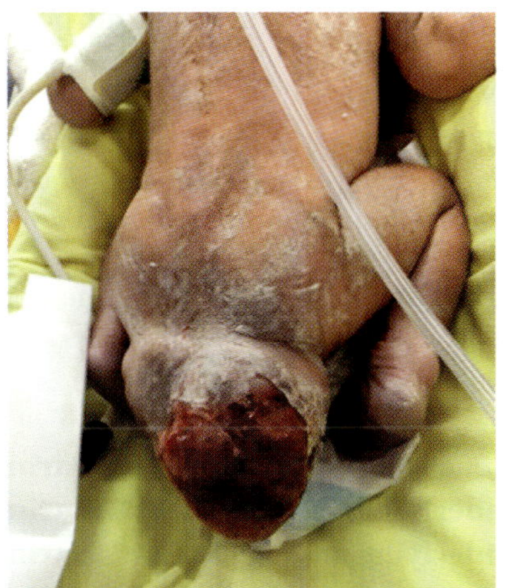

1. **Identify the above fetal condition that can lead to fetal nonimmune hydrops.**
2. **What are the prenatal markers of poor prognosis in this disorder?**
3. **What is the prenatal classification of this disorder? Does it carry prognostic significance?**
4. **What prenatal evaluation is warranted in this case?**
5. **What is the differential diagnosis?**
6. **What are the obstetric concerns of this case?**

Ans.

1. Sacrococcygeal teratoma (SCT)
2. High tumor volume index (TVI) = total tumor volume/estimated fetal weight (EFW) >0.16, total tumor volume to head volume ratio >1, fast growth rate, and predominantly solid tumors with high vascularity gestational age at prenatal diagnosis <30 weeks
3. *Altman classification type I:* Tumors predominantly external (45%); type II: tumors presenting externally but with a significant intrapelvic portion (35%); type III: tumors predominantly intrapelvic (10%); type IV: presacral tumors without an external component (10%). No.
4. Assess tumor volume, its relation to head volume or EFW, and vascularization index. Assess for signs of fetal hydrops (high output cardiac failure due to shunting of blood), fetal anemia (due to intratumor hemorrhage), rate of growth of the tumor, placentomegaly, and polyhydramnios.
5. Spinal dysraphism. Mass of SCT is usually placed more caudally between the coccyx and the anus displacing the latter anteriorly. Mass of spinal dysraphism is placed between sacrum and coccyx.

6. Preterm labor, cesarean births in order to deliver the tumor unruptured (sometimes classical cesarean), and traumatic postpartum hemorrhage.

SUGGESTED READING

1. Özsürmeli M, Büyükkurt S, Sucu M, Arslan E, Mısırlıoğlu S, Akçabay Ç, et al. Evaluation of prenatally diagnosed fetal sacrococcygeal teratomas: A case series of seventeen pregnancies from South-central Turkey. Turk J Obstet Gynecol. 2020;17(3):170-4.
2. Phi JH. Sacrococcygeal Teratoma: A Tumor at the Center of Embryogenesis. J Korean Neurosurg Soc. 2021;64(3):406-13.

STATION 8.

1. **Most common underlying etiology for NIH in trimester 1 is________.**
2. **Most common underlying etiology for NIH in trimester 2 is________.**
3. **Most common underlying etiology for NIH in trimester 3 is________.**
4. **The single most important predictor of live birth in NIH is ________.**

Ans.

1. Chromosomal abnormalities
2. Congenital infections
3. Cardiac malformations
4. *Gestational age at presentation:* More the gestational age at presentation, more the live birth rate (LBR).

SUGGESTED READING

1. Sileo FG, Kulkarni A, Branescu I, Homfray T, Dempsey E, Mansour S, et al. Non-immune fetal hydrops: etiology and outcome according to gestational age at diagnosis. Ultrasound Obstet Gynecol. 2020;56(3):416-21.

STATION 9. **A 34-year-old, G4P3L1, at 22 weeks. Parents first cousins. History of two prior pregnancy losses at 24 and 26 weeks respectively to fetal hydrops (karyotype normal in both). Her maternal mean corpuscular volume (MCV) is 74 fL. She has pericardial effusion, ascites, pleural effusion, and skin edema in the fetus. No gross malformation. Indirect Coombs test (ICT) and serology for TORCH (toxoplasmosis, other infections, rubella, cytomegalovirus, herpes simplex), parvovirus, and syphilis are negative. FISH and CMA are normal.**

1. **What should be the next investigation in this case?**
2. **What abnormality can be suspected in the fetus with maternal MCV shown above?**
3. **What therapeutic intervention can potentially salvage the baby?**
4. **What prenatal genetic test should be offered to clinch the diagnosis in this case?**
5. **What are the postnatal management options for babies with this disorder?**

Ans.

1. Middle cerebral artery (MCA) peak systolic velocity (PSV)
2. α-thalassemia. With a microcytic hypochromic blood picture in the absence of iron deficiency and normal HbA2 in HPLC in both parents of offsprings with recurrent hydrops should incite molecular testing for α-thalassemia.
3. Intrauterine transfusion
4. Mutation testing of both parents for α-thalassemia gene mutation followed by chorionic villus sampling (CVS) at 11–13 weeks gestation.
5. Hematopoietic stem cell transplant (HSCT) and serial blood transfusions

SUGGESTED READING

1. Akar M, Dilli D, Dilmen U. A Case of Nonimmune Hydrops Fetalis Caused by Homozygous α-Thalassemia. Turk J Haematol. 2013;30(1):63-6.

STATION 10.

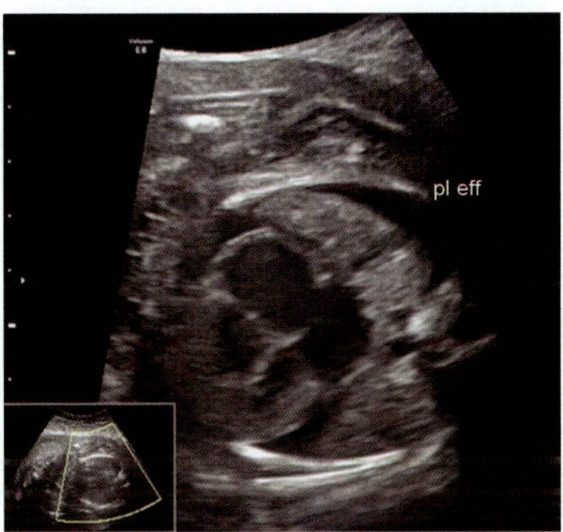

A 25-year-old, G3P1L0A1, Rh negative nonisoimmunized pregnancy, presented at 28 weeks with scalp edema + bilateral pleural effusion/ progressive ascites (AC 14 cm)/pericardial effusion. The couple were in a second-degree consanguineous alliance. There is a history of preterm vaginal delivery of a live baby at 32 weeks with history of exchange transfusion. T1: Dual low risk; No NTNB; mid-trimester anomaly scan performed at 20 weeks shows no abnormality. Echo: NAD.

1. **What investigation should be offered next to decipher the cause of hydrops if karyotype and CMA are normal?**
2. **What will be the finding if inborn errors of metabolism (IEM) are suspected to be the cause?**
3. **What will be the most appropriate genetic test for amniotic fluid analysis in this case?**

4. What is the most important differential diagnosis in second or third trimester NIH in the absence of structural abnormalities after intrauterine infections?

Ans.

1. Ascitic tap and analysis
2. Vacuolated lymphocytes in ascitic tap
3. Whole exome sequencing (WES) or targeted gene panel for NIH
4. In born errors—most commonly lysosomal storage disorders

SUGGESTED READING

1. Mone F, Eberhardt RY, Hurles ME, Mcmullan DJ, Maher ER, Lord J, et al. Fetal hydrops and the Incremental yield of Next-generation sequencing over standard prenatal Diagnostic testing (FIND) study: prospective cohort study and meta-analysis. Ultrasound Obstet Gynecol. 2021;58(4):509-18.

STATION 11.

1. **What is the modality and cut-off for the diagnosis of fetal anemia?**
2. **How should fetal anemia be quantified on Doppler?**
3. **What tests should be offered for infective causes of fetal anemia?**
4. **What noninfective causes of fetal anemia should be considered in the differential diagnosis?**

Ans.

1. MCA-PSV MoM (multiple of the median) >1.5
2. Circle of Willis should be focused in the base of skull view and zoomed such that it occupies at least two-thirds of the screen. MCA Doppler performed keeping the angle of insonation <20°, as close to zero degrees as possible, keeping the sweep speed such that 4–5 wave forms appear on the screen at a time. The maximum PSV of the wave form should be noted. This measurement is repeated three times and the maximum value taken in cm/sec. This value is then converted to MoM from the Mari's chart.
3. PCR for cytomegalovirus (CMV), parvovirus, and toxoplasmosis
4. Rh blood group alloimmunization:
   - Inherited conditions, e.g., hemoglobinopathies like α-thalassemia
   - Acquired conditions, e.g., hemolysis, fetomaternal hemorrhage, or red cell aplasia
   - *IEM:* Glucose-6-phosphate dehydrogenase (G6PD) deficiency, erythrocyte enzymopathies such as pyruvate kinase deficiency, lysosomal storage disorders.

SUGGESTED READING

1. Society for Maternal-Fetal Medicine (SMFM); Norton ME, Chauhan SP, Dashe JS. Society for maternal-fetal medicine (SMFM) clinical guideline #7: nonimmune hydrops fetalis. Am J Obstet Gynecol. 2015;212(2):127-39.

STATION 12.

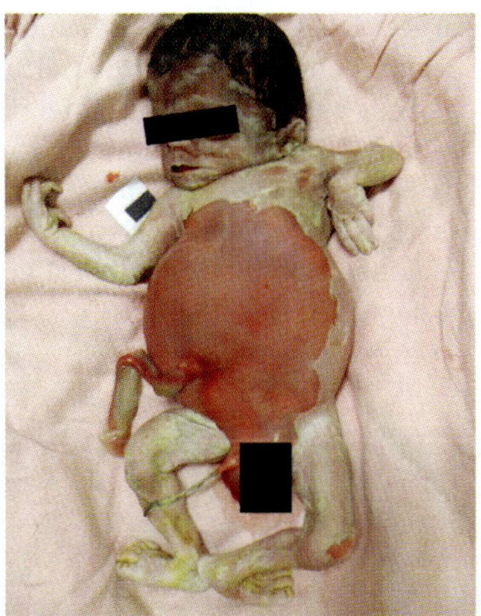

A 26-year-old G2P1L1 nonconsanguineous, in vitro fertilization (IVF) conceived pregnancy (self-gametes), presents with NIH at 31 weeks gestation. There is history of fever without rash 2 months back. Past pregnancy and family history are uneventful. Her combined first trimester screen is low risk and midtrimester anomaly scan is normal.

1. **What is the most likely cause of NIH presenting in this case?**
2. **What should the workup include?**
3. **If the infection screen is positive on maternal serology, what tests should be performed further for fetal infection.**
4. **What are the transplacental therapies available for fetal infections?**

Ans.

1. Infections
2. Detailed anomaly scan along with fetal echocardiography to rule out structural malformations. MCA-PSV to rule out fetal anemia. Infection screen especially TORCH immunoglobulin M (IgM), IgG, and avidity if IgG is positive. FISH and CMA to complete the workup even though genetic abnormalities are relatively rare at this gestation.
3. If maternal serology is positive for recent infection (IgM/IgG positive with low avidity, or evidence of seroconversion then maternal serum PCR and PCR on amniotic fluid specimen for the same infection should be offered. It must be understood that fetal infection can be absent even with a positive amniotic fluid PCR and vice versa.
4. *Toxoplasma:* Tablet pyrimethamine 25 mg OD/sulphadiazine 1 g QID with folinic acid rescue.
   CMV: Tablet valacyclovir 8 g/day in case primary maternal infection is diagnosed in first trimester, until amniocentesis to rule out fetal infection draws results.

SUGGESTED READING

1. Leruez-Ville M, Chatzakis C, Lilleri D, Blazquez-Gamero D, Alarcon A, Bourgon N, et al. Consensus recommendation for prenatal, neonatal and postnatal management of congenital cytomegalovirus infection from the European congenital infection initiative (ECCI). Lancet Reg Health Eur. 2024;40:100892. Erratum in: Lancet Reg Health Eur. 2024;42:100974.
2. Society for Maternal-Fetal Medicine (SMFM); Norton ME, Chauhan SP, Dashe JS. Society for maternal-fetal medicine (SMFM) clinical guideline #7: nonimmune hydrops fetalis. Am J Obstet Gynecol. 2015;212(2):127-39.

STATION 13.

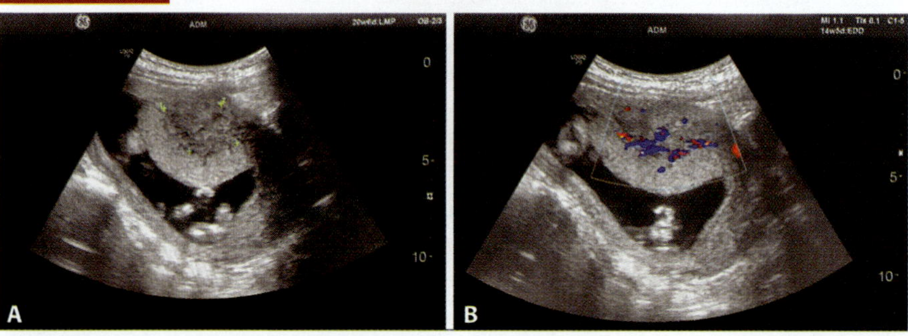

A 25-year-old primigravida presented with a hypoechoic mass in the placenta at the cord insertion site 4 × 3 cm at 14 weeks. Her NT was normal. On serial monitoring the mass grew in size to 9 × 9 cm and the fetus developed hydrops.

1. **Describe the lesion seen in the images A and B and the provisional diagnosis.**
2. **What is the differential diagnosis for the placental pathology shown? What are the features differentiating one from the other?**
3. **What are the histological types of this pathology?**
4. **What intervention can be offered for this placental pathology?**

Ans.

1. Gray-scale findings are well-defined complex echogenic mass different from the rest of placenta. On Doppler, the mass has vascularity. Most likely placental chorioangioma.
2. Placental teratoma, blood clot, and leiomyoma. Chorioangioma is differentiated from the rest by demonstration of vascular channels similar to fetal vessels. Echo pattern of blood clot differs with time, while chorioangioma remains same. Myoma is seen in maternal surface
3. Angiomatous, cellular, and degenerate
4. Laser photocoagulation of the feeding vessel

SUGGESTED READING

1. Kodandapani S, Shreshta A, Ramkumar V, Rao L. Chorioangioma of placenta: a rare placental cause for adverse fetal outcome. Case Rep Obstet Gynecol. 2012;2012:913878.

STATION 14.

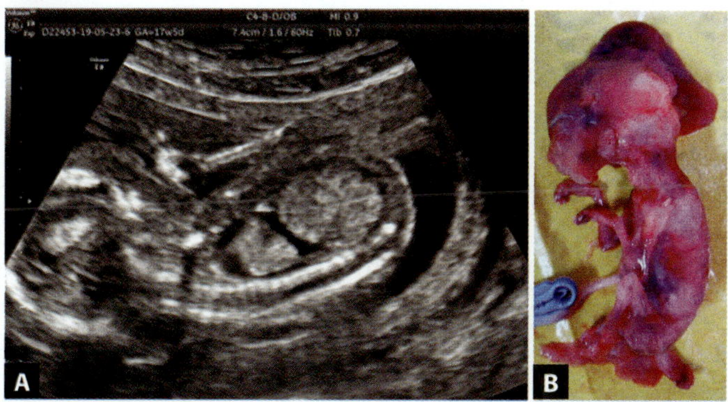

A G3 A2 presented at 17+5 weeks with history of recurrent NIH and absent fetal movements. At the NT scan, NT was 3.9 mm; nasal bone was present and DV showed reversal of "a" wave. No biochemical screen. At the time of the 17 weeks evaluation the baby was found to have pleural effusion, diffuse subcutaneous edema; and no movements despite good cardiac activity. Enzyme levels, quantitative fluorescent polymerase chain reaction (QF-PCR), MCA-PSV, and fetal Echo were normal. Along with features of NIH, both USG and MRI were suggestive of absent stomach bubble. Parents opted for termination of pregnancy. Gross examination as above.

There was history of a previous baby with absent stomach on USG and polyhydramnios.

1. **What are the findings in the images A and B? Possible etiology in view of recurrent NIH.**
2. **What is the prenatal ultrasound classification of this disorder?**
3. **What would be the best strategy for genetic evaluation of this case?**
4. **What investigation can best clinch the diagnosis if parents decline prenatal testing?**
5. **How should these findings be worked up to find the etiology?**

Ans.

1. Loss of muscle mass and contractures. Multiple pterygium syndrome
2. Munich classification:
    - Type I, the most common, with joint affliction is the most common
    - Type II with associated anomalies

- Type III with neuromuscular involvement. These are likely to be life threatening and associated with intellectual disability like fetal akinesia deformation sequence (FADS)

3. Amniocentesis followed by FISH, which if normal followed by CMA, which if abnormal followed by trio WES on stored DNA after thorough genetic counseling.
4. FISH followed by CMA on products of conception
5. If termination of pregnancy is opted: Autopsy
   If prenatal diagnosis is sought: USG (for uterine anomalies, associated fetal abnormalities), 2D and 3D USG (for assessment of lung volume, joint contractures, polyhydramnios, etc.), and fetal MRI to corroborate these findings and for brain abnormalities. Detailed maternal assessment for antibodies suggestive of myasthenia gravis, myotonic dystrophy 1 or drug exposure, and infections. Amniocentesis/CVS (based on gestational age at presentation) followed by tests as above.

SUGGESTED READING

1. Niles KM, Blaser S, Shannon P, Chitayat D. Fetal arthrogryposis multiplex congenita/fetal akinesia deformation sequence (FADS)-Aetiology, diagnosis, and management. Prenat Diagn. 2019;39(9):720-31.

STATION 15. A 23-year-old primigravida with nonconsanguineous alliance presented with progressive fetal pleural and pericardial effusion with diffuse skin edema at 22 weeks gestation. Biometry, measurements in the image above at 16 weeks gestation. The femur length was <2nd centile and thoracic circumference <5th centile. MCA PSV was normal. Her combined first trimester scan was low risk and infection screen was negative.

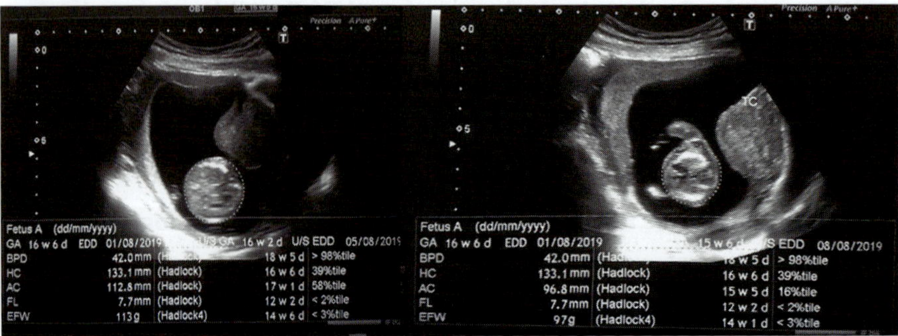

1. **What is the most likely etiology for NIH in this case?**
2. **What parameters are markers of guarded prognosis in this case?**
3. **Should invasive testing be offered in this case?**
4. **If yes, which genetic tests should be offered?**

Ans.

1. Lethal skeletal dysplasia
2. Thoracic circumference to abdominal circumference <0.6, femur length-to-abdominal circumference ratio of <0.16
3. Amniocentesis, if diagnosed in the second trimester
4. A panel should be ordered when the differential diagnosis includes more than one type of skeletal dysplasia. Targeted testing for a specific gene variant can be ordered when a causative variant has been identified in an affected family member or the suspicion of certain skeletal dysplasia is very high on imaging. In case of equivocal results whole exome/genome should be offered.

SUGGESTED READING

1. Savarirayan R, Rossiter JP, Hoover-Fong JE, Irving M, Bompadre V, Goldberg MJ, et al. Best practice guidelines regarding prenatal evaluation and delivery of patients with skeletal dysplasia. Am J Obstet Gynecol. 2018;219(6):545-62.

STATION 16.

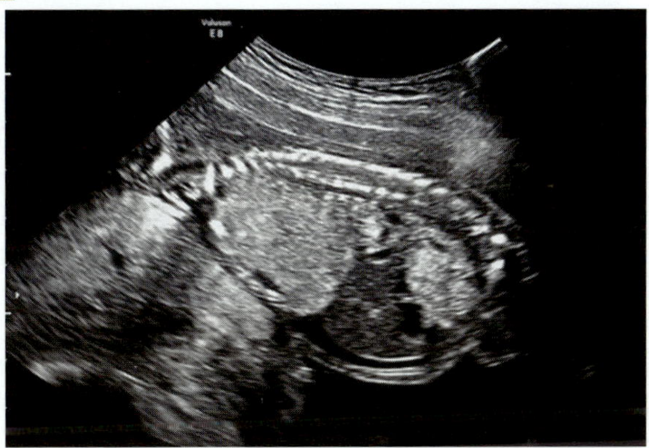

A G2P1L1 19 weeks 2 days pregnancy presents with above ultrasound findings.

1. **What classification can be used to prognosticate the pulmonary lesion shown in the above image?**
2. **What measurements can guide the frequency of surveillance?**
3. **What are the factors determining prognosis in this case?**
4. **What modalities of imaging can be used for prenatal identification of these lesions?**

Ans.

1. Adzick et al: This classification based on size of cysts has prognostic significance.
   - *<5 mm:* Microcysts; homogeneous echogenic appearance, with no visible cystic spaces; when large and grow rapidly, they are

frequently associated with a mediastinal shift, pulmonary hypoplasia, polyhydramnios, and hydrops.
- *>5 mm:* Macrocysts, slow growing, and good prognosis

2. Congenital pulmonary airway malformation (CPAM) volume ratio or CVR
3. *Factors determining prognosis:*
    - The size of the lesion and its secondary effects (mediastinal shift, the extent of pulmonary hypoplasia, polyhydramnios, and cardiovascular compromise)
    - The degree of development of the unaffected lung
    - The presence or absence of other congenital anomalies, such as extralobar sequestration, diaphragmatic hernia, pulmonary hypoplasia, cardiovascular malformation, hydrocephalus, skeletal malformation, jejunal atresia, bilateral renal agenesis/dysgenesis, and Pierre Robin syndrome
4. *Prenatal diagnosis:*
    - *USG*: Screening—hyperechoic, heterogeneous tissue with multiple hypoechoic cysts that may differ in size and number.
    - *MRI*: For morphological and volumetric evaluation of the fetal lung. Homogeneous or heterogeneous T2-hyperintense lesion containing cystic spaces and vascular architectural distortion
    - *Color Doppler:* To differentiate between CPAM and bronchopulmonary sequestration (BPS). The former derives its blood supply from the pulmonary circulation, the latter from the systemic circulation. 2D color Doppler is not 100% sensitive to pick up this detail.

SUGGESTED READING

1. Grewal DS, Singh AK. Congenital cystic adenomatoid malformation: Antenatal ultrasonography features. Med J Armed Forces India. 2018;74(2):177-9.

STATION 17.

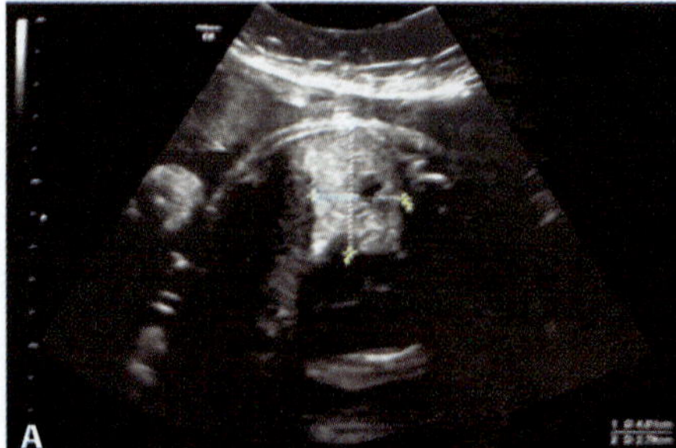

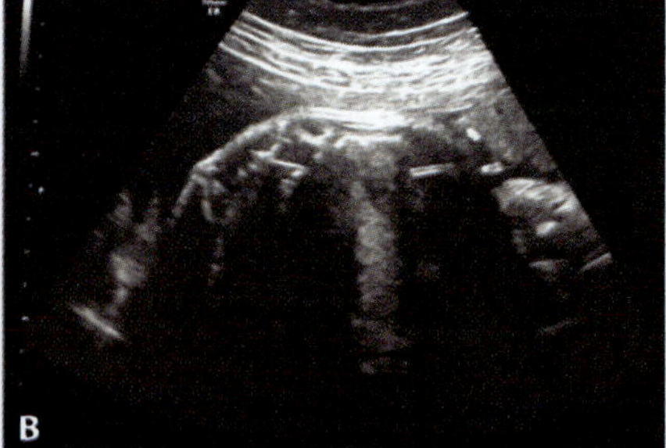

1. **Identify the pulmonary lesion shown in image A and the intervention shown in image B.**
2. **What are the indications of the above intervention?**

3. What is the most common complication of this intervention?

4. What are the other management options for these lesions?

Ans.

1. Image A: CPAM. Image B: Thoracoamniotic shunt (TAS)
2. The criteria for TAS placement are:
   a. Gestational age >20 and <32 weeks (if performed at <20 weeks, it may increase the risks of chest wall deformity)
   b. Nonimmune hydrops
   c. Lesions causing mediastinal deviation, rapidly increasing in size or being associated with increasing polyhydramnios, or rapidly reaccumulating after thoracocentesis
   d. Large bilateral pulmonary embolism (PE) with a suspicion of pulmonary hypoplasia
   e. Macrocystic CPAM with a dominating cyst with CVR >1.6
   f. Absence of other associated major fetal anomalies detected by USG
3. Fetal or uterine trauma, shunt occlusion or displacement, amniotic fluid leakage, sepsis, preterm birth, and intrauterine fetal death
4. A course of maternal steroids, EXIT procedure, thoracocentesis, and maternal-fetal surgery (thoracotomy followed by lobectomy)

SUGGESTED READING

1. David M, Lamas-Pinheiro R, Henriques-Coelho T. Prenatal and Postnatal Management of Congenital Pulmonary Airway Malformation. Neonatology. 2016;110(2):101-15.

STATION 18.

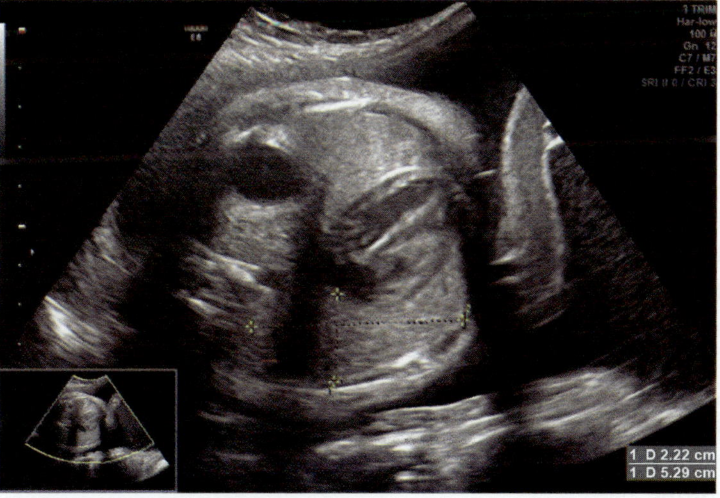

1. **Identify the lesion in the above image and also the measurement taken.**
2. **What is the significance of the measurement taken in the above image?**
3. **What prenatal tests should be offered in this case?**
4. **What intervention can be potentially lifesaving and the trial that proved its efficacy?**
5. **What is the rationale underlying this intervention?**

Ans.

1. Congenital diaphragmatic hernia; contralateral lung dimensions
2. As part of observed to expected lung-to-head ratio to prognosticate CDH
3. Amniocentesis followed by FISH and chromosomal microarray
4. Fetoscopic endotracheal occlusion (FETO) performed between 26 and 30 weeks. TOTAL trial in which neonatal survival was 40% in the FETO group and 15% in the expectant management group.
5. Tracheal occlusion leads to lung growth. Removal of occlusion after a certain period stimulates lung maturation (stimulates type II pneumocytes). Therefore, FETO is offered around 26–30 weeks and the balloon deflated and removed at 34 weeks.

SUGGESTED READING

1. Deprest JA, Nicolaides KH, Benachi A, Gratacos E, Ryan G, Persico N, et al. Randomized Trial of Fetal Surgery for Severe Left Diaphragmatic Hernia. N Engl J Med. 2021;385(2):107-18.

STATION 19. A 34-year-old G2A1 patient presented with an 11 weeks scan report suggestive of single fetal demise. Her prior scan was suggestive of a twin gestation. On scanning at 12 weeks and 3 days, she appears to have two babies in utero one apparently with only the lower half of the body visible but moving, and the other apparently healthy cotwin.

1. **What is your provisional diagnosis for this case?**
2. **What in your opinion should be the chorionicity of this case?**
3. **What complications do you expect in the healthy twin in this case?**
4. **What intervention can help achieve an improved perinatal outcome in this case and when should it be offered?**
5. **What complications should the prospective parents be counseled about prior these interventions?**

Ans.

1. Twin reversed arterial perfusion (TRAP) sequence
2. Monochorionic
3. Hydrops

4. Radiofrequency ablation, intrafetal laser or bipolar cord coagulation, performed at 16–26 weeks gestation. The size of the acardiac twin is prognostic abdominal circumference ratio >50% is one of the determinant factors for fetal intervention besides features of early hydrops in the donor twin or polyhydramnios.
5. Risk of preterm premature rupture of membranes (PPROM), preterm birth, and pregnancy loss

SUGGESTED READING

1. Alshanafey S, Al-Nemer M, Tulbah M, Khan RM, Sahan NA, Mugbel MA, et al. Management of twin reversed arterial perfusion sequence: eight cases over 13 years. Ann Saudi Med. 2023;43(4):199-203.

SECTION 5

Fetal Interventions

19. **Fetal Interventions in Singleton Pregnancies**
Vandana Chaddha

20. **Fetal Interventions in Multifetal Gestations**
Vandana Chaddha

21. **Medical Transplacental Therapy**
K Manikandan, Arpit Jindal

22. **Prophylactic Interventions**
Preeti Parekh Tomar

CHAPTER 19

Fetal Interventions in Singleton Pregnancies

Vandana Chaddha

STATION 1.

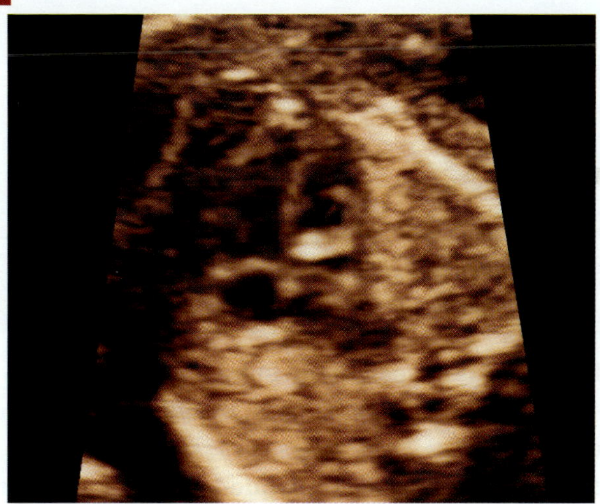

1. **What is the soft marker seen in the image?**
2. **Would you offer invasive testing if it is isolated?**
3. **If the background quadruple test is showing high risk and couple opts for ensuring 100%, that there is no aneuploidy—what would be your intervention of choice at 20 weeks?**
4. **If the above patient is 23 weeks at presentation which genetic test would you definitely like to do?**

Ans.

1. Echogenic foci
2. An isolated echogenic foci in the background of normal biochemical screening may not be significant clinically. However, if they are multiple, biventricular echogenic foci, or have other accompanying soft markers, then further testing may be approached.
3. Intervention of choice at 20 weeks is amniocentesis.
4. Genetic test of choice at 23 weeks is amnio followed by fluorescent in situ hybridization (FISH) or quantitative fluorescent polymerase chain reaction (QF-PCR) so an early report is reassuring. Microarray can also be done as an accompanying test.

SUGGESTED READING

1. American College of Obstetricians and Gynecologists' Committee on Practice Bulletins—Obstetrics, Committee on Genetics, Society for Maternal-Fetal Medicine. Practice Bulletin No. 162: Prenatal Diagnostic Testing for Genetic Disorders. Obstet Gynecol. 2016;127:e108.

STATION 2.

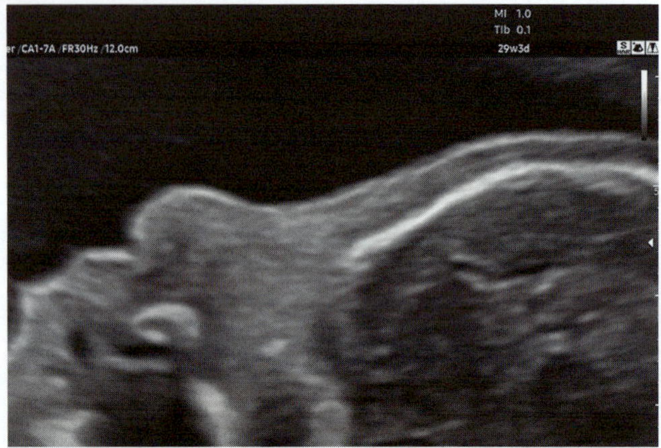

1. **What is the soft marker seen in the image?**
2. **Which is the trimester where it would be of higher significance—first or second trimester?**
3. **If unossified nasal bone is accompanied by aberrant right subclavian artery (ARSA) and increased nuchal fold at 24 weeks—which is the procedure of choice?**
4. **In scenario 3 above, what is the test of choice—FISH/microarray/ both?**

Ans.

1. Soft marker seen in the image is hypo-ossified nasal bone.
2. Higher significance of this soft marker is in the second trimester.
3. The procedure of choice is amniocentesis.
4. Both

SUGGESTED READING

1. American College of Obstetricians and Gynecologists' Committee on Practice Bulletins—Obstetrics, Committee on Genetics, Society for Maternal-Fetal Medicine. Practice Bulletin No. 162: Prenatal Diagnostic Testing for Genetic Disorders. Obstet Gynecol. 2016;127:e108.

STATION 3.

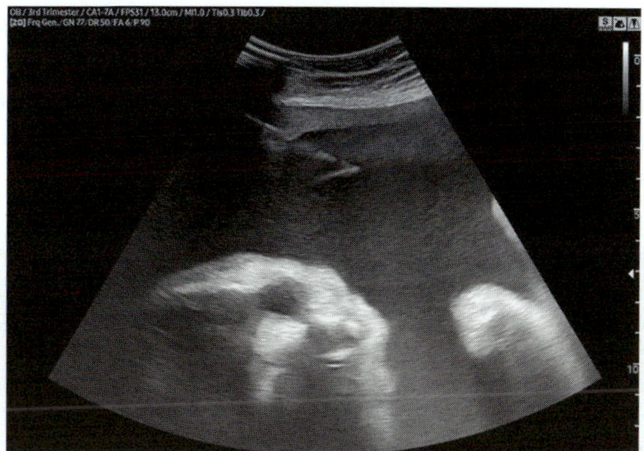

1. **What is the ideal gestation at which amniocentesis is done?**
2. **What is the anesthesia given for amniocentesis?**
3. **How much sample is typically taken for a microarray/FISH?**
4. **What is the turnaround time for microarray/FISH?**

Ans.

1. Above 16 weeks and close to 17 weeks for DNA-based testing.
2. None
3. 20 mL
4. The turnaround time is 2 weeks for microarray and 2–3 days for FISH.

SUGGESTED READING

1. RCOG. Amniocentesis and Chorionic Villus Sampling (Green-top Guideline No. 8). [online] Available from https://content.sph.harvard.edu/wwwhsph/sites/2413/2014/08/Amniocentesis_RoyalCollege_ResArt_2010.pdf 2021 [Last accessed May, 2025].

STATION 4.

1. **What is the risk for repeat sampling after amniocentesis?**
2. **What is the risk for blood stained sample?**
3. **What is the risk for maternal cell contamination?**
4. **What is the risk for confined placental mosaicism?**

Ans.

1. 6%
2. 0.8%
3. 1–2%
4. None

SUGGESTED READING

1. RCOG. Amniocentesis and Chorionic Villus Sampling (Green-top Guideline No. 8). [online] Available from https://content.sph.harvard.edu/wwwhsph/sites/2413/2014/08/Amniocentesis_RoyalCollege_ResArt_2010.pdf 2021 [Last accessed May, 2025].

STATION 5.

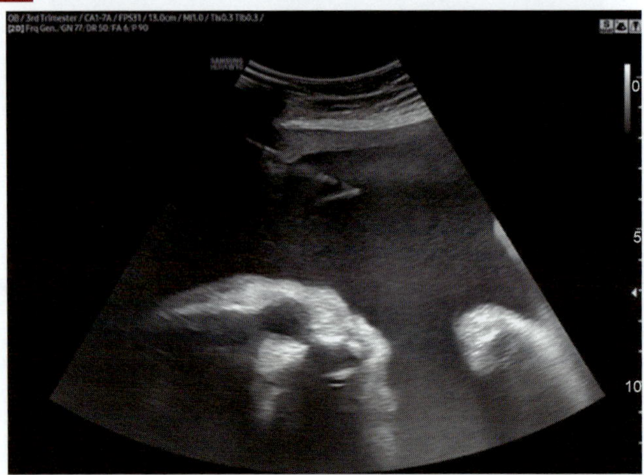

1. **What are the diagnostic indications to do amniocentesis in the third trimester?**
2. **What are the therapeutic indications to do amniocentesis in the third trimester?**
3. **What is the risk for preterm labor?**
4. **What is the risk for culture failure?**

Ans.

1. Fetal structural anomalies, suspected fetal infection, and severe early onset fetal growth restriction.
2. Polyhydramnios
3. 3–4%
4. 10%, increases with gestation

SUGGESTED READING

1. Bardin R, Hadar E, Haizler-Cohen L, Gabbay-Benziv R, Meizner I, Kahana S, et al. Cytogenetic analysis in fetuses with late onset abnormal sonographic findings. J Perinat Med. 2018;46(9):975-82.

2. Daum H, Ben David A, Nadjari M, Zenvirt S, Helman S, Yanai N, et al. Role of late amniocentesis in the era of modern genomic technologies. Ultrasound Obstet Gynecol. 2019;53(5):676-85.
3. O'Donoghue K, Giorgi L, Pontello V, Pasquini L, Kumar S. Amniocentesis in the third trimester of pregnancy. Prenat Diagn. 2007;27(11):1000-4.

STATION 6.

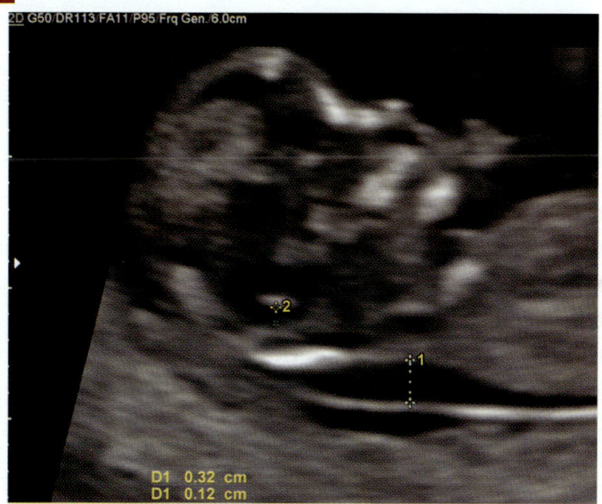

1. **What are the soft markers seen in the image?**
2. **Which is the intervention of choice in the first trimester?**
3. **What is the gestation in which chorionic villous sampling (CVS) is done?**
4. **What is the complication which could happen if done before 10 weeks?**

Ans.

1. Increased nuchal translucency (>95th centile)
2. Chorionic villous sampling
3. 11–13 weeks
4. Limb reduction defects

SUGGESTED READING

1. RCOG. Amniocentesis and Chorionic Villus Sampling (Green-top Guideline No. 8). [online] Available from https://content.sph.harvard.edu/wwwhsph/sites/2413/2014/08/Amniocentesis_RoyalCollege_ResArt_2010.pdf 2021 [Last accessed May, 2025].

STATION 7.

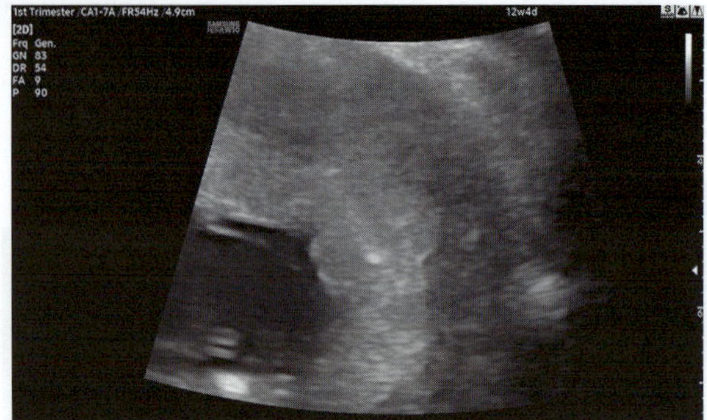

1. **What is the risk for repeat sampling after CVS?**
2. **What is the minimum amount of chorionic villi needed for analysis of a CVS sample?**
3. **What is the risk of maternal cell contamination?**
4. **What is the risk of confined placental mosaicism?**

Ans.

1. 6%
2. 20 µg
3. 1–2%
4. <2%

SUGGESTED READING

1. RCOG. Amniocentesis and Chorionic Villus Sampling (Green-top Guideline No. 8). [online] Available from https://content.sph.harvard.edu/wwwhsph/sites/2413/2014/08/Amniocentesis_RoyalCollege_ResArt_2010.pdf 2021 [Last accessed May, 2025].

STATION 8.

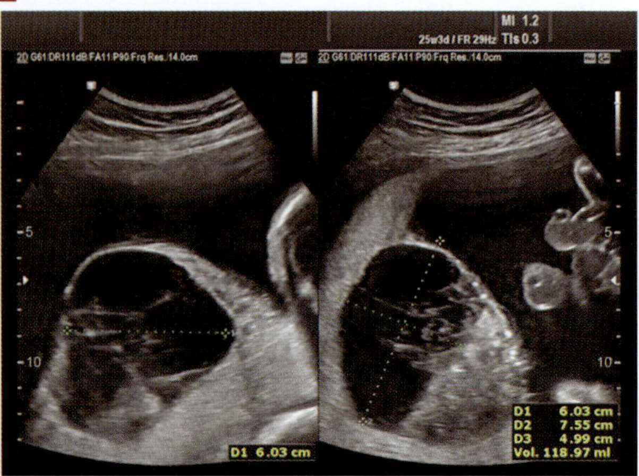

1. **What is the pathology seen in the above image? Why could it lead to hydrops?**
2. **What is the potential complication and the objective measure at which you would intervene?**
3. **What is the intervention of choice if hydrops begins?**
4. **What are the complications involved in these interventions?**

Ans.

1. The pathology seen in the above image is a placental vascular tumor. It can lead to nonimmunological hydrops (NIHF) due to high output heart failure from arteriovenous shunting.
2. The potential complication at which to intervene is hydrops, the risk increases with increasing size of the chorioangioma. For chorioangiomas ≥2, ≥4, ≥6, ≥8, ≥10 cm, the frequency of fetal hydrops was approximately 15, 16, 20, 28, and 52%.
3. Intrauterine embolization, endoscopic laser coagulation of the feeding vessels (when there is adequate distance between the tumor location and the cord insertion), and insertion of coils or plugs to diminish or eliminate flow in the chorioangioma have been successful in pilot studies.
4. The complications involved in these interventions are—fetal bleeding, exsanguination, and fetal death.

SUGGESTED READING

1. Buca D, Iacovella C, Khalil A, Rizzo G, Sirotkina M, Makatsariya A, et al. Perinatal outcome of pregnancies complicated by placental chorioangioma: systematic review and meta-analysis. Ultrasound Obstet Gynecol. 2020;55(4):441-9.
2. Mathis J, Raio L, Baud D. Fetal laser therapy: applications in the management of fetal pathologies. Prenat Diagn. 2015;35(7):623-36.

STATION 9.

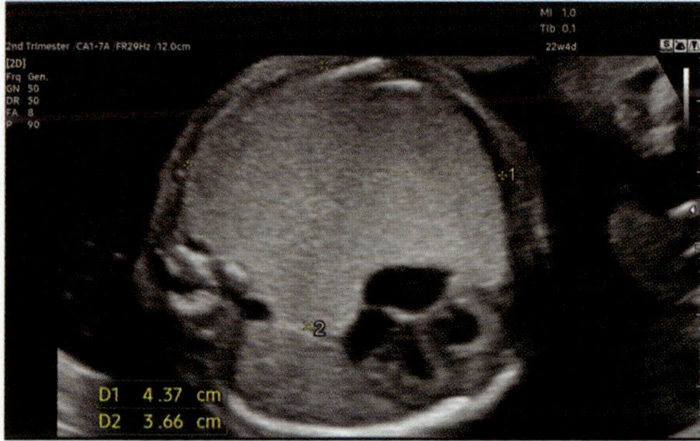

1. **What are the differentials of large white lung?**
2. **Which is the trimester where it would be typically diagnosed first or second?**

3. **Would you give steroids before or after 32 weeks?**
4. **Would you give steroids for cyst volume ratio (CVR) > or < 1.6?**

Ans.

1. Solid congenital pulmonary airway malformation, bronchial obstruction
2. Second trimester
3. Steroids would be given to resolve before 32 weeks.
4. CVR > 1.6

SUGGESTED READING

1. Lecomte B, Hadden H, Coste K, Gallot D, Laurichesse H, Lemery D, et al. Hyperechoic congenital lung lesions in a non-selected population: from prenatal detection till perinatal management. Prenat Diagn. 2009;29(13): 1222-30.
2. Witlox RS, Lopriore E, Oepkes D. Prenatal interventions for fetal lung lesions. Prenat Diagn. 2011;31(7):628-36.

STATION 10.

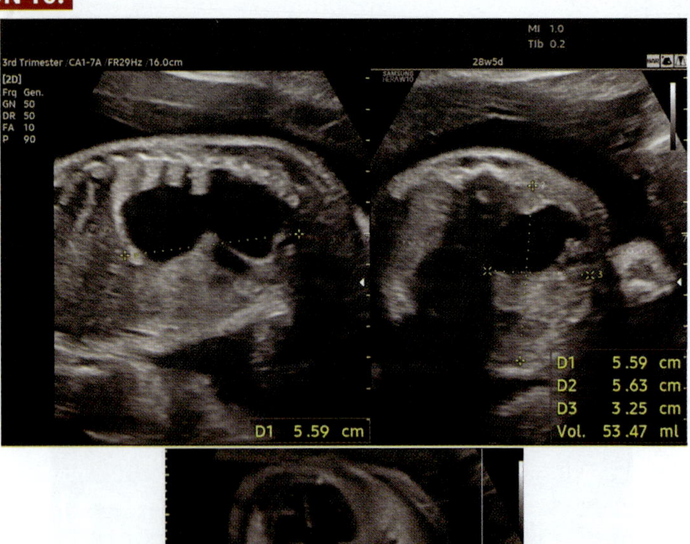

1. **What is the pathology seen in the above image?**
2. **What is the basis of the pathology?**
3. **What is the potential complication and the objective measure at which you would intervene?**
4. **What is the intervention of choice if hydrops begins?**

Ans.

1. Macrocystic congenital cystic adenomatoid malformation (CCAM)
2. Intrapulmonary cystic mass due to overgrowth of terminal bronchioles.
3. Hydrops, CVR > 1.6
4. Thoracoamniotic shunt

SUGGESTED READING

1. Yinon Y, Grisaru-Granovsky S, Chaddha V, Windrim R, Seaward PG, Kelly EN, et al. "Perinatal outcome following fetal chest shunt insertion for pleural effusion." Ultrasound Obstet Gynecol. 2010;36(1):58-64.

STATION 11.

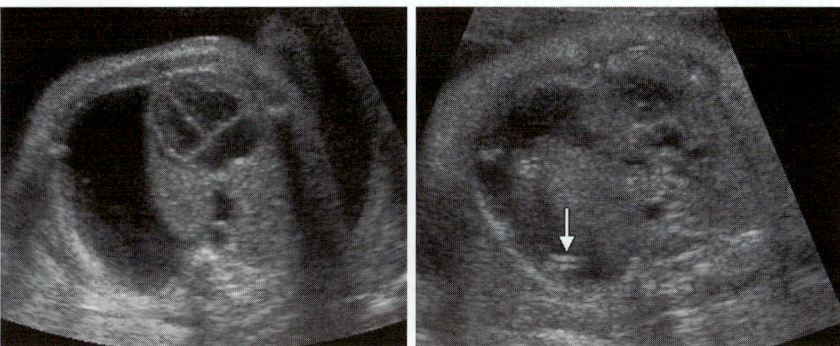

1. **What is the pathology seen in the above image?**
2. **What are the investigations of the above pathology?**
3. **What is the intervention of choice?**
4. **How to follow-up the case?**

Ans.

1. Unilateral pleural effusion
2. Amnio-FISH, microarray, whole exome, cytomegalovirus (CMV) PCR, and pleural fluid analysis for lymphocytes.
3. Drain at the time of pleurocentesis, follow-up thoracoamniotic shunt using double pigtail catheter if reaccumulating in isolated pleural effusion.
4. Close ultrasound surveillance to look for shunt displacement and reaccumulation of fluid.

SUGGESTED READING

1. Yinon Y, Grisaru-Granovsky S, Chaddha V, Windrim R, Seaward PG, Kelly EN, et al. "Perinatal outcome following fetal chest shunt insertion for pleural effusion." Ultrasound Obstet Gynecol. 2010;36(1):58-64.

STATION 12.

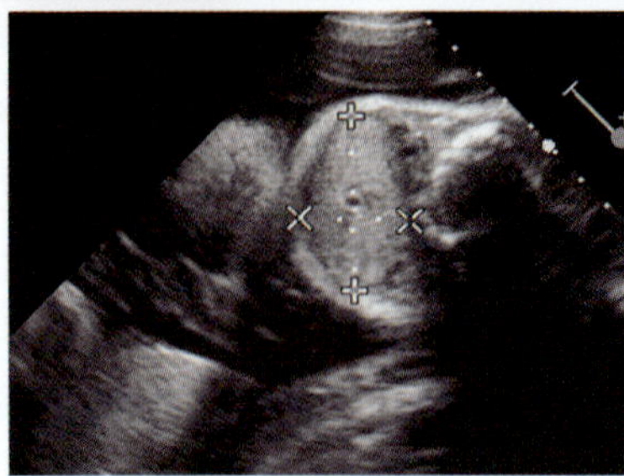

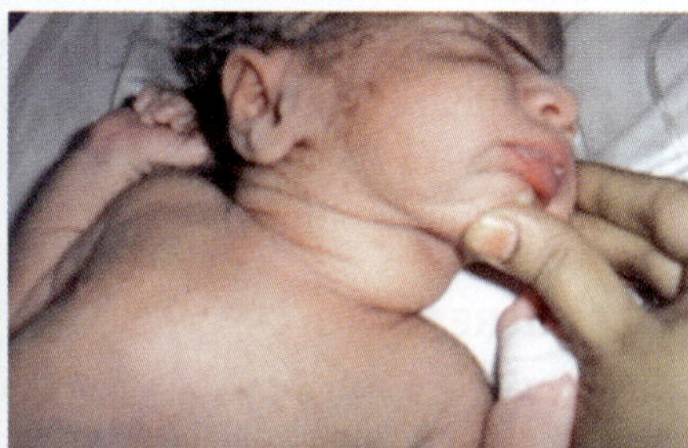

1. **What is the pathology seen in the above image?**
2. **What is the basis of the pathology?**
3. **What are the complications of fetal goiter?**
4. **What is the intervention of choice to look at fetal thyroid-stimulating hormone (TSH)?**

Ans.

1. Uniform echogenicity in neck of fetus—both lobes of fetal thyroid are enlarged. This neck mass is suggestive of goiter. Multiple causes must be considered in fetal neck masses investigation, such as cystic hygroma, teratoma, angioma, lymphangioma, and goiter, among others.
2. Iodine deficiency, overtreatment of maternal Graves' disease, inappropriate maternal thyroid replacement, and rarely, congenital hypothyroidism.
3. Fetal goiter is often associated with a retroflexed neck and polyhydramnios, raising concerns regarding airway obstruction in such cases.
4. Cordocentesis

SUGGESTED READING

1. Blumenfeld YJ, Davis A, Milan K, Chueh J, Hudgins L, Barth RA, et al. "Conservatively managed fetal goiter: an alternative to in utero therapy." Fetal Diagn Ther. 2013;34(3):184-7.

STATION 13.

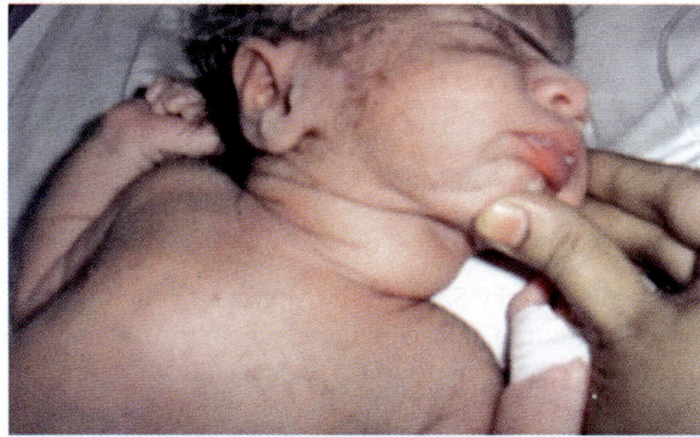

1. **What is the treatment for the pathology seen in the above image?**
2. **What is the basis of the treatment of fetal goiter?**
3. **What is the primary goal of treatment?**
4. **Do we need to treat all goiters?**

Ans.

1. Intraamniotic injections of LT4 to resolve mass suggestive of goiter.
2. Fetus swallows amniotic fluid, LT4 does not cross placenta.
3. Reducing goiter size.
4. Small goiters can be managed conservatively.

SUGGESTED READING

1. Mastrolia SA, Mandola A, Mazor M, Hershkovitz R, Mesner O, Beer-Weisel R, et al. "Antenatal diagnosis and treatment of hypothyroid fetal goitre in an euthyroid mother: a case report and review of literature." J Matern Fetal Neonatal Med. 2015;28(18):2214-20.

STATION 14.

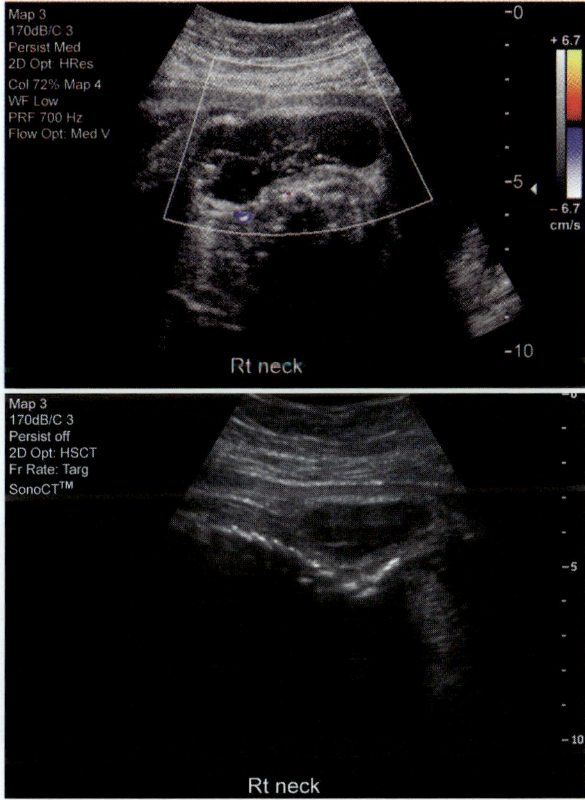

1. **What is the pathology seen in the above image?**
2. **What is an EXIT procedure?**

3. **Why is tocolysis important for the EXIT procedure?**
4. **Can you perform neonatal surgery in an EXIT procedure?**

Ans.

1. Fetal neck mass which can cause tracheal obstruction after birth.
2. The principle of an exit procedure is to continue to maintain placental circulation after birth and establish the neonatal airway and then cut the placental supply. In EXIT, the fetus is partially delivered and intubated without clamping the umbilical cord. Uteroplacental blood flow and gas exchange are maintained by using inhalational agents to provide uterine relaxation and amnioinfusion to maintain uterine volume and to avoid uterine collapse that could result in placental separation and/or cord compression. This provides time for cannulation for extracorporeal membrane oxygenation (ECMO) and chest decompression before delivery of the fetus.
3. Tocolysis maintains the uterine tone and prevents placental separation. However, one has to be better prepared for postpartum hemorrhage and inversion of uterus. 13% of mothers need transfusion.
4. In rare instances, the neck or lung mass can be excised before completing delivery.

SUGGESTED READING

1. Shamshirsaz AA, Aalipour S, Erfani H, Nassr AA, Stewart KA, Kravitz ES, et al. Obstetric outcomes of ex-utero intrapartum treatment (EXIT). Prenat Diagn. 2019;39(8):643-6.

STATION 15.

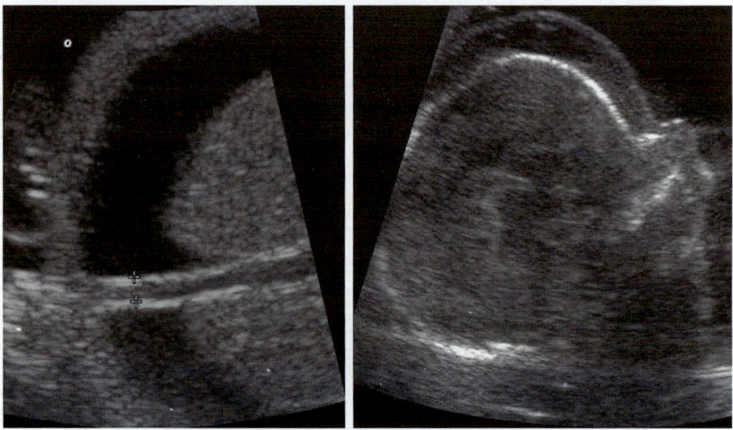

1. **What is the common cause of fetal anemia?**
2. **What are the infections that can cause fetal anemia?**

3. **What are the genetic syndromes that can cause fetal anemia?**
4. **What is the placental pathology that can cause fetal anemia?**

Ans.

1. Maternal isoimmunization—Rh antigens, atypical antigens
2. Parvovirus, cytomegalovirus, toxoplasmosis, rubella
3. Lysosomal storage disease, Fanconi anemia, α-thalassemia
4. Chorioangioma

SUGGESTED READING

1. Mari G, Deter RL, Carpenter RL, Rahman F, Zimmerman R, Moise KJ Jr, et al. Noninvasive diagnosis by Doppler ultrasonography of fetal anemia due to maternal red-cell alloimmunization. Collaborative Group for Doppler Assessment of the Blood Velocity in Anemic Fetuses. N Engl J Med. 2000;342(1):9-14.
2. Society for Maternal-Fetal Medicine (SMFM), Norton ME, Chauhan SP, Dashe JS. Society for maternal-fetal medicine (SMFM) clinical guideline #7: nonimmune hydrops fetalis. Am J Obstet Gynecol. 2015;212(2):127-39.

STATION 16.

1. **What is the blood test which is offered to a pregnant woman to screen for Rh isoimmunization?**
2. **Which is the critical titer for indirect Coombs test?**
3. **What are the rare antigens which can cause isoimmunization?**
4. **Will repeating ICT titers be helpful when it has exceeded the critical titers?**

Ans.

1. Indirect Coombs test [In the first alloimmunized pregnancy with a RhD-positive fetus, the maternal indirect Coombs titer (i.e., indirect antiglobulin test) is monitored monthly until 24 weeks and then every 2 weeks, as long as it remains stable. Rising titers should be repeated weekly until the titer reaches the "critical" level].
2. 1:16–1:32
3. Kell, Duffy, Kidd, MNS
4. Once the critical titers of ICT have been exceeded, repeating titers will not be helpful.

SUGGESTED READING

1. Markham KB, Moise KJ Jr. Anti-Rh(D) Alloimmunization: Outcomes at a single institution. Am J Obstet Gynecol. 2017;218:S318.
2. Markham KB, Rossi KQ, Nagaraja HN, O'Shaughnessy RW. Hemolytic disease of the fetus and newborn due to multiple maternal antibodies. Am J Obstet Gynecol. 2015;213(1):68.e1.

STATION 17.

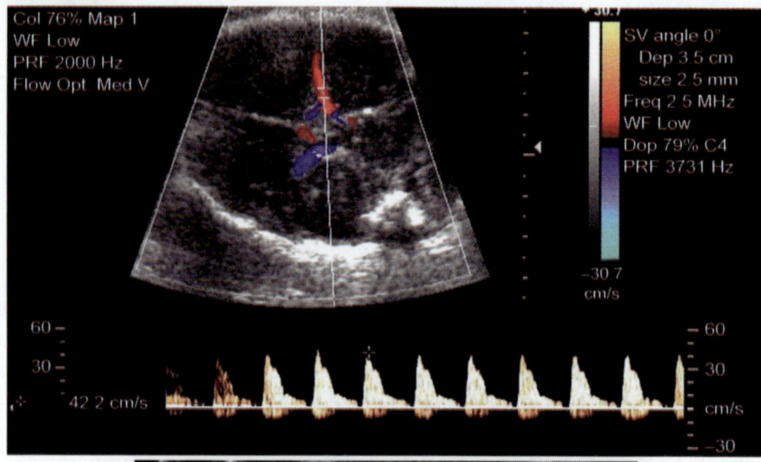

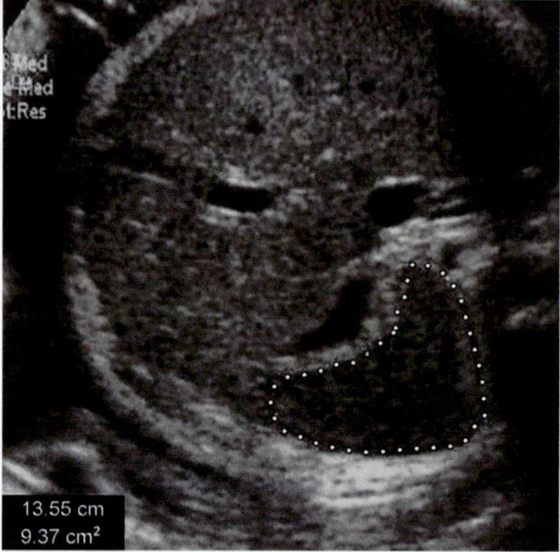

1. **What are the ultrasound parameters which help in detecting fetal anemia?**
2. **What is the most useful of them?**
3. **What are the graphs available to plot the middle cerebral artery peak systolic velocity?**
4. **What is the sensitivity and specificity of above curves?**

Ans.

1. Middle cerebral artery peak systolic velocity, liver length, spleen perimeter, umbilical vein velocity, placental thickness, and polyhydramnios.
2. Middle cerebral artery peak systolic velocity

3. *Mari et al. 2000:* Curves for middle cerebral artery peak systolic velocity (MCA PSV)
4. 100% sensitivity, 88% specificity, 12% FPR

SUGGESTED READING

1. Mari G, Abuhamad AZ, Cosmi E, Segata M, Altaye M, Akiyama M. Middle cerebral artery peak systolic velocity: technique and variability. J Ultrasound Med. 2005; 24(4):425-30.

STATION 18.

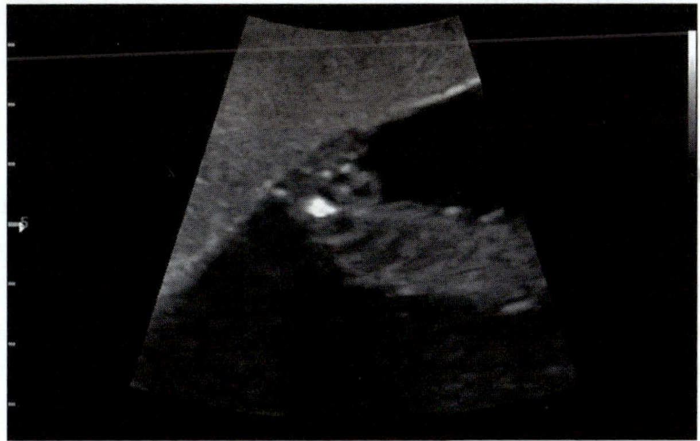

1. **What is the formula for intravenous transfusion?**
2. **What is a transfusion coefficient for calculating transfusion volume?**
3. **What is the choice of site for doing the transfusion?**
4. **How is the blood prepared for the fetus? Mention three criteria?**

Ans.

1. Fetoplacental volume* [expected hematocrit – current fetal hematocrit]/ hematocrit of bag (60–70%), fetoplacental volume is fetal weight* 0.14
2. As an example to increase the hematocrit volume of a 1,000 g fetus from 20 to 40% one multiplies the transfusion coefficient 0.04 (coefficient to raise hematocrit by 20) by the weight 1,000 g to yield 40 mL.
3. Intravascular in cord, intrahepatic umbilical vein, intraperitoneal
4. O negative blood, gamma irradiated, high hematocrit, leukodepleted, CMV negative

SUGGESTED READING

1. Donepudi R, Antolin E, Molina F, Sananes N, Khalil A, Abbasi N, et al. Practice patterns amongst fetal centers performing intrauterine transfusions (PACT): An international survey study. Eur J Obstet Gynecol Reprod Biol. 2022;274:171-4.

STATION 19.

1. **What are the goals of in utero repair of spina bifida?**
2. **What are the benefits of in utero rather than postnatal repair?**
3. **What are the pregnancy complications of in utero repair?**
4. **What is the preoperative fetal evaluation?**

Ans.

1. The technical goal of in utero spina bifida repair is to create complete, water-tight coverage of the defect, with the objective of halting progressive intrauterine neuronal injury.
2. The benefits of in utero rather than postnatal repair are:
   - Decreased need for cerebrospinal fluid (CSF) shunting
   - Improved motor development and function
   - Possible improvement in bladder function
   - Modest improvements in quality of life and impact on family
3. Chorioamniotic separation (CAS), chorioamnionitis, uterine bleeding, preterm prelabor rupture of membranes (PPROM), preterm labor, placental abruption, fetal injury, uterine dehiscence, or rupture.
4. Preoperative fetal evaluation should include a detailed ultrasound examination and/or magnetic resonance imaging (MRI) to confirm open spinal bifida and evaluate the defect, associated brain findings, and neurologic implications. The key inclusion criteria are:
   a. Open spina bifida with the upper boundary between T1 and S1
   b. Hindbrain herniation
   c. Gestational age 19 + 0 to 25 + 6 weeks of gestation at the time of the procedure.
   d. Chromosomal microarray (CMA) to rule out microdeletions and microduplications.

SUGGESTED READING

1. Moldenhauer JS, Bahtiyar MO, Bennett KA, Emery SP, Lillegard JB, Fisher A, et al. Open maternal-fetal surgery for myelomeningocele closure: Outcomes from the Fmmc consortium registry sponsored by NAFTnet. Los Cabos, Mexico: 40th International Fetal Medicine and Surgery Society Annual Meeting; 2022.
2. Molina-Giraldo S, Zapata Salcedo R, Rojas Arias JL, Acuña Osorio E, Pinto Quiñones ML, Restrepo HF, et al. Open surgery for in utero repair of spina bifida: Microneurosurgery versus standard technique - A systematic review. Prenat Diagn. 2021;41(13):1615-23.

STATION 20.

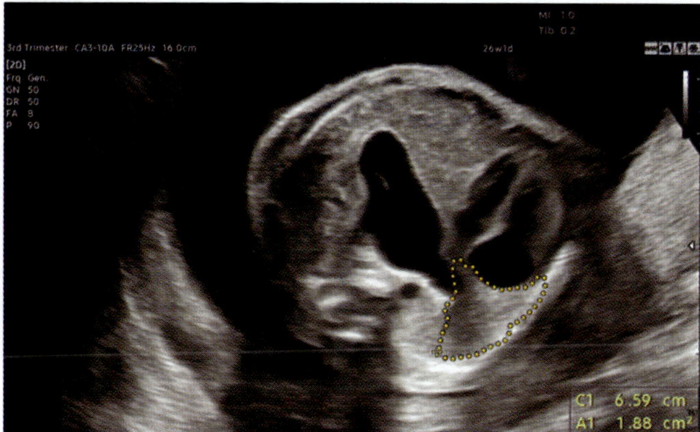

1. **What is the pathology in the above image? What are the goals and appropriate timing of in utero repair of this pathology by fetal endoscopic tracheal occlusion (FETO)?**
2. **What are the pregnancy complications of in utero repair?**
3. **What are the weaknesses of the TOTAL (tracheal occlusion to accelerate lung growth) trial?**
4. **What are the strengths of the TOTAL trial?**

Ans.

1. The pathology seen in the image is congenital diaphragmatic hernia (CDH). FETO appears to be effective to reduce mortality, rate of pulmonary hypertension, and use of ECMO in severe CDH. Prenatal FETO obstructs the normal egress of lung fluid during pulmonary development, thereby increasing transpulmonic pressure and resulting in large fluid-filled lungs. A percutaneous procedure using a balloon for FETO under maternal local anesthesia, with fetal analgesia and immobilization, has been developed. The optimal timing, duration, and release of the occlusion are not known. In left-sided CDH, one experienced group inserts the balloon at 27 + 0–29 + 6 weeks in severe cases [observed/expected lung to head ratio (O/E) LHR <25%] because earlier occlusion has a high complication rate. In moderate cases (O/E LHR: 25–35% with liver in any position, 35–45% with liver herniation), the procedure was performed later in gestation, at 30 + 0–31 + 6 weeks.
2. FETO is associated with a high risk of membrane rupture and preterm delivery. Though maternal risks are limited, balloon removal can be

challenging and lethal to the neonate. Ideally, the occlusion is reversed at 34 weeks, usually by fetoscopy or ultrasound-guided puncture, and the pregnancy is allowed to continue, but reversal can also be performed after partial fetal delivery with the fetus still on placental circulation. All of the above would require a strong logistic fetal medicine support. Long-term outcomes of the impact of prematurity are not available.

3. The weaknesses of the TOTAL trial are—numbers still small, no medium or long-term results, and centers not blinded to treatment.
4. The strengths of the TOTAL trial are—largest trial in history, large numbers, sufficient power, and reference data for other studies, virtually no missing data, outcomes in line, with other nonintervention studies.

SUGGESTED READING

1. Deprest JA, Benachi A, Gratacos E, Nicolaides KH, Berg C, Persico N, et al. Randomized trial of fetal surgery for moderate left diaphragmatic hernia. N Engl J Med. 2021;385(2):119-29.
2. Deprest JA, Nicolaides KH, Benachi A, Gratacos E, Ryan G, Persico N, et al. Randomized trial of fetal surgery for severe left diaphragmatic hernia. N Engl J Med. 2021;385(2):107-18.

Fetal Interventions in Multifetal Gestations

Vandana Chaddha

STATION 1.

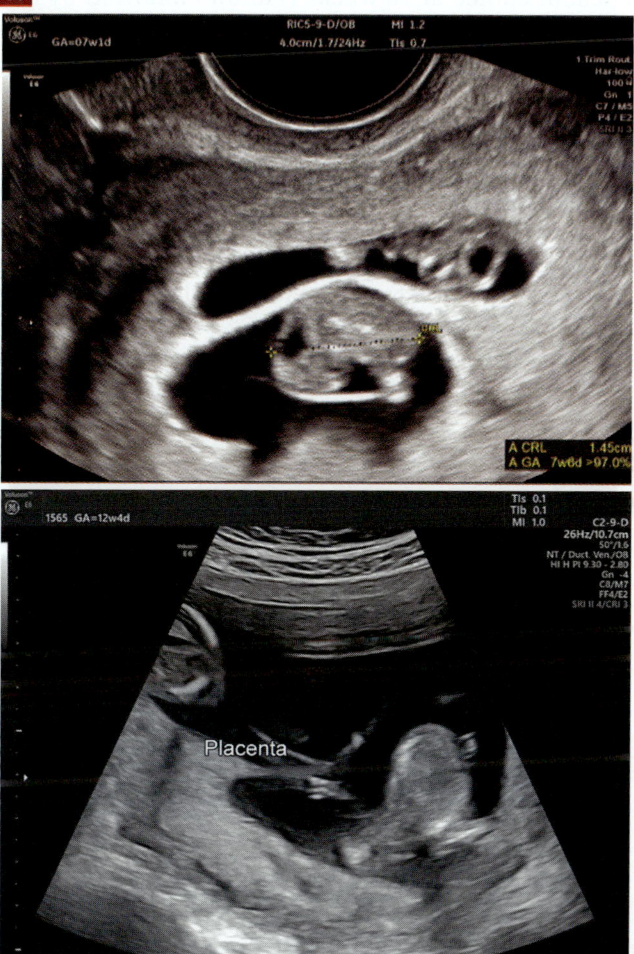

1. **What is the chorionicity of the twins seen in the image?**
2. **Would you offer diagnostic invasive testing to one or both?**
3. **If the background of first trimester screen test is showing high risk and couple opts for ensuring 100% results, that there is no aneuploidy—what would be your intervention of choice at 12 weeks?**

4. If the above patient is 16 weeks at presentation which intervention would you offer?

Ans.

1. The above image shows a set of dichorionic diamniotic twins.
2. Invasive testing would be offered to both as they have separate genetic make-up.
3. Intervention of choice at 12 weeks is chorionic villous sampling for both the twins.
4. Genetic test of choice at 16 weeks is amnio followed by fluorescent in situ hybridization (FISH) or quantitative fluorescent polymerase chain reaction (QF-PCR), so an early report is reassuring. Microarray can also be done as an accompanying test. Ideally, the test should be done for both twins.

SUGGESTED READING

1. American College of Obstetricians and Gynecologists' Committee on Practice Bulletins—Obstetrics, Committee on Genetics, Society for Maternal-Fetal Medicine. Practice Bulletin No. 162: Prenatal Diagnostic Testing for Genetic Disorders. Obstet Gynecol. 2016;127:e108.
2. De Catte L, Liebaers I, Foulon W. Outcome of twin gestations after first trimester chorionic villus sampling. Obstet Gynecol. 2000;96(5 Pt 1):714-20.

STATION 2.

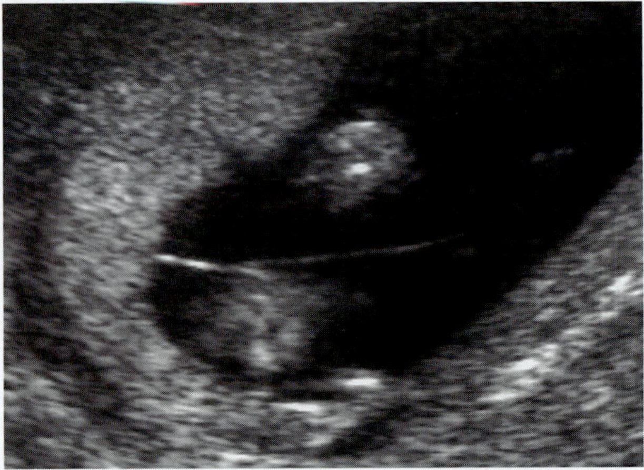

1. What is the chorionicity of the twins seen in the image?

2. Would you offer invasive testing to one or both?

3. If the background of first trimester screen test is showing high risk and couple opts for ensuring 100% results, that there is no aneuploidy—what would be your intervention of choice at 12 weeks?

4. If the above patient is 16 weeks at presentation and the monochorionic diamniotic (MCDA) twins are discordant anomalous, which diagnostic intervention would you offer?

Ans.

1. The above image shows a set of MCDA twins.
2. Invasive testing would be offered to one as they have same genetic make-up.
3. Intervention of choice at 12 weeks is chorionic villous sampling of common placenta.
4. Genetic test of choice at 16 weeks, especially in the setting of a discordant anomalous twin is amnio followed by FISH or QF-PCR, so an early report is reassuring. Microarray can also be done as an accompanying test.

SUGGESTED READING

1. American College of Obstetricians and Gynecologists' Committee on Practice Bulletins—Obstetrics, Committee on Genetics, Society for Maternal-Fetal Medicine. Practice Bulletin No. 162: Prenatal Diagnostic Testing for Genetic Disorders. Obstet Gynecol. 2016;127:e108.
2. Weisz B, Rodeck CH. Invasive diagnostic procedures in twin pregnancies. Prenat Diagn. 2005;25(9):751-8.

STATION 3.

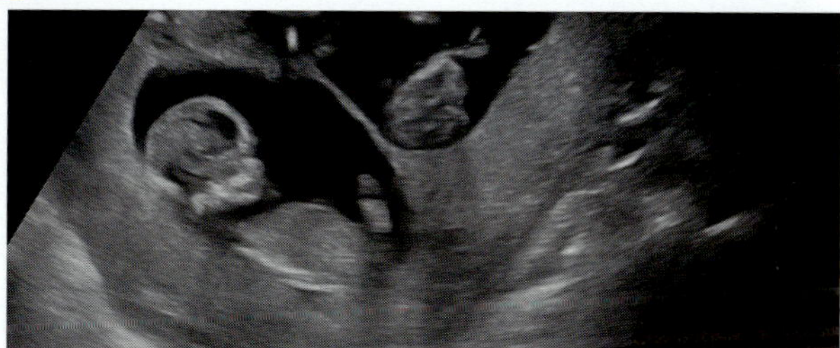

1. **What is the most appropriate method of labeling twins?**
2. **Why is it of utmost importance in twin interventions?**
3. **Which is the preferred technique—separate puncture or single needle?**
4. **What is the disadvantage of single-needle technique in twins?**

Ans.

1. Consistent strategy should be applied for identifying and labeling each twin over serial examinations. In general, twins can be labeled in the following ways:
   - Twin A is the presenting twin, and twin B is the nonpresenting twin.
   - Placental position of each twin.

- Each twin may be identified based on its orientation relative to the other twin: Left or right lateral for twins positioned next to each other and top (fundal) or bottom (cervical) for twins positioned vertically.
- Documenting the sites of placental implantation (anterior, posterior, lateral) and the sites and types of placental cord insertion (e.g., marginal versus central, normal versus velamentous) is also useful.

2. It is of utmost importance to correctly label the twins in a diagnostic intervention, so we can plan a subsequent selective feticide carefully.
3. Separate puncture of each sac is preferred in dichorionic as well as discordant monochorionic twins.
4. Theoretical concerns with this procedure include the potential for mixing the two fluids, leading to inaccurate interpretation of genetic tests, and shearing of the dividing membrane, resulting in a functionally monoamniotic pregnancy with its attendant risks.

SUGGESTED READING

1. Simonazzi G, Curti A, Farina A, Pilu G, Bovicelli L, Rizzo N. Amniocentesis and chorionic villus sampling in twin gestations: which is the best sampling technique? Am J Obstet Gynecol. 2010;202:365.e1.
2. Weisz B, Rodeck CH. Invasive diagnostic procedures in twin pregnancies. Prenat Diagn. 2005;25(9):751-8.

STATION 4.

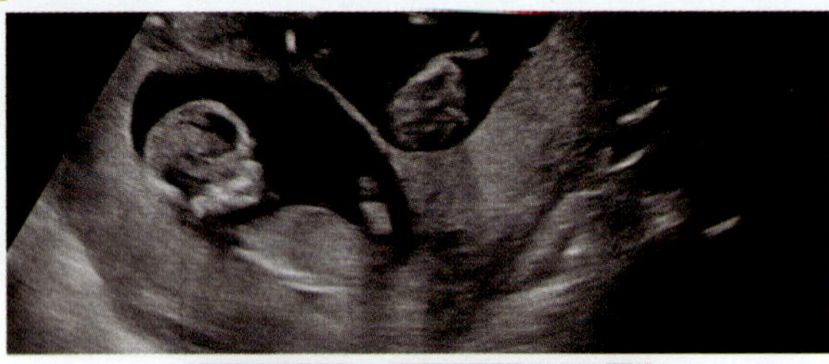

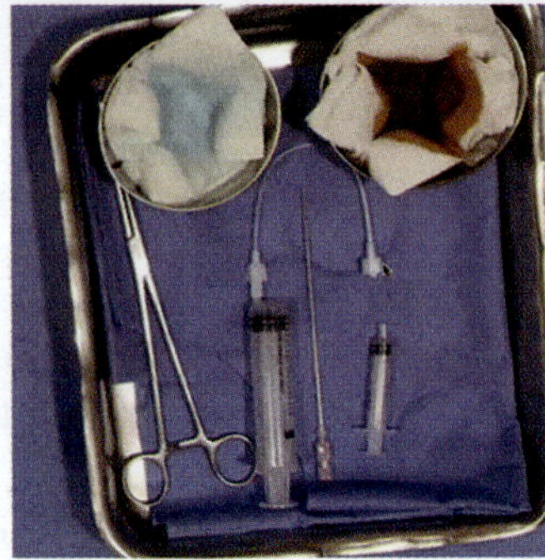

1. **Where should the tip of the aspirating device be placed in twin chorionic villus sampling (CVS)?**

2. **How do you differentiate between the samples?**
3. **What is the next step if the samples seem to be the same DNA?**
4. **What is the possibility of follow-up amniocentesis in twin CVS?**

Ans.

1. If the placentas are fused and either dichorionic or of uncertain chorionicity, the tip of the aspirating device should be inserted either close to the insertion of the umbilical cord or at the placental margin, far away from the other placenta.
2. The cytogenetic results and DNA polymorphism may permit differentiation between the samples.
3. If the results are identical and chorionicity remains uncertain, confirmation that each fetus has been sampled is advisable; this can be achieved by amniocentesis later in pregnancy.
4. Follow-up amniocentesis is required in up to 6% of cases.

SUGGESTED READING

1. Pergament E, Schulman JD, Copeland K, Fine B, Black SH, Ginsberg NA, et al. The risk and efficacy of chorionic villus sampling in multiple gestations. Prenat Diagn. 1992;12(5):377-84.
2. Wapner RJ, Johnson A, Davis G, Urban A, Morgan P, Jackson L. Prenatal diagnosis in twin gestations: a comparison between second-trimester amniocentesis and first-trimester chorionic villus sampling. Obstet Gynecol. 1993;82(1):49-56.

STATION 5.

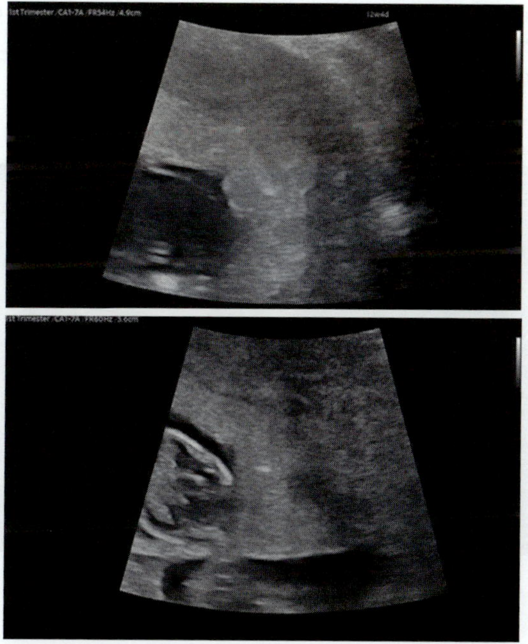

1. **What are the peculiar complications which could happen in twin CVS?**
2. **What is the risk of a sampling error in twin gestation?**
3. **What is the risk of a sampling error in higher order multiple gestation?**
4. **What is the advantage of earlier CVS versus late amniocentesis in twins?**

Ans.

1. Uncertain results requiring further investigation (such as sampling one fetus twice, cross contamination due to mixed sampling, and maternal cell contamination) are more frequent in multiple gestations assessed by CVS than by amniocentesis.
2. The risk of a sampling error in twin gestation is small (0.6–0.8%).
3. The risk of a sampling error in triplets and higher order gestations (1.2%)
4. CVS offers the advantage of earlier selective fetal reduction, if requested, because of abnormal results.

SUGGESTED READING

1. Agarwal K, Alfirevic Z. Pregnancy loss after chorionic villus sampling and genetic amniocentesis in twin pregnancies: a systematic review. Ultrasound Obstet Gynecol. 2012;40(2):128-34.
2. De Catte L, Liebaers I, Foulon W. Outcome of twin gestations after first trimester chorionic villus sampling. Obstet Gynecol. 2000;96(5 Pt 1):714-20.
3. RCOG. Amniocentesis and Chorionic Villus Sampling (Green-top Guideline No. 8). [online] Available from https://content.sph.harvard.edu/wwwhsph/sites/2413/2014/08/Amniocentesis_RoyalCollege_ResArt_2010.pdf 2021 [Last accessed May, 2025].

STATION 6.

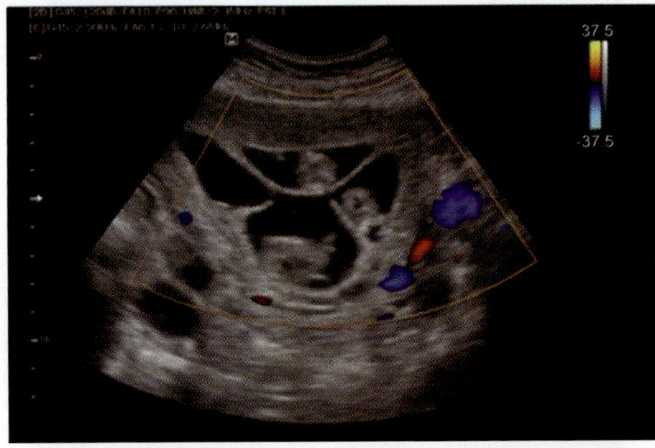

1. **What is multifetal pregnancy reduction (MPR)?**
2. **What is the primary justification for MPR?**
3. **The risk of which potential maternal complications are concomitantly reduced in multifetal gestation when multifetal reduction is offered?**
4. **When can the procedure be offered in twin pregnancies?**

Ans.

1. Multifetal pregnancy reduction is a procedure in which the overall number of fetuses in the gestation is reduced by terminating one or more fetuses mostly chosen randomly, but with consideration of technical factors.
2. The primary justification for MPR is that the "take home" baby rate per pregnancy is increased by increasing the gestational age at birth and birth weight, thus reducing morbidity and mortality from preterm birth.
3. The risks for some maternal complications, such as preeclampsia and preterm births are also reduced. Economic and psychological impacts of multiple gestation on families also play a role.
4. It may be mulled over in twin pregnancies, where a reduction in primarily late preterm birth has been demonstrated. Reduction to a singleton may have additional advantages for women with comorbidities or a history of adverse pregnancy outcomes.

SUGGESTED READING

1. Committee opinion No. 719: Multifetal pregnancy reduction. Obstet Gynecol. 2017;130(3):e158-63.
2. Zipori Y, Haas J, Berger H, Barzilay E. Multifetal pregnancy reduction of triplets to twins compared with non-reduced triplets: a meta-analysis. Reprod Biomed Online. 2017;35(3):296-304.

STATION 7.

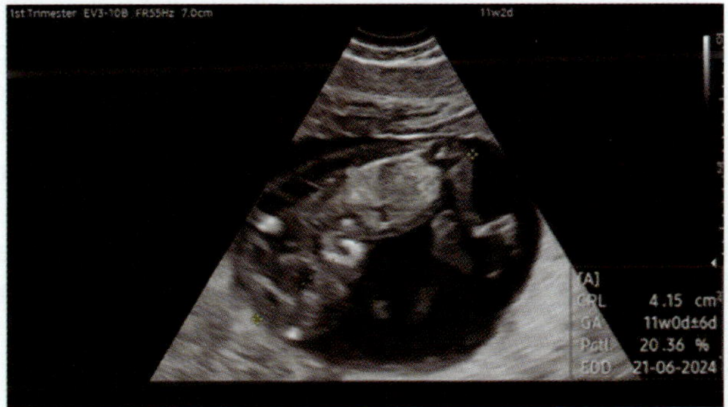

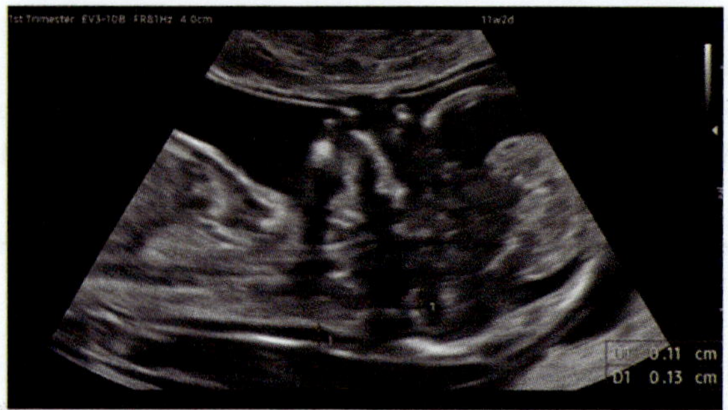

1. **What is selective termination (ST) or selective feticide? Could it be offered to the dichorionic diamniotic (DCDA) twins in the above case scenario where there is a discordance of anomaly?**
2. **What is the most critical aspect of selective feticide?**
3. **What is the technique offered for selective feticide?**
4. **What is the postprocedural follow-up protocol immediately after selective feticide?**

Ans.

1. Selective termination refers to a procedure in which one or more specific fetuses of a multifetal gestation are terminated due to a known or suspected fetal abnormality, including a chromosomal, structural, genetic, or growth abnormality. This is in contrast to MPR, in which the fetus(es) is chosen randomly, but with consideration of technical factors. Yes, the anomalous twin could be selectively reduced in the above case scenario.
2. The first step is to correctly identify the fetus to be terminated. Previously diagnosed fetal abnormalities, particularly genetic disorders in which the fetus may appear sonographically normal, are not always obvious at the time of ST. Correct identification of the affected fetus can be made by ultrasound detection of a structural abnormality (if present); by gender (if discordant); or by previously documented fetal, gestational sac, and/or placental position. Therefore, precise in utero mapping of fetal and placental positioning at the time of prenatal diagnosis is critical.
3. Potassium chloride is injected into the thoracic cavity (ideally intracardiac) of the affected fetus under ultrasound guidance until asystole is confirmed, similar to the technique used for MPR.
4. Perform an ultrasound 1 hour after the procedure to ensure asystole of the terminated fetus and normal cardiac activity of the remaining fetus.

SUGGESTED READING

1. Bigelow CA, Factor SH, Moshier E, Bianco A, Eddleman KA, Stone JL. Timing of and outcomes after selective termination of anomalous fetuses in dichorionic twin pregnancies. Prenat Diagn. 2014;34(13):1320-5.

2. Eddleman KA, Stone JL, Lynch L, Berkowitz RL. Selective termination of anomalous fetuses in multifetal pregnancies: two hundred cases at a single center. Am J Obstet Gynecol. 2002;187(5):1168-72.

STATION 8.

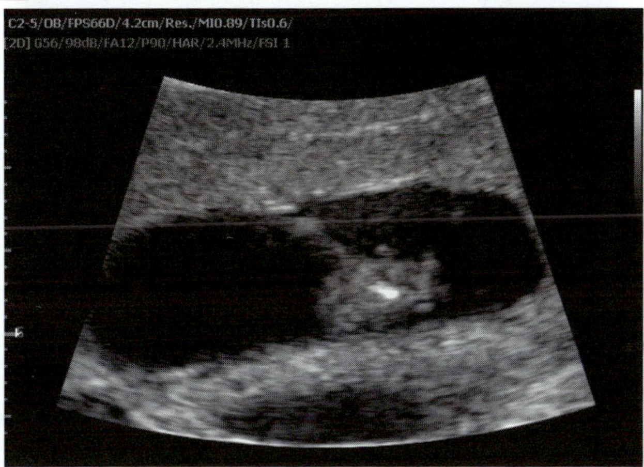

1. **Which biochemical marker is typically elevated for several weeks after any fetal reduction procedure?**
2. **What is the elevation probably caused by?**
3. **What would be the best modality to identify neural tube defects in the pregnancies that have undergone fetal reduction?**
4. **Have cases of clinically evident disseminated intravascular coagulation been reported after medical fetal reduction (MFR)?**

Ans.

1. The maternal serum α-fetoprotein (MSAFP) concentration is typically elevated for several weeks after any fetal reduction procedure and is not necessarily indicative of fetal defects.
2. The elevation is probably caused by release of tissue or serum from the reduced fetus(es).
3. Since MSAFP is always elevated, it should not be used to screen for neural tube defects. Detailed ultrasound should be performed to rule out neural tube defects.
4. No cases of clinically evident disseminated intravascular coagulation have been reported.

SUGGESTED READING

1. Grau P, Robinson L, Tabsh K, Crandall BF. Elevated maternal serum alpha-fetoprotein and amniotic fluid alpha-fetoprotein after multifetal pregnancy reduction. Obstet Gynecol. 1990;76(6):1042-5.

STATION 9.

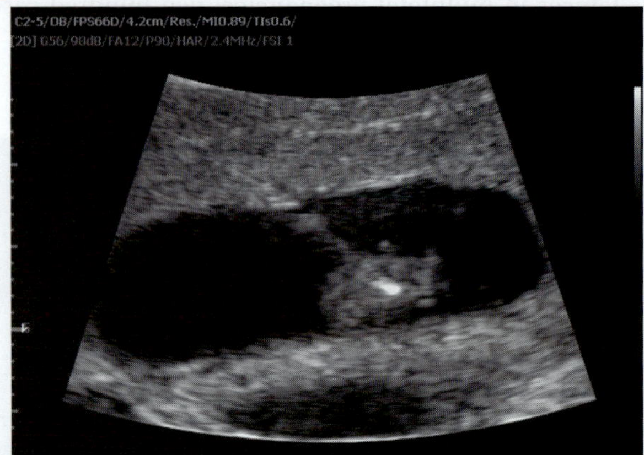

1. **Can maternal serum screening tests for Down syndrome be offered after MFR/ST?**
2. **Should noninvasive prenatal diagnostic tests, which assess cell-free DNA in the maternal circulation, be avoided after MFR/ST?**
3. **Can diagnostic testing performed on amniotic fluid or chorionic villi be *altered* following MFR/ST?**
4. **What is the best modality for detailed assessment of fetal development after MFR?**

Ans.

1. No. Maternal serum screening tests for Down syndrome, such as the dual marker or the quad screen, should not be performed after such procedures, as the presence of reduced fetuses will result in a high rate of abnormal results.
2. Noninvasive prenatal diagnostic tests, which assess cell-free DNA in the maternal circulation, should also be generally avoided because DNA from the reduced fetuses can be present in the maternal circulation.
3. Diagnostic testing performed on amniotic fluid or chorionic villi can also be used since neither are affected by a history of MPR or ST.
4. Detailed assessment of fetal development by ultrasound remains the preferred means to screen nonreduced fetuses for neural tube defects and markers associated with aneuploidy.

SUGGESTED READING

1. Chen M, Su F, Wang J, Zhou L, Liu Q, Chai X, et al. Temporal persistence of residual fetal cell-free DNA from a deceased cotwin after selective fetal reduction in dichorionic diamniotic twin pregnancies. Prenat Diagn. 2021;41(12):1602-10.
2. Grau P, Robinson L, Tabsh K, Crandall BF. Elevated maternal serum alpha-fetoprotein and amniotic fluid alpha-fetoprotein after multifetal pregnancy reduction. Obstet Gynecol. 1990;76(6):1042-5.

STATION 10.

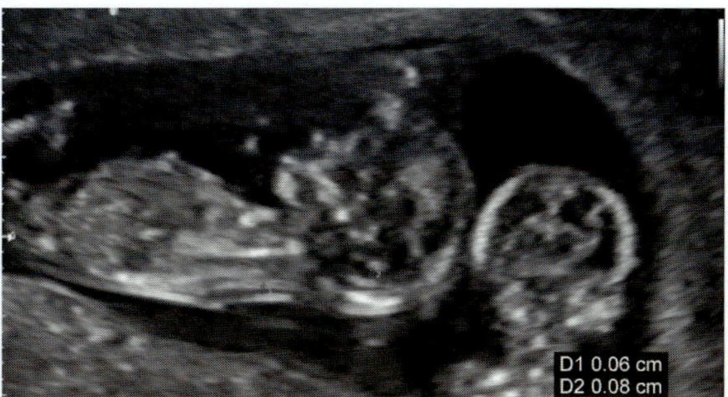

1. **Why is accurate determination of chorionicity crucial before performing ST?**
2. **Is it advisable to use the same modality for fetal reduction in monochorionic twins as is in dichorionic ones? Give reasons for your answer. What is the risk in one twin demise if the two fetuses are monochorionic?**
3. **What are the adverse hemodynamic changes that could occur in the survivor in cases of single fetal demise in monochorionic gestations?**
4. **What is the difference in the termination techniques in dichorionic versus monochorionic pairs?**

Ans.

1. Accurate determination of chorionicity is crucial before performing ST, as termination techniques are different for dichorionic versus monochorionic pairs.
2. If two fetuses are monochorionic and thus have a shared circulation, and if one is reduced by injection of a toxin, then there is a chance that the toxin will also enter the co-twin's circulation and cause fetal death.
3. Hypotension could occur in the survivor, due to blood loss into the vascular system of the terminated fetus and could result in neurologic injury.
4. Termination techniques are different for dichorionic versus monochorionic pairs (intrathoracic potassium chloride injection versus cord occlusion). The most common method for ST is cord occlusion, because it decreases the risk to the co-twin since it separates the vascular systems of the fetuses.

SUGGESTED READING

1. Alphathanasiadis AP, Zafrakas M, Tarlatzis BC, Vaitsi V, Mikos T, Bontis J. Multifetal pregnancy reduction in pregnancies with a monochorionic component. Fertil Steril. 2005;83(2):474-6.
2. Denbow ML, Overton TG, Duncan KR, Cox PM, Fisk NM. High failure rate of umbilical vessel occlusion by ultrasound-guided injection of absolute alcohol or enbucrilate gel. Prenat Diagn. 1999;19(6):527-32.

STATION 11.

1. **What are the various clinical situations in which selective feticide may be offered in monochorionic twins?**
2. **What are the types of interventions offered in twins for selective feticide?**
3. **What are the preparatory techniques involved in the same?**
4. **What are the complications involved in these interventions?**

Ans.

1. The acardiac twins, severe twin-to-twin transfusion syndrome (TTTS), discordant anomalous, selective fetal growth restriction (FGR)
2. Radiofrequency ablation (RFA), Nd:YAG/Diode laser ablation, ligation, cautery—bipolar/unipolar
3. Intravenous antibiotics, intravenous sedation, preparation of abdomen using povidone iodine, local anesthesia infiltration, and puncture site identified in maternal abdomen.
4. Chorioamnionitis, preterm labor, premature rupture of membranes, abruption, maternal bleed, co-twin demise, and co-twin survival with morbidity.

SUGGESTED READING

1. Mathis J, Raio L, Baud D. Fetal laser therapy: applications in the management of fetal pathologies. Prenat Diagn. 2015;35(7):623-36.
2. Shevell T, Malone FD, Weintraub J, Thaker HM, D'alton ME. Radiofrequency ablation in a monochorionic twin discordant for fetal anomalies. Am J Obstet Gynecol. 2004;190(2):575-6.

STATION 12.

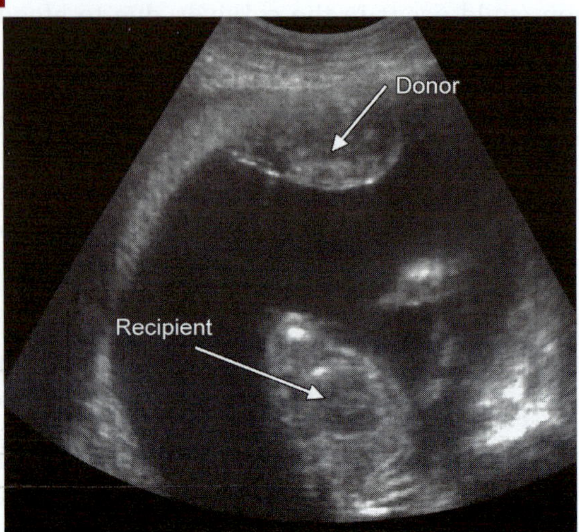

1. **What is the pathology seen in the above image?**
2. **What is the basis of the pathology?**
3. **Describe the staging used for this disorder in monochorionic twins?**
4. **Does the clinical presentation of a particular case always follow an orderly progression?**

Ans.

1. Twin-twin transfusion syndrome
2. The TTTS phenotype results from unbalanced flow through placental intertwin vascular anastomoses that lead to hypovolemia in one twin (donor twin) and hypervolemia in the other (recipient twin).
3. Quintero staging:

Stage I	Oligohydramnios and polyhydramnios sequence • The bladder of the donor twin is visible • Doppler indices [umbilical artery (UA), umbilical vein (UV), and ductus venosus (DV)] in both twins are normal
Stage II	Oligohydramnios and polyhydramnios sequence • Bladder of the donor is not visualized • Doppler indices (UA, UV, DV) in both twins are normal
Stage III	Oligohydramnios and polyhydramnios sequence • *Abnormal Doppler indices:* At least one of the following is present in either twin: absent or reversed end-diastolic velocity in the UA, reversed flow in a-wave of the DV, or pulsatile flow in the UV
Stage IV	Oligohydramnios and polyhydramnios sequence • One or both fetuses show signs of hydrops
Stage V	Oligohydramnios and polyhydramnios sequence • One or both fetuses are dead

4. The five classic stages of TTTS are based on findings from two-dimensional ultrasound and Doppler velocimetry of the umbilical artery, umbilical vein, and ductus venosus. Higher stages, which are characterized by abnormal Dopplers with or without hydrops, are generally associated with a worsening perinatal prognosis, but the clinical presentation of a particular case does not always follow an orderly progression of stages.

SUGGESTED READING

1. Quintero RA, Morales WJ, Allen MH, Bornick PW, Johnson PK, Kruger M. Staging of twin-twin transfusion syndrome. J Perinatol. 1999;19(8 Pt 1):550-5.
2. Taylor MJ, Govender L, Jolly M, Wee L, Fisk NM. Validation of the Quintero staging system for twin-twin transfusion syndrome. Obstet Gynecol. 2002;100(6):1257-65.

STATION 13.

1. **Is fetal intervention offered for Quintero stage 1?**
2. **What is the optimal therapy for Quintero stage 2 and above and why?**
3. **Why is laser ablation preferred over amnioreduction?**
4. **What is the technique employed for laser ablation?**

Ans.

1. For patients with stage I TTTS with no or tolerable symptoms it is suggested to undergo expectant management rather than invasive therapy (laser coagulation of placental intertwin vascular anastomoses).
2. Laser coagulation of placental intertwin vascular anastomoses leads to resolution of the intertwin volume imbalance and secretion and exchange of vasoactive mediators.
3. Laser ablation results in greater prolongation of gestational age, higher neonatal survival, and improved long-term neurologic outcome.
4. Sequential selective technique followed by the "Solomon" method to assure complete dichorionization of the placenta. Single amnioreduction after removing the fetoscope to relieve maternal symptoms can be done.

SUGGESTED READING

1. Roberts D, Neilson JP, Kilby MD, Gates S. Interventions for the treatment of twin-twin transfusion syndrome. Cochrane Database Syst Rev. 2014;2014(1): CD002073.
2. van Klink JM, Koopman HM, van Zwet EW, Oepkes D, Walther FJ, Lopriore E. Cerebral injury and neurodevelopmental impairment after amnioreduction versus laser surgery in twin-twin transfusion syndrome: a systematic review and meta-analysis. Fetal Diagn Ther. 2013;33(2):81-9.

STATION 14.

1. **When is selective reduction performed for treatment of TTTS?**
2. **What is the technical difficulty if the stuck twin lies along the vascular equator?**
3. **Which fetus is selected oligohydramnios or polyhydramnios for selective reduction?**
4. **Which is the preferred modality for selective reduction of monochorionic twins?**

Ans.

1. Selective reduction has been performed for treatment of TTTS when one fetus has a very poor prognosis—life-threatening malformation, severe growth restriction, severe cardiac failure, and evidence of brain injury.

2. Laser ablation may not be possible when a stuck twin overlies the site of the placental anastomoses. Selective reduction is an option in these cases.
3. The fetus predicted to have the least chance for survival is usually selected for the reduction procedure. For example, a recipient with advanced cardiac findings or hydrops or a donor that is growth restricted with discordant fetal weight >30% and abnormal umbilical artery Doppler.
4. Selective reduction of one twin is an option that may improve the prognosis of the co-twin if a technique is used that does not impact its circulation. While perinatal outcomes are comparable among the various procedures (bipolar cord coagulation, laser cord coagulation, and RFA), RFA is the preferred technique for selective reduction of monochorionic twins because the smaller device reduces maternal morbidity.

SUGGESTED READING

1. Moise KJ Jr, Johnson A, Moise KY, Nickeleit V. Radiofrequency ablation for selective reduction in the complicated monochorionic gestation. Am J Obstet Gynecol. 2008;198(2):198.e1-198.e5.
2. Yinon Y, Ashwal E, Weisz B, Chayen B, Schiff E, Lipitz S. Selective reduction in complicated monochorionic twins: prediction of obstetric outcome and comparison of techniques. Ultrasound Obstet Gynecol. 2015;46(6):670-7.

STATION 15.

1. **What is the advantage of doing amnioreduction in TTTS?**
2. **Where should the needle be placed in the maternal abdomen for amnioreduction and why?**
3. **How much fluid can be removed in one setting?**
4. **What is the complication encountered in *amniodrainage?* Name two.**

Ans.

1. Amnioreduction reduces uterine overdistention, which is a risk factor for preterm labor and preterm prelabor rupture of membranes (PPROM). It also decreases pressure inside the amniotic cavity and may thus improve uteroplacental perfusion.
2. The needle is placed as close to the midline of the uterus as possible with a slight angulation toward the maternal xiphoid to reduce the risk of needle displacement as the uterine size diminishes with drainage of amniotic fluid.
3. It is recommended to remove fluid until polyhydramnios is no longer present (maximum vertical pocket <8 cm); others suggest removing no >3 liters of amniotic fluid over approximately an hour.
4. Decompression of the uterus with rapid removal of a large volume of fluid may cause placental abruption or fetal bradycardia.

SUGGESTED READING

1. Leung WC, Jouannic JM, Hyett J, Rodeck C, Jauniaux E. Procedure-related complications of rapid amniodrainage in the treatment of polyhydramnios. Ultrasound Obstet Gynecol. 2004;23(2):154-8.
2. Mari G, Roberts A, Detti L, Kovanci E, Stefos T, Bahado-Singh RO, et al. Perinatal morbidity and mortality rates in severe twin-twin transfusion syndrome: results of the International Amnioreduction Registry. Am J Obstet Gynecol. 2001;185(3):708-15.

STATION 16.

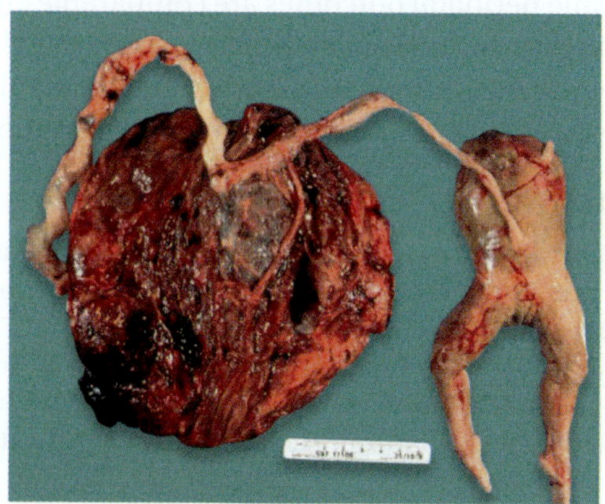

1. **What is pathology seen in the above image?**
2. **What are the management options for the above pathology?**
3. **What is the advantage of intervention at 12 weeks?**
4. **Name three poor prognostic factors for this pathology if managed conservatively.**

Ans.

1. Twin reversed arterial perfusion sequence.
2. Conservative, intervention at 12 weeks, intervention beyond 16 weeks.
3. Intervention at 12 weeks avoids risk of death of the pump twin.
4. Poor prognostic factors:
   - High-output heart failure. Signs of developing or overt heart failure can include cardiomegaly, tricuspid regurgitation, diminished contractility, and/or reversed a-wave in the ductus venosus or umbilical vein pulsations on Doppler studies and echocardiography.
   - Hydrops fetalis
   - Pump twin abnormal Doppler studies showing persistent absent or reversed end-diastolic velocity in the umbilical artery [absent end-diastolic velocity (AEDV), reversed end-diastolic velocity (REDV)], pulsatile blood flow in the umbilical vein, and/or reversed a-wave in the ductus venosus Doppler waveform (which may be indicative of evolving or overt cardiac failure).

- Acardiac twin weight to pump twin weight ratio >0.70.
- Polyhydramnios
- Monoamniotic pregnancy

SUGGESTED READING

1. Quintero RA, Chmait RH, Murakoshi T, Pankrac Z, Swiatkowska M, Bornick PW, et al. Surgical management of twin reversed arterial perfusion sequence. Am J Obstet Gynecol. 2006;194(4):982-91.

STATION 17.

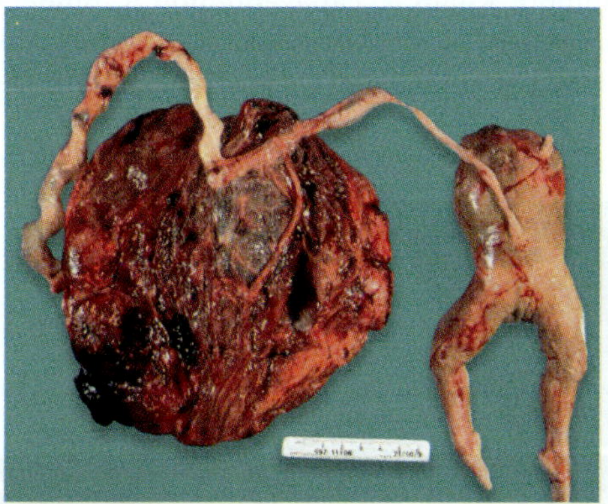

1. **What is the treatment for the pathology seen in the above image?**
2. **What is the rationale for the treatment?**
3. **What are the modalities which can be proposed for the same?**
4. **When should delivery be planned after treatment of pathology shown above?**

Ans.

1. Cord occlusion interrupts the vascular communication(s) between twins, thereby relieving the pump twin of the hemodynamic burden of supporting its acardiac co-twin. Because all of the blood is being supplied by the pump twin and the cord is occluded, this twin is not at increased risk of adverse effects from demise of the acardiac twin, in contrast to the sequelae of monochorionic twins with one natural demise.
2. The rationale is to optimize the outcome of the pump twin since the acardiac twin has no potential for independent survival.
3. The choice of cord occlusion technique for a specific pregnancy should be individualized based on operator experience, center resources/procedural availability, clinical presentation, gestational age, and patient preference. Contemporary cord occlusion techniques include:
   - Radiofrequency ablation
   - Bipolar cord coagulation
   - Laser photocoagulation

4. Pregnancies not undergoing cord occlusion, plan delivery at 34 + 0–36 + 6 weeks of gestation, but deliver sooner if pump twin compromise or a standard obstetric indication for preterm birth develops.

SUGGESTED READING

1. Jelin E, Hirose S, Rand L, Curran P, Feldstein V, Guevara-Gallardo S, et al. Perinatal outcome of conservative management versus fetal intervention for twin reversed arterial perfusion sequence with a small acardiac twin. Fetal Diagn Ther. 2010;27(3):138-41.
2. Pagani G, D'Antonio F, Khalil A, Papageorghiou A, Bhide A, Thilaganathan B. Intrafetal laser treatment for twin reversed arterial perfusion sequence: cohort study and meta-analysis. Ultrasound Obstet Gynecol. 2013;42(1):6-14.

STATION 18.

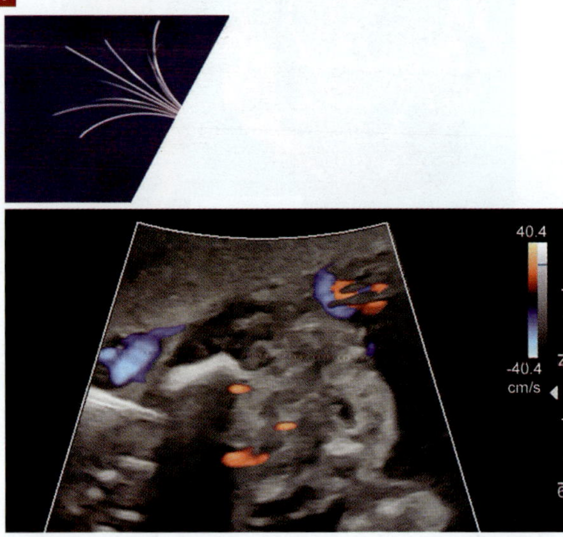

1. **What is the gauge of lumbar puncture (LP) needle through which an RFA needle can pass?**
2. **How many mm beyond the targets is the RFA needle passed before the trienes are opened?**
3. **What are the settings of the RFA machine during fetal cord ablation procedure?**
4. **What are the tissue changes visible on screen as the coagulation happens?**

Ans.

1. 17 gauge
2. 5–6 mm
3. 150 watts, 100°, and 2–3 minutes
4. The tissue becomes echogenic or white.

SUGGESTED READING

1. Lee H, Bebbington M, Crombleholme TM, North American Fetal Therapy Network. The North American Fetal Therapy Network Registry data on outcomes of radiofrequency ablation for twin-reversed arterial perfusion sequence. Fetal Diagn Ther. 2013;33(4):224-9.
2. Moldenhauer J, Lim F-Y, Miller R, Johnson A, Emery S, Moon-Grady A, et al. 180: North American fetal therapy network: selective reduction in complicated monochorionic twins. Am J Obstet Gynecol. 2017;216(1):S118-S119.

STATION 19.

1. **For a woman undergoing amniocentesis, what would be the investigations mandatary preoperatively?**
2. **What gauge needle would be required for this procedure?**
3. **What should be done to avoid maternal cell contamination?**
4. **What factors increase the chances of maternal contamination in amniocentesis?**

Ans.

1. Prerequisite investigations would be:
   - Blood group and Rh
   - Detailed ultrasound to look for any fetal anomalies/soft markers.
   - Placental localization to identify the most appropriate window for needle entry.
   - Cervical length assessment
   - Confirming chorionicity and mapping the fetuses in case of multifetal gestation.
2. 20–22 gauge spinal needle
3. Discard first 2 mL of amniotic fluid.
4. Multiple pricks and needle traversing the placenta leading to a bloody tap.

SUGGESTED READING

1. Ghi T, Sotiriadis A, Calda P, Da Silva Costa F, Raine-Fenning N, Alfirevic Z, et al. ISUOG Practice Guidelines: invasive procedures for prenatal diagnosis. Ultrasound Obstet Gynecol. 2016;48(2):256-68.

CHAPTER 21

Medical Transplacental Therapy

K Manikandan, Arpit Jindal

STATION 1.

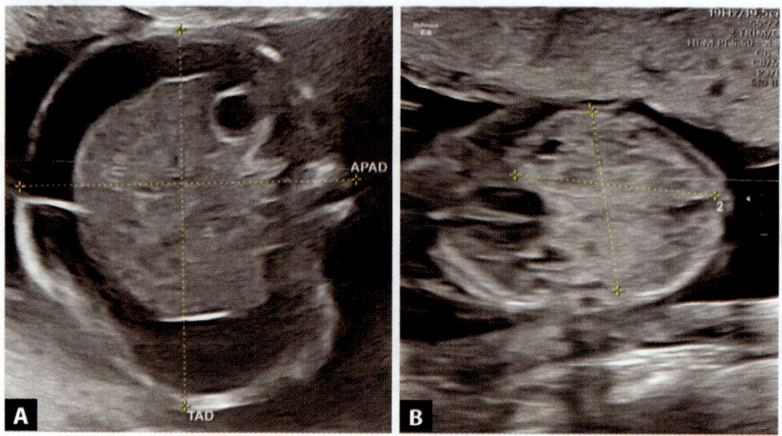

A 26-year-old patient, G2P1L0, with previous intrapartum stillbirth presents with the above images A and B at 21–22 weeks. Given in the images above are the axial sections of the fetal abdomen (Image A) and the fetal thorax (Image B).

1. **What is the primary diagnosis?**
2. **What is the complication seen?**
3. **What is the prenatal prognostication parameter?**
4. **What is the therapeutic intervention in this fetus now, including the dose and regimen?**
5. **What is the success rate of such therapy?**

Ans.

1. Congenital pulmonary airway malformation, solid type
2. Ascites and subcutaneous edema or hydrops fetalis
3. Congenital pulmonary airway malformation (CPAM) volume ratio or CVR
4. *Maternal corticosteroid:* Injection betamethasone 12 mg two doses 24 hours apart
5. 80% survival after two courses

SUGGESTED READING

1. Fortes IMLP, Junior JRB. Use of Corticosteroids in Prenatal Treatment of Congenital Pulmonary Adenomatoid Malformation: Integrative Review. Rev Bras Ginecol Obstet. 2022;44(3):304-10.

STATION 2. A second gravida presents for booking visit. She is 6 weeks from last menstrual period (LMP). In her previous pregnancy, the child was born with ambiguous genitalia and spent 3 weeks in neonatal intensive care unit (NICU) due to poor feeding, vomiting, and dehydration. Neonatal clinical charts have documented hypoglycemia, hyponatremia, hyperkalemia, and elevated 17OH progesterone levels in serum. The child is now 9 months and is attending pediatric surgery for evaluation of ambiguous genitalia.

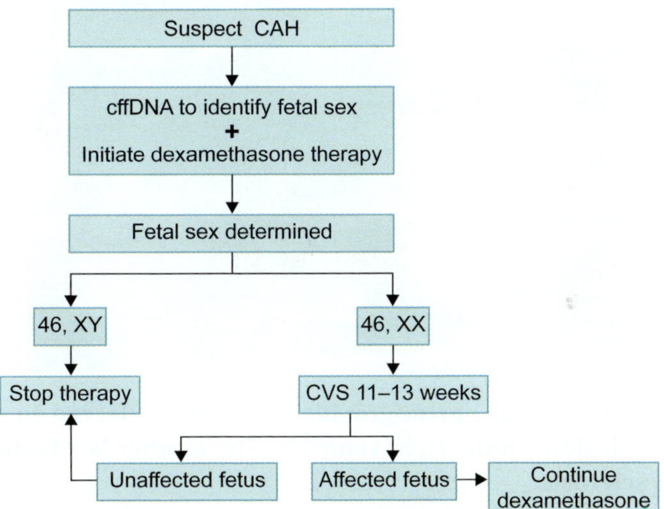

1. **What is the diagnosis based on the given history?**
2. **What are the two broad clinical categories of the disease based on the time of presentation? What is the most common etiology for the clinical presentation shown in the above image?**
3. **What is the transplacental therapy that can prevent the recurrence of ambiguous genitalia in the current pregnancy—mention the starting gestational age, dose, and total duration of therapy?**
4. **How do you offer prenatal diagnosis for this case and what is the mode of inheritance of this disorder?**
5. **What is the premise of the above therapy?**

Ans.

1. Congenital adrenal hyperplasia
2. Classic and nonclassic; 21-α-hydroxylase enzyme deficiency

3. Dexamethasone, orally started before 7 weeks, dose 20 μg/kg maternal body weight, stop by 16 weeks
4. Chorionic villous sampling for the mutation of congenital adrenal hyperplasia (CAH); autososmal recessive
5. To prevent virilization of the female fetus.

SUGGESTED READING

1. Okpaise OO, Ahn H, Tonni G, Ruano R. Prenatal diagnosis and in utero treatment of congenital adrenal hyperplasia: an up-to-date comprehensive review. Prenat Diagn. 2024;44(5):635-64.

STATION 3.

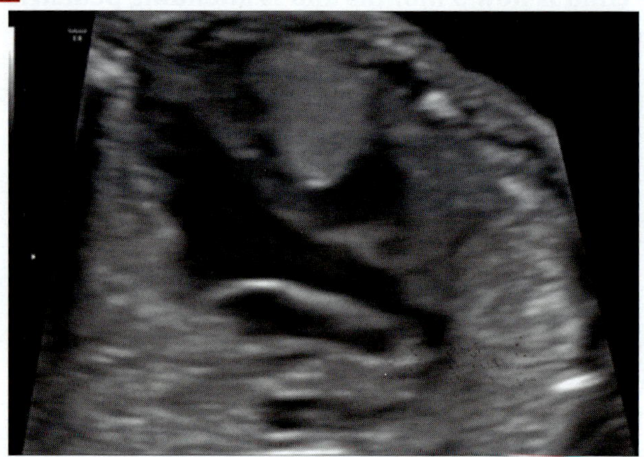

A 21-year-old woman, primigravida, has been referred in view of a "echogenic lesion" in the right ventricle. The mother is a known case of tuberous sclerosis.

1. **What is the diagnosis of cardiac lesion?**
2. **Mention the indications for treating this cardiac lesion in utero.**
3. **What is the drug that can be used to treat this lesion?**
4. **What is the usual natural history of this cardiac lesion?**
5. **What factor is believed to be responsible for regression of the rhabdomyomas at birth?**

Ans.

1. Cardiac rhabdomyoma
2. Outflow tract obstruction; arrhythmia
3. Sirolimus
4. Spontaneous regression in 50% of cases by the age of 2 years.
5. Rhabdomyomas are believed to regress owing to the mitotic potential of maternal estrogens being lost at birth.

SUGGESTED READING

1. Kıztanır H, Sulu A, Akin T, Kosger P, Ucar B. Fetal and postnatal diagnosis and management of cardiac rhabdomyomas and association with tuberous sclerosis complex. Cir Cardiov. 2023;30(5):294-99.
2. Park H, Chang CS, Choi SJ, Oh SY, Roh CR. Sirolimus therapy for fetal cardiac rhabdomyoma in a pregnant woman with tuberous sclerosis. Obstet Gynecol Sci. 2019;62(4):280-4.

STATION 4.

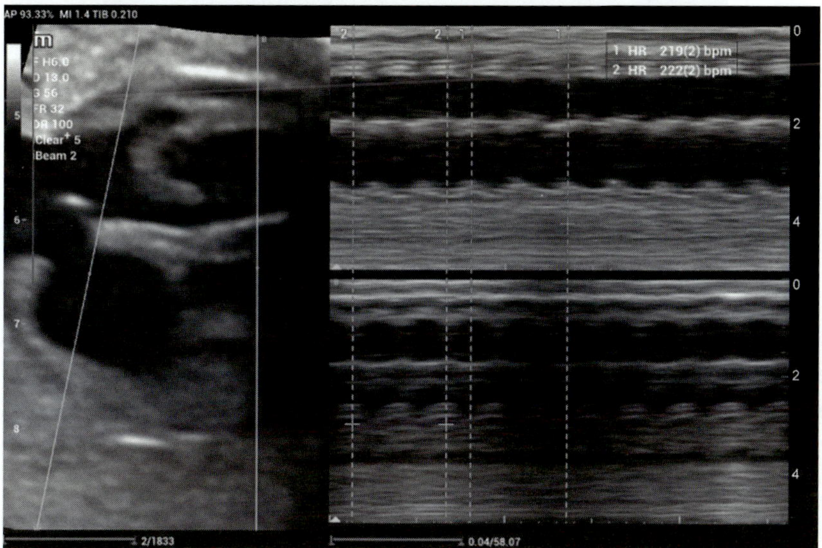

A 20-year-old woman, primigravida, Rh negative pregnancy, came for routine growth scan at 32 weeks. There is normal intracardiac segmental anatomy. Her atrial rate is 219 beats/min and ventricular rate is 222 beats/min.

1. **What is the diagnosis based on the given history and imaging?**
2. **What can be the complication if left untreated?**
3. **List three first-line drugs that can be used to treat this transplacentally.**
4. **What is the most important concern during fetal treatment?**

Ans.

1. Supraventricular tachycardia
2. Hydrops and fetal demise
3. Digoxin, flecainide, and sotalol
4. Maternal drug toxicity

SUGGESTED READING

1. Wacker-Gussmann A, Strasburger JF, Cuneo BF, Wakai RT. Diagnosis and treatment of fetal arrhythmia. Am J Perinatol. 2014;31(7):617-28.

STATION 5.

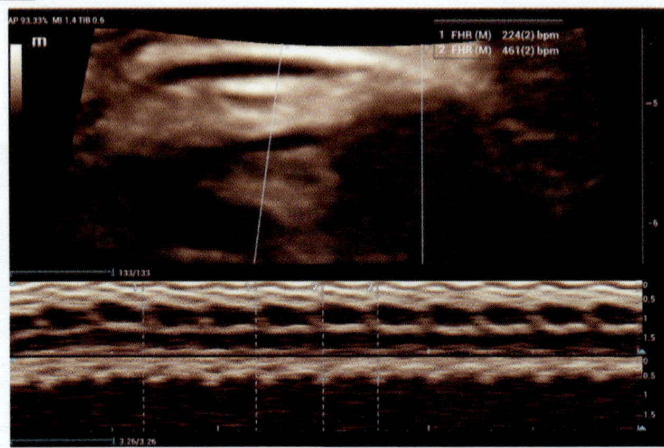

A 28-year-old patient, G2P1, came for growth scan at 32 weeks 3 days. Her atrial rate was 461 beats/min and ventricular rate was 224 beats/min. There is normal intracardiac segmental anatomy and no features of hydrops.

1. **What is the diagnosis based on the given history and imaging?**
2. **Which of the given parameters is essential in differentiating this from supraventricular tachycardia?**
3. **Of the available drugs for transplacental therapy, which can result in cardioversion than simple rate control?**
4. **What are the parameters to be monitored in the mother?**

Ans.

1. Atrial flutter
2. Atrial rate
3. Sotalol; digitalis
4. ECG, electrolytes

SUGGESTED READING

1. Wacker-Gussmann A, Strasburger JF, Cuneo BF, Wakai RT. Diagnosis and treatment of fetal arrhythmia. Am J Perinatol. 2014;31(7):617-28.

STATION 6.

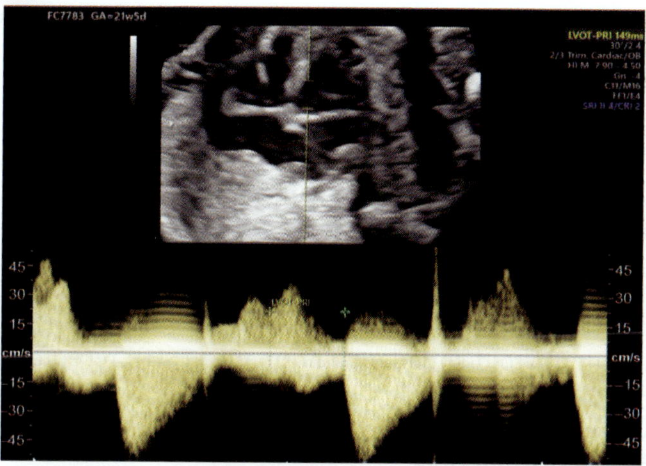

A 25-year-old patient, primigravida, at 21 weeks 5 days period of gestation, is anti-Ro strongly positive. On detailed fetal echocardiography, there is diffuse echogenicity of anterior papillary muscle of right ventricle and left ventricle with increased echogenicity of aortic root annulus. mPR interval is 149 s (>99th for the gestational age). Atrial heart rate is 143 beats/min and ventricular heart rate 143 beats/min.

1. **What is the diagnosis based on the given history and imaging?**
2. **Mention the landmarks for measuring the mechanical PR interval in the fetus.**
3. **What can be the complication if left untreated?**
4. **What drug given transplacentally can potentially revert the finding?**
5. **What is a potential complication of the therapy given in question 4 above?**

Ans.

1. First-degree heart block
2. Beginning of "A" wave to beginning of ventricular ejection (V wave)
3. Complete (third degree) heart block
4. Tablet dexamethasone 4–8 mg OD
5. Fetal growth restriction (FGR)

SUGGESTED READING

1. Melim C, Pimenta J, Areias JC. Congenital atrioventricular heart block: From diagnosis to treatment. Rev Port Cardiol. 2022;41(3):231-40.

STATION 7. **A 26-year-old patient, G2A1, 26 weeks 1 day, recently diagnosed with hyperthyroidism. On ultrasound examination of the fetus, there are features of anterior neck mass and fetal heart rate of 190 beats/min. She is currently not on any medication.**

1. **What is the cause of fetal goiter?**
2. **Which maternal antibody is responsible for the fetal condition?**
3. **What is the test to confirm the fetal diagnosis?**
4. **First-line drug of treatment.**

Ans.

1. Fetal hyperthyroidism
2. Thyrotropin [thyroid-stimulating hormone (TSH)] receptor antibodies (TRAb)
3. Fetal blood sampling
4. Methimazole/carbimazole

SUGGESTED READING

1. Alexander EK, Pearce EN, Brent GA, Brown RS, Chen H, Dosiou C, et al. 2017 Guidelines of the American Thyroid Association for the Diagnosis and Management of Thyroid Disease During Pregnancy and the Postpartum. Thyroid. 2017;27(3):315-89.

STATION 8.

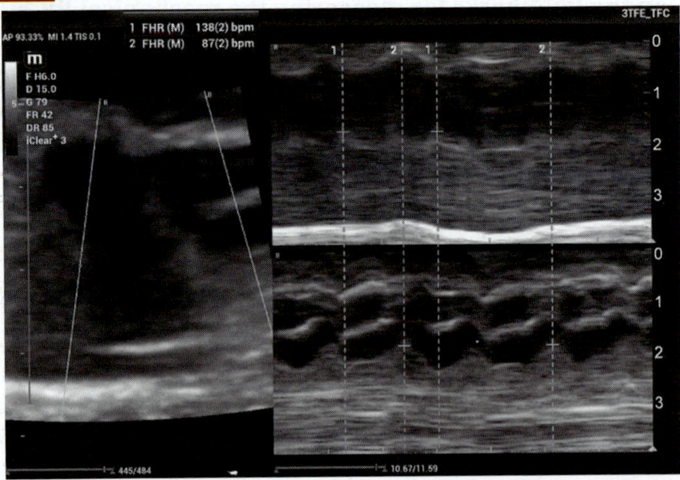

A 21-year-old woman, primigravida, at 21 weeks 1 day period of gestation. She is strongly positive for anti-Ro antibodies. The atrial rate is 138 beats/min and regular and ventricular rate is 87 beats/min and

regular. The intracardiac segmental anatomy is normal. No features of hydrops.

1. **What is fetal cardiac diagnosis?**
2. **What other potential cardiac pathology can happen?**
3. **What is the risk of recurrence of this condition in a subsequent pregnancy?**
4. **What drug has shown promise in reducing the risk of recurrence of this condition in such mothers?**

Ans.

1. Congenital heart block (or congenital atrioventricular block)
2. Myocarditis
3. 18%
4. Hydroxy chloroquine

SUGGESTED READING

1. Melim C, Pimenta J, Areias JC. Congenital atrioventricular heart block: From diagnosis to treatment. Rev Port Cardiol. 2022;41(3):231-40.

STATION 9.

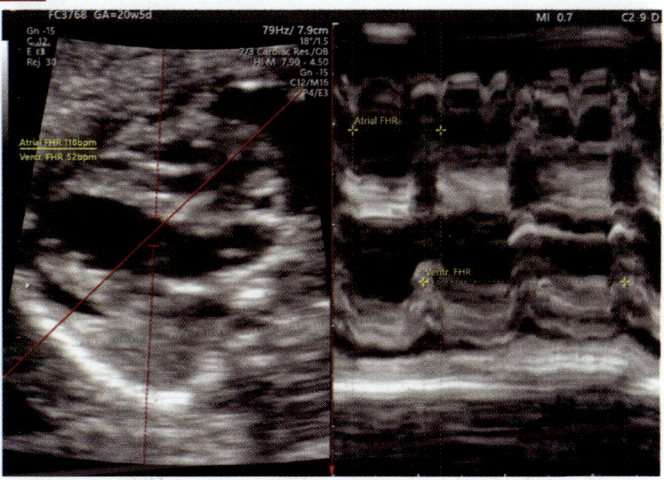

A 20-year-old woman, primigravida, is strongly positive for anti-Ro. Her atrial rate is 118 beats/min and ventricular rate is 52 beats/min. There is associated pericardial effusion and mild ascites and normal intracardiac segmental anatomy.

1. **What are the findings in the above image?**
2. **What is the diagnosis based on history and image findings?**

3. **She has been started on oral dexamethasone. What additional drug may be considered to improve cardiac rate?**
4. **Mention any two poor prognostic factors in this condition?**

Ans.

1. Atrial contractions and ventricular contractions are independent of each other.
2. Third-degree heart block; complete atrioventricular block
3. Salbutamol (oral 2 mg OD)
4. Hydrops; ventricular rate <55 beats/min; endocardial fibroelastosis

SUGGESTED READING

1. Melim C, Pimenta J, Areias JC. Congenital atrioventricular heart block: From diagnosis to treatment. Rev Port Cardiol. 2022;41(3):231-40.

STATION 10.

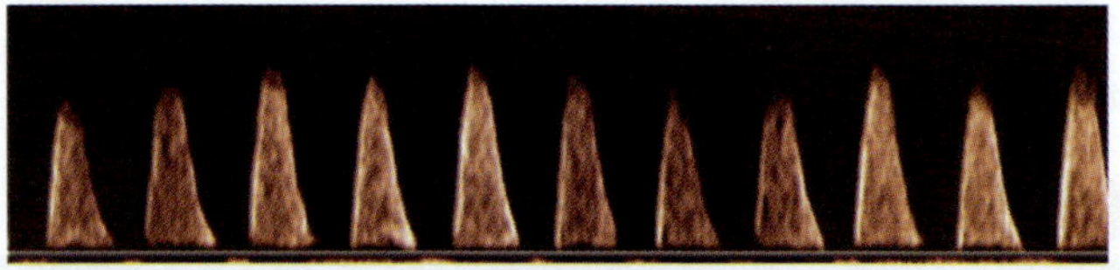

A 35-year-old patient, primigravida, with gestational hypertension presented for fetal growth assessment at 31 weeks 1 day period of gestation. The estimated fetal weight (EFW) is 1st centile (890 g) with absent end diastolic flow in umbilical artery and high resistance flow in ductus venosus.

1. **What is the stage of the fetal condition?**
2. **What drug can be given to mother to decrease the mortality and morbidity of the newborn?**
3. **What is the mechanism of action?**
4. **What is the ideal time interval to deliver after giving the drug?**

Ans.

1. Stage III FGR
2. Fluorinated corticosteroids (dexamethasone/betamethasone)
3. Surfactant production; gene expression
4. Between 2 and 7 days after initiation of the treatment course

SUGGESTED READING

1. Brownfoot FC, Gagliardi DI, Bain E, Middleton P, Crowther CA. Different corticosteroids and regimens for accelerating fetal lung maturation for women at risk of preterm birth. Cochrane Database Syst Rev. 2013;(8):CD006764.

STATION 11. **A 32-year-old woman, G2A1, with hypothyroidism, came for fetal growth assessment at 31 weeks 1 day period of gestation. The EFW is 800 g (<1st centile) with oligohydramnios. Umbilical artery Doppler shows reversed end diastolic flow, with normal flow in ductus venosus.**

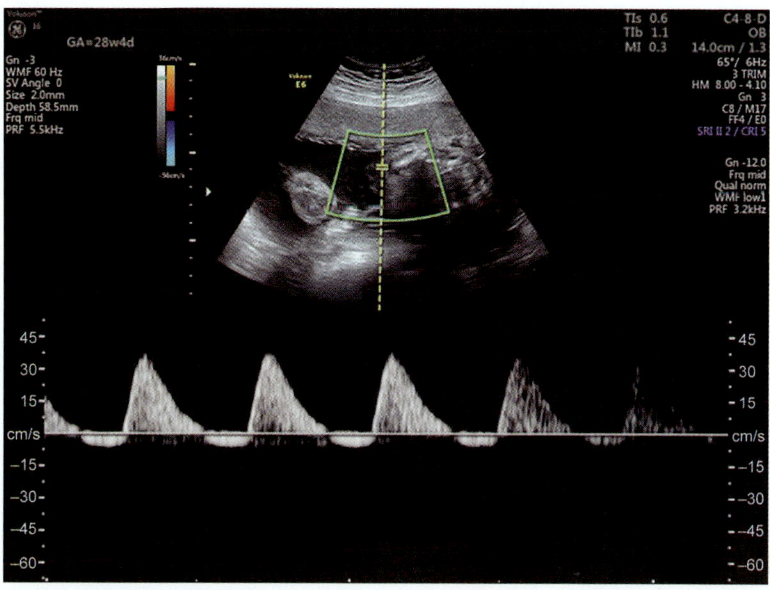

1. **When should you plan delivery of this fetus?**
2. **The parents are concerned about cerebral palsy in the premature infant. What drug has been shown to reduce the risk of this condition?**
3. **What is the mechanism of action?**
4. **What is the dose regimen for the above mentioned drug?**

Ans.

1. Delivery after steroids
2. $MgSO_4$
3. Membrane stabilization; prevention of damage by free radicals
4. 4 g IV over 30 minutes, followed by IV infusion of 1 g/h until delivery; to be started at least 4 hours before expected delivery, and not before 24 hours of expected delivery

SUGGESTED READING

1. Luyt K. Antenatal magnesium sulphate reduces cerebral palsy after preterm birth, implementation into clinical practice needs to be accelerated globally to benefit preterm babies. Cochrane Database Syst Rev. 2024;9(9):ED000168.

STATION 12. **A 32-year-old patient, primigravida, delivered at 37 weeks 5 days following induction for gestational hypertension. The newborn was hydropic, pale, and required resuscitation. Neonatal abdomen ultrasound revealed ascites and hepatomegaly. Infection screening and inborn errors of metabolism screening returned negative, while serum ferritin was highly elevated. Liver biopsy was indicative of neonatal hemochromatosis, and a final diagnosis of gestational autoimmune liver disease was established. Unfortunately, the newborn expired.**

1. **What is the recurrence risk in subsequent pregnancy?**
2. **What drug can be given to the mother antenatally to prevent this disease?**
3. **Mention the dose and schedule of the drug.**
4. **What condition must be excluded in the mother before starting therapy as it can cause anaphylaxis to the treatment drug?**

Ans.

1. 95%
2. Intravenous immunoglobulin
3. Start by 18 weeks; 1 g/kg body weight; weekly once
4. IgA deficiency

SUGGESTED READING

1. Louis D, More K, Oberoi S, Shah PS. Intravenous immunoglobulin in isoimmune hemolytic disease of newborn: an updated systematic review and meta-analysis. Archives of Disease in Childhood-Fetal and Neonatal Edition. 2014; 99(4):F325-31.

STATION 13. **A 31-year-old patient, G2P1, presented at 13 weeks 2 days for combined first trimester screening. Her first baby was postnatally diagnosed to have fetal and neonatal alloimmune thrombocytopenia (FNAIT) and had suffered intraventricular hemorrhage in the newborn period.**

1. **What is the principal drug therapy to prevent FNAIT in the current fetus?**
2. **What is the additional drug to be used to reduce the need for high dose of the principal drug?**
3. **When should the treatment start in high-risk groups?**
4. **What should the fetus be monitored for during the pregnancy?**

Ans.

1. Intravenous immunoglobulin (IVIg)
2. Prednisone
3. 12–16 weeks
4. Intraventricular hemorrhage/intracranial hemorrhage

SUGGESTED READING

1. Wabnitz H, Khan R, Lazarus AH. The use of IVIg in fetal and neonatal alloimmune thrombocytopenia—Principles and mechanisms. Transfus Apher Sci. 2020; 59(1):102710.

STATION 14.

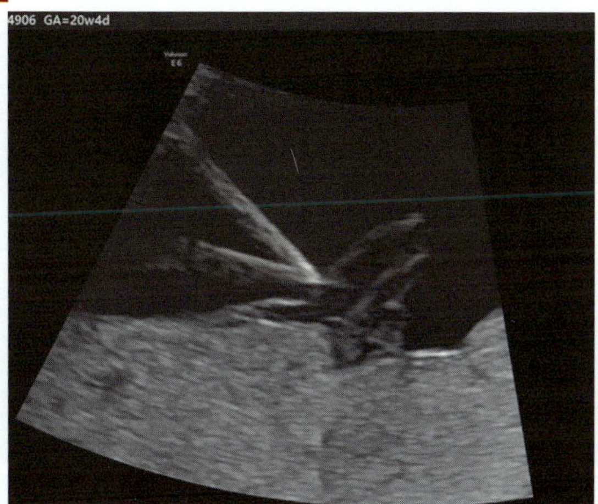

A 26-year-old woman, fourth gravida, underwent intrauterine transfusions four times in the current pregnancy for Rh isoimmunized pregnancy. Her first child is alive and healthy. The second born child has bilirubin-induced neurological damage and has developed features spasticity of upper limbs. The third pregnancy ended in fetal demise after hydrops fetalis was detected at 29 weeks. In the current pregnancy, the last transfusion was given at 34 weeks 5 days.

1. **When is she best delivered?**
2. **The parents are anxious about the neonatal jaundice that complicated their second child. What drug given to the mother can decrease the risk of exchange transfusion in such pregnancies?**
3. **What is the mechanism of action?**
4. **What is the dose?**

Ans.

1. 37–38 weeks
2. Phenobarbital
3. Hepatic induction of enzymes
4. 30 mg tid for the last 7–10 days before birth

SUGGESTED READING

1. Thomas JT, Muller P, Wilkinson C. Antenatal phenobarbital for reducing neonatal jaundice after red cell isoimmunization. Cochrane Database Syst Rev. 2007;2007(2):CD005541.

2. Trevett TN Jr, Dorman K, Lamvu G, Moise KJ Jr. Antenatal maternal administration of phenobarbital for the prevention of exchange transfusion in neonates with hemolytic disease of the fetus and newborn. Am J Obstet Gynecol. 2005;192(2):478-82.

STATION 15.

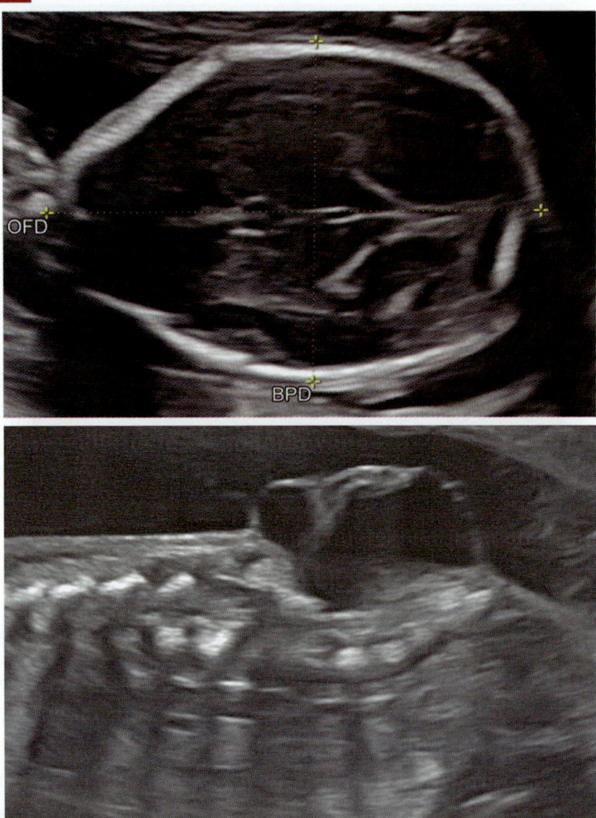

A 33-year-old female, G2A1, working in a coal factory came for pre-pregnancy counseling. Her previous fetus had the findings seen in the above image.

1. **What is the diagnosis?**
2. **What should be given as a prophylaxis that can decrease the chance of recurrence in the next pregnancy?**
3. **Mention the dose.**
4. **Mention the starting period of prophylaxis that can effectively prevent the recurrence.**

Ans.

1. Open neural tube defect (Arnold-Chiari malformation/Chiari II malformation)

2. Folic acid/folate
3. 4 mg or 5 mg
4. 3 months prior to conception

SUGGESTED READING

1. Folic acid for the prevention of neural tube defects. American Academy of Pediatrics. Committee on Genetics. Pediatrics. 1999;104(2 Pt 1):325-7.

STATION 16. **A 26-year-old woman, primigravida, presents at 14 weeks with a scan report suggestive of hepatic calcifications. Her cytomegalovirus (CMV) serology tested positive for both immunoglobulin G (IgG) and IgM.**

Please answer the following questions:

1. **Name one single test that could confirm that this is a recent infection. How would you interpret the report?**
2. **How would you confirm fetal affliction and when?**
3. **How can sequelae to the neonate be prevented following seroconversion in pregnancy?**
4. **How will the fetus be followed up?**

Ans.

1. CMV IgG avidity if <60% is suggestive of recent infection within the past 3 months.
2. Amniocentesis followed by CMV polymerase chain reaction (PCR) on the amniotic fluid sample. The test should be performed at or after 17 weeks gestation provided >8 weeks have elapsed since serological conversion.
3. By offering tablet valacyclovir 2 g four times a day starting as early as maternal infection is diagnosed and continuing until the results of amniotic fluid PCR have been obtained.
4. With USG and MRI in the third trimester to rule out sequelae.

SUGGESTED READING

1. Leruez-Ville M, Chatzakis C, Lilleri D, Blazquez-Gamero D, Alarcon A, Bourgon N, et al. Consensus recommendation for prenatal, neonatal and postnatal management of congenital cytomegalovirus infection from the European congenital infection initiative (ECCI). Lancet Reg Health Eur. 2024;40:100892. Erratum in: Lancet Reg Health Eur. 2024;42:100974.

STATION 17. **In the above scenario say whether the following statements (1–3) regarding neonatal follow-up are right or wrong. Please correct if wrong.**

1. **Congenital CMV infection in the neonate should be confirmed using IgM CMV testing.**

2. **Congenital CMV should be tested for within first 6 weeks of life.**
3. **All neonates diagnosed as late onset FGR secondary to utero-placental insufficiency should be tested for congenital CMV.**
4. **What assessments should the neonate be offered at birth in a case of suspected congenital CMV infection?**

Ans.

1. No. It should be tested using salivary or urinary CMV PCR. If the salivary test is positive, it is mandatory to confirm with a urinary CMV PCR.
2. No. It should be tested within first 3 weeks.
3. No. All neonates diagnosed as early onset FGR of unknown etiology should be investigated for congenital CMV infection.
4. Anthropometric, ophthalmological, audiometry assessment, complete blood count, and liver function tests should be performed

SUGGESTED READING

1. Leruez-Ville M, Chatzakis C, Lilleri D, Blazquez-Gamero D, Alarcon A, Bourgon N, et al. Consensus recommendation for prenatal, neonatal and postnatal management of congenital cytomegalovirus infection from the European congenital infection initiative (ECCI). Lancet Reg Health Eur. 2024;40:100892. Erratum in: Lancet Reg Health Eur. 2024;42:100974.

CHAPTER 22

Prophylactic Interventions

Preeti Parekh Tomar

STATION 1.

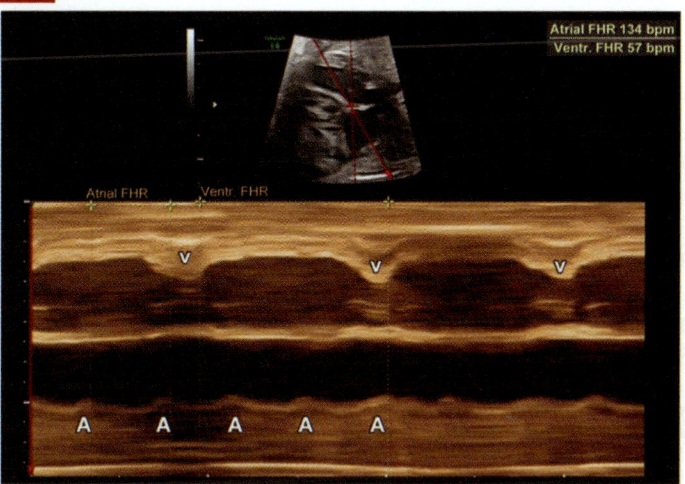

Mrs X, a 25-year-old P1L0, comes to your OPD for prenatal counselling. In her last pregnancy, the fetus was diagnosed to have a complete heart block, following which the fetus developed hydrops and she had an intrauterine demise at 30 weeks. The mother was worked up and was found to be positive for anti-Sjögren's syndrome-related antigen A (anti-SSA)/Ro antibodies.

1. **What is the risk of having recurrent congenital heart block in subsequent pregnancies in this patient?**
2. **Which drug can be offered to this patient for prevention of recurrent congenital heart block (CHB)?**
3. **What is the risk of recurrent heart block after initiation of the aforementioned drug?**
4. **What is the mechanism of action by which this drug works in prevention of CHBs in women who test positive for anti-SSA/Ro antibodies.**
5. **Name the trial that has studied the drug and its use in prevention of CHB in women with anti SSA/Ro antibodies.**

Ans.

1. The risk of congenital heart block in a fetus exposed to maternal anti-SSA/Ro antibodies is approximately 2% if the mother has never had an affected child and 18% if she has.
2. Hydroxychloroquine 400 mg, initiated at or before 10 weeks of period of gestation.
3. After initiation of hydroxychloroquine (HCQ), the risk of recurrent CHB decreased to half, from 18 to 7.4%.
4. Immune complexes containing SSA/Ro antibodies bind to toll-like receptors on macrophages which lead to secretion of cytokines that cause endomyocardial fibrosis. This inflammatory response is suppressed by HCQ, which acts as a TLR antagonist, by activation of endosomal acidification or by directly binding to nucleic acids.
5. Preventive Approach to Congenital Heart Block with Hydroxychloroquine (PATCH) study

SUGGESTED READING

1. Izmirly P, Kim M, Friedman DM, Costedoat-Chalumeau N, Clancy R, Copel JA, et al. Hydroxychloroquine to prevent recurrent congenital heart block in fetuses of anti-SSA/Ro-positive mothers. J Am Coll Cardiol. 2020;76(3):292-302.

STATION 2.

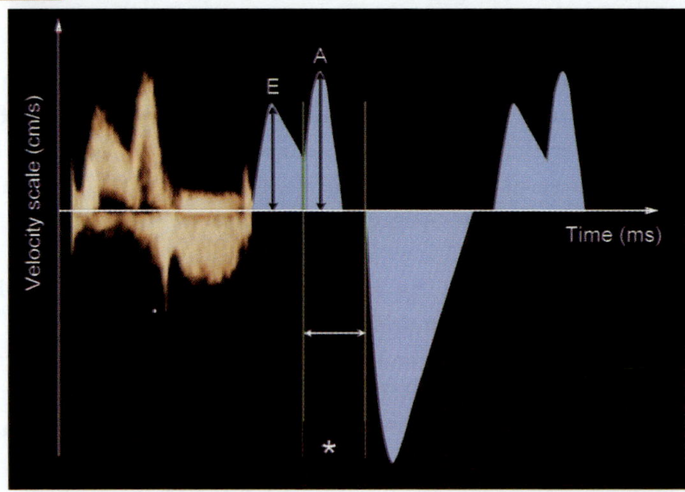

1. **Identify the echocardiography parameter that is being measured here (labeled by *).**
2. **Which fetuses would require monitoring of the above parameter?**
3. **What is the cutoff of the above parameter when it is said to be prolonged?**
4. **How would you manage a fetus which has a normal heart rate, but a prolongation of the above mentioned parameter?**

Ans.

1. Mechanical PR interval
2. Fetuses where the mother has history of recurrent congenital heart block in previous pregnancy/mothers who are positive for anti-SSA (Ro) and anti-SSB (La) antibodies.
3. Mechanical PR interval >150 ms is prolonged, however gestation specific reference charts should be used.
4. Initiation of dexamethasone therapy

SUGGESTED READING

1. De Carolis S, Garufi C, Garufi E, De Carolis MP, Botta A, Tabacco S, et al. Autoimmune congenital heart block: a review of biomarkers and management of pregnancy. Front Pediatr. 2020;8:607515.
2. Wojakowski A, Izbizky G, Carcano ME, Aiello H, Marantz P, Otaño L. Fetal Doppler mechanical PR interval: correlation with fetal heart rate, gestational age and fetal sex. Ultrasound Obstet Gynecol. 2009;34(5):538-42.

STATION 3.

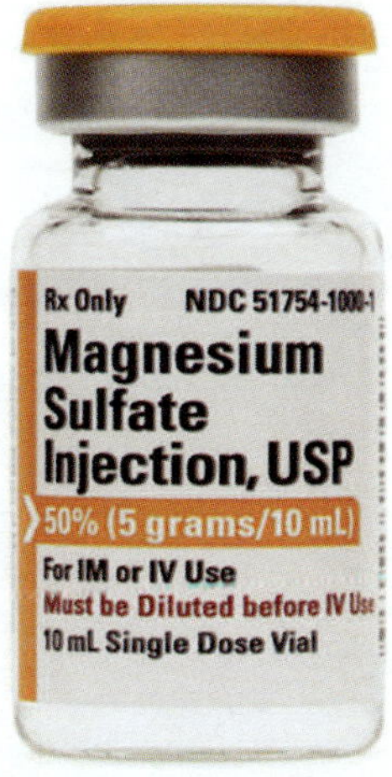

1. **What is the use of the above drug in preventive fetal medicine?**
2. **At what gestational age is the above drug recommended?**
3. **What is the optimal dose and timing of its administration for fetal indication?**
4. **Name the trials that have studied the use of $MgSO_4$ for fetal indications.**

Ans.

1. Neuroprotection in extreme preterm neonates
2. From viability till 32 weeks of gestation
3. In women at risk of early preterm birth, use magnesium sulfate for neuroprotection of the fetus—intravenously with a 4 g loading dose

(administered slowly over 20–30 minutes) followed by 1 g/hour maintenance dose via the intravenous route and continue regimen until birth, but stop after 24 hours if undelivered
4. PREMAG trial, BEAM trial

SUGGESTED READING

1. Marret S, Marpeau L, Zupan-Simunek V, Eurin D, Lévêque C, Hellot MF, et al. Magnesium sulphate given before very-preterm birth to protect infant brain: the randomised controlled PREMAG trial*. BJOG. 2007;114(3):310-8.
2. Rouse DJ, Hirtz DG, Thom E, Varner MW, Spong CY, Mercer BM, et al. A Randomized, Controlled Trial of Magnesium Sulfate for the Prevention of Cerebral Palsy. NEJM. 2008;359(9):895-905.
3. Shennan A, Suff N, Jacobsson B, FIGO Working Group for Preterm Birth. FIGO good practice recommendations on magnesium sulfate administration for preterm fetal neuroprotection. Intern J Gynecol Obstet. 2021;155(1):31-3.

STATION 4.

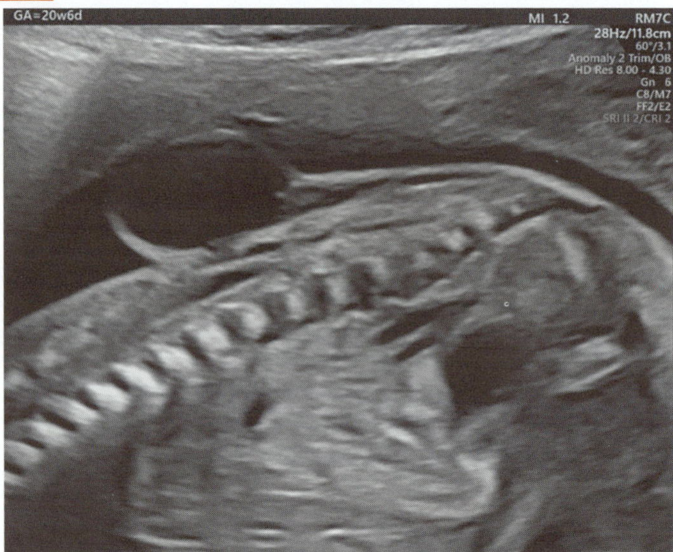

1. **Identify the above condition.**
2. **What are the ultrasound signs in the brain that are associated with this condition in the second trimester?**
3. **How early can this be diagnosed and how?**
4. **Which drug is known to prevent this condition?**

Ans.

1. Open spina bifida
2. Lemon sign, Banana sign, ventriculomegaly
3. 11–13 weeks scan—obliteration of intracranial translucency, crash sign
4. Folic acid starting from the periconceptional period

SUGGESTED READING

1. Chaoui R, Benoit B, Mitkowska-Wozniak H, Heling KS, Nicolaides KH. Assessment of intracranial translucency (IT) in the detection of spina bifida at the 11-13-week scan. Ultrasound Obstet Gynecol. 2009;34(3):249-52.
2. Recommendations for the use of folic acid to reduce the number of cases of spina bifida and other neural tube defects. MMWR Recomm Rep. 1992;41(RR-14):1-7.

STATION 5.

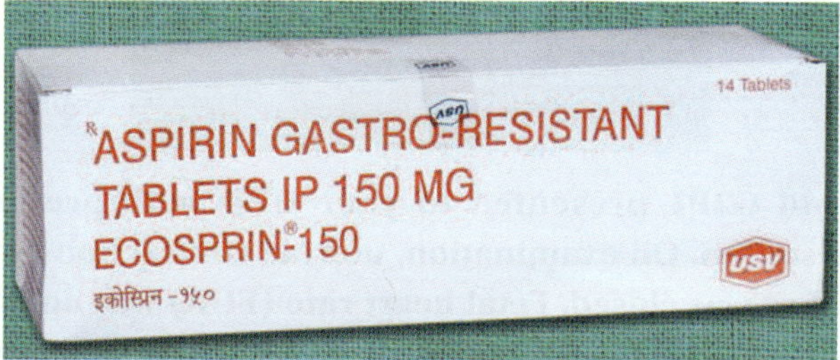

1. **What is this drug used to prevent in pregnancy?**
2. **What is the best time to screen for preeclampsia?**
3. **What is the optimal dosage of this drug?**
4. **Name the study which studies the effect of aspirin on preeclampsia prevention.**

Ans.

1. Preterm preeclampsia and fetal growth restriction
2. 11 - 13 + 6 weeks
3. 150 mg given at bedtime prior to 16 weeks
4. ASPRE

SUGGESTED READING

1. Rolnik DL, Wright D, Poon LCY, Syngelaki A, O'Gorman N, de Paco Matallana C, et al. ASPRE trial: performance of screening for preterm pre-eclampsia. Ultrasound Obstet Gynecol. 2017;50(4):492-5.

STATION 6.

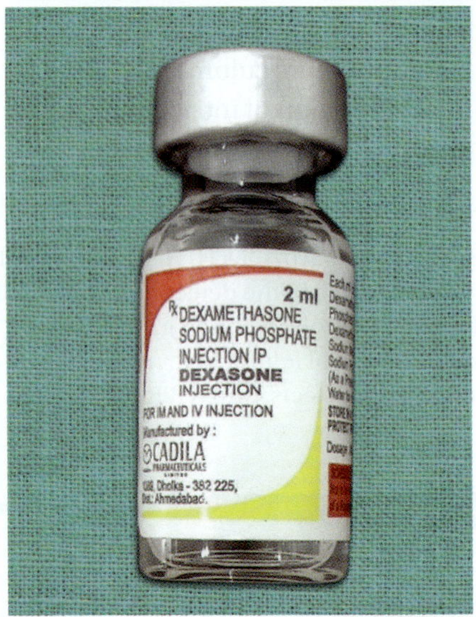

A 34-year-old G2P1 presented to your OPD with preterm pain at 30 weeks' gestation. On examination, uterine contractions were present and external os was closed. Fetal heart rate (FHR) was normal. Despite tocolytic therapy, the contractions progressed and after 24 hours, cervix dilated to 1 cm.

1. **Which drug can be used to prevent respiratory distress syndrome?**
2. **What is the optimal dosage of the drug?**
3. **Which salt is used in India for the above purpose?**
4. **What is the consensus on repeat dose if previous dose is given few weeks earlier?**

Ans.

1. Corticosteroids—betamethasone and dexamethasone
2. Betamethasone—two 12 mg boluses given intramuscularly 24 hours apart (total 24 mg)
   Dexamethasone—four doses of 6 mg given intramuscularly (IM) 12 hours apart (total 24 mg)
3. Dexamethasone—four doses of 6 mg given IM 12 hours apart (total 24 mg) as betamethasone sulphate is not available in India.
4. A single rescue course of antenatal corticosteroids if women remain at high risk of preterm birth and >7 days have lapsed since previous treatment.

SUGGESTED READING

1. Stock SJ, Thomson AJ, Papworth S; The Royal College of Obstetricians, Gynaecologists. Antenatal corticosteroids to reduce neonatal morbidity and mortality. BJOG. 2022;129:e35-60.

STATION 7.

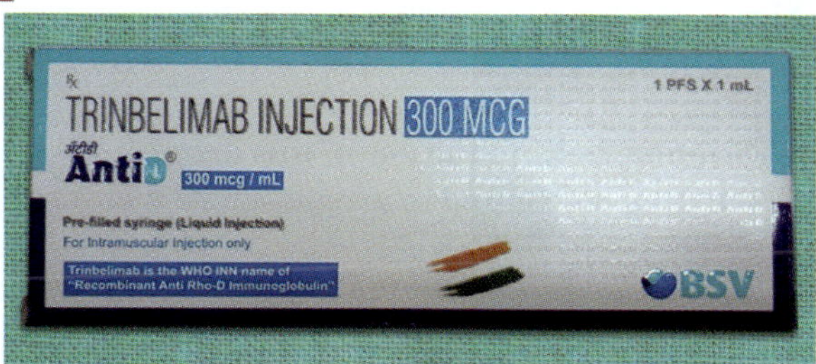

G3P1L1A1, Rh-negative (husband Rh-positive), comes to your antenatal clinic at 22 weeks of gestation with Rh titers of 1:64. Her ultrasound reveals single live intrauterine gestation corresponding to the period of gestation.

1. **What complications do we expect in the fetus of an isoimmunized mother?**
2. **What is the principal physiological rationale for increased fetal middle cerebral artery-peak systolic velocity (MCA-PSV) in anemic states?**
3. **Which is the method of choice to monitor the babies for fetal anemia in Rh-negative mothers?**
4. **If the indirect Coombs test (ICT) titers were negative, what measures would be indicated to prevent sensitization in pregnancy?**

Ans.

1. Fetal hemolytic disease with anemia
2. *Fetal anemia:* Increased flow of low viscosity blood preserves brain oxygenation
3. Serial sonographic surveillance every 1–2 weeks for fetal risk of anemia using MCA-PSV. MCA-PSV >1.5 multiples of the median (MoM) for gestational age is used as a cutoff for moderate-to-severe fetal anemia requiring cordocentesis and possible intrauterine transfusion.
4. Routine prophylactic antenatal administration of anti-D immunoglobulin in the absence of new-onset D-sensitization by 28 weeks' gestation

SUGGESTED READING

1. Qureshi H, Massey E, Kirwan D, Davies T, Robson S, White J, et al. BCSH guideline for the use of anti-D immunoglobulin for the prevention of haemolytic disease of the fetus and newborn. Transfusion Med. 2014;24:8-20.

STATION 8. A 28-year-old G2P1L1 patient comes to your clinic for counselling. Her previous child is 4 years old affected with congenital adrenal hyperplasia.

1. **What is the genetic basis of the disease, and which antenatal test can help in detecting congenital adrenal hyperplasia (CAH) in the ongoing pregnancy?**
2. **Which drug is given in pregnancy in mothers with previous child with CAH?**
3. **What is the rationale behind the use of this drug?**
4. **How long is the drug continued in pregnancy?**

Ans.

1. A total of 95% of CAH cases are caused by *21-hydroxylase (OH)* deficiency coded by the gene *CYP21A2* on chromosome 6. The second most common enzyme deficiency leading to CAH is 11 β-hydroxylase (*11 β-OH*) deficiency, which makes up 5–8% of CAH cases and is encoded by the *CYP11B2* gene located on chromosome 8q21.
   Chorionic villous sampling for direct DNA analysis of the *CYP21A2* gene
2. Low-dose dexamethasone is started before the 7th–8th weeks' gestation
3. Low-dose dexamethasone may prevent virilization of the developing female genitalia.
   As the adrenal glands have not started to secrete androgen and fetal labioscrotal folds are yet to close.
4. Low-dose dexamethasone dosing is continued throughout the pregnancy until fetal sex is determined to be male or if the female fetus is deemed not to have CAH.

SUGGESTED READING

1. Okpaise OO, Ahn H, Tonni G, Ruano R. Prenatal diagnosis and in utero treatment of congenital adrenal hyperplasia: an up-to-date comprehensive review. Prenat Diagn. 2024;44(5):635-43.

SECTION 6

Completing the Jigsaw

23. **Drugs and Radiation**
    Malathi Prasad, Pooja Vaziraani

24. **Fetal Autopsy**
    Manisha Kumar

Drugs and Radiation

Malathi Prasad, Pooja Vaziraani

STATION 1.

1. **What is a teratogen?**
2. **What are the key factors that determine whether an agent is teratogenic?**
3. **What is the most critical period of fetal development in terms of teratogenic effects?**

Ans.

1. A teratogen is any substance, organism, or physical agent that can cause developmental abnormalities or birth defects in a fetus when a pregnant woman is exposed to it during pregnancy.
2. The key factors include the timing of exposure (e.g., during specific stages of organ development), the dose of the teratogen, and the genetic susceptibility of the fetus.
3. The most critical period is during the first trimester, especially between weeks 3 and 8, when organogenesis occurs and the fetus is highly vulnerable to developmental disruptions.

SUGGESTED READING

1. Winterstein AG, Wang Y, Smolinski NE, Thai TN, Ewig C, Rasmussen SA. Prenatal Care initiation and exposure to teratogenic medications. JAMA Netw Open. 2024;7(2):e2354298.

STATION 2.

Case scenario: **A pregnant woman (12 weeks) has been prescribed valproate for epilepsy.**

1. **What are the major categories of drugs in terms of their safety during pregnancy?**
2. **What would you advise her regarding its use in pregnancy?**
3. **A pregnant woman asks if drinking alcohol during pregnancy is safe. What would you advise her?**

Ans.

1. The major categories include:
   - *Category A:* Drugs that are considered safe during pregnancy (no risk to the fetus in well-controlled studies).

- *Category B:* Drugs that have not shown a risk to the fetus in animal studies, but no adequate studies in pregnant women.
- *Category C:* Drugs that may have adverse effects on the fetus based on animal studies, but their benefits might outweigh the risks in some cases.
- *Category D:* Drugs that show evidence of human fetal risk but may be prescribed in life-threatening situations when the benefits outweigh the risks.
- *Category X:* Drugs that should not be used during pregnancy as they have been shown to cause harm to the fetus.

2. Valproate is classified as Category D, which means there is evidence of harm to the fetus. It can cause neural tube defects, cognitive impairments, and other birth defects. If she has already been taking valproate, she should not stop it abruptly without medical guidance, as this can lead to seizures, which may also harm the fetus.
3. Alcohol consumption during pregnancy is not safe and can lead to fetal alcohol spectrum disorders (FASD), which can cause physical, behavioral, and cognitive impairments. There is no known safe level of alcohol during pregnancy.

SUGGESTED READING

1. Genetic Alliance; District of Columbia Department of Health. Appendix D, Teratogens/Prenatal Substance Abuse. Understanding Genetics: A District of Columbia Guide for Patients and Health Professionals. Washington (DC): Genetic Alliance; 2010.
2. Ornoy A, Koren G, Yanai J. Is post exposure prevention of teratogenic damage possible: Studies on diabetes, valproic acid, alcohol and anti folates in pregnancy: Animal studies with reflection to human. Reproductive Toxicology. 2018;80:92-104.

STATION 3.

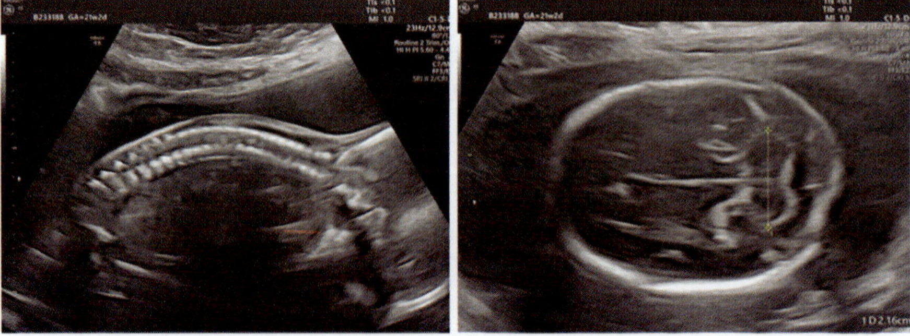

***Case scenario:* A 37-year-old pregnant patient with 22 weeks of gestation and uncontrolled diabetes mellitus (DM) has come for a 2nd opinion for spinal deformity.**

1. **Please see the images and give your diagnosis.**
2. **What is the etiology in such cases and how will you counsel this couple?**
3. **What are the preventive strategies for next pregnancy?**
4. **How will this pregnancy be followed-up if the couple opts to continue?**

Ans.

1. Sacral agenesis type-1. Conus medullaris seen at L5 level (tethered cord).
2. Multifactorial, folic acid deficiency, uncontrolled maternal DM, and syndromes.
3. Sacral agenesis is likely due to diabetes as HBA1C is high (9.4) at the time of organogenesis. Child will have disability due to motor, sensory, neural involvement, and bladder/bowel dysfunction.
4. If they plan to continue pregnancy, follow-up and pediatric neurosurgeon opinion suggested.

If the couple opt to discontinue the pregnancy it is suggested to send fetus and placenta in 10% formalin (1 part formalin in 9 parts water) for detail histopathological examination (HPE) and autopsy. This will help in confirming the diagnosis and to rule out other anomalies which cannot be evident on ultrasound. The information thus gained will help in the next pregnancy.

SUGGESTED READING

1. Gajagowni S, Nair P, Bapat A, Vachharajani AJ. Diabetic Embryopathies. NeoReviews. 2022;23(10):e677-88.

STATION 4.

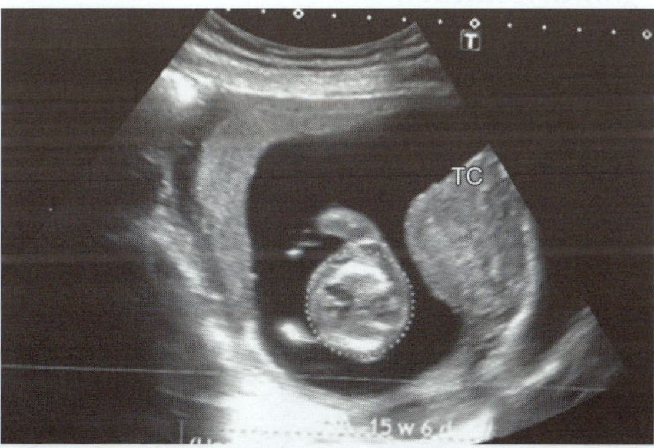

Courtesy: Dr K Aparna Sharma.

1. **This is an axial image at the level of the four-chamber view of the heart. Please identify the limb anomaly shown here.**
2. **Name one possible teratogenic drug causing this condition.**
3. **Give the associated fetal malformations seen with the use of this drug.**
4. **Name one differential diagnosis of this condition.**

Ans.

1. Phocomelia and micromelia—upper limb of the fetus is markedly short with complete or partial absence of bones.
2. Thalidomide
3. Thalidomide exposure notably affects limb development but can affect a wide range of systems. These include:
   - Limb abnormalities
     - Phocomelia
     - Amelia
     - Clubfeet
     - Polydactyly
     - Radial ray anomalies
   - Facial abnormalities
     - Microtia
     - Congenital facial palsy
     - Abnormal lacrimation
     - Orofacial clefts
     - Microphthalmia
   - Congenital cardiac anomalies
     - Ventricular septal defects
     - Atrial septal defects
     - Conotruncal defects
   - Growth
     - Fetal growth restriction
4. *Differential diagnosis:* Roberts syndrome (pseudothalidomide syndrome) an autosomal recessive condition.

SUGGESTED READING

1. Vargesson N. Thalidomide-induced teratogenesis: history and mechanisms. Birth Defects Res C Embryo Today. 2015;105(2):140-56.

STATION 5.

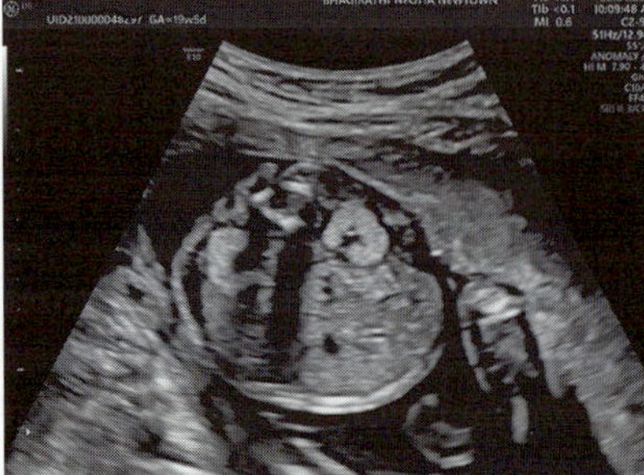

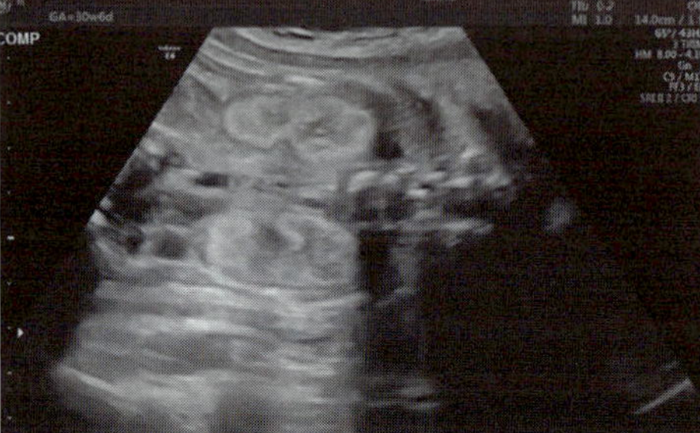

1. **Identify the ultrasound finding.**
2. **Name the antihypertensive drugs associated with this condition.**
3. **What are other common ultrasound findings seen with the use of this drug?**
4. **How will you follow-up?**

Ans.

1. Bilateral echogenic kidneys
2. Angiotensin-converting enzyme (ACE) inhibitors and angiotensin receptor blockers
3. Associated with renal dysgenesis, fetal oliguria (and oligohydramnios), skull defects, fetal growth restriction, and death.
4. Serial fetal sonograms for amniotic fluid volume and fetal growth are indicated for exposures during pregnancy.

SUGGESTED READING

1. Cooper WO, Hernandez-Diaz S, Arbogast PG, Dudley JA, Dyer S, Gideon PS, et al. Major congenital malformations after first-trimester exposure to ACE inhibitors. N Engl J Med. 2006;354(23):2443-51.

STATION 6.

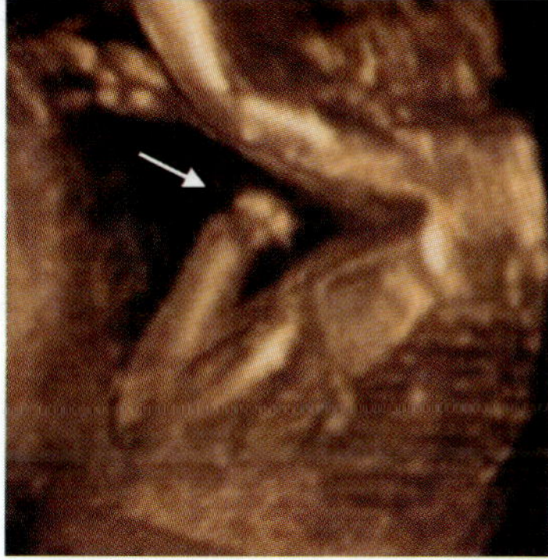
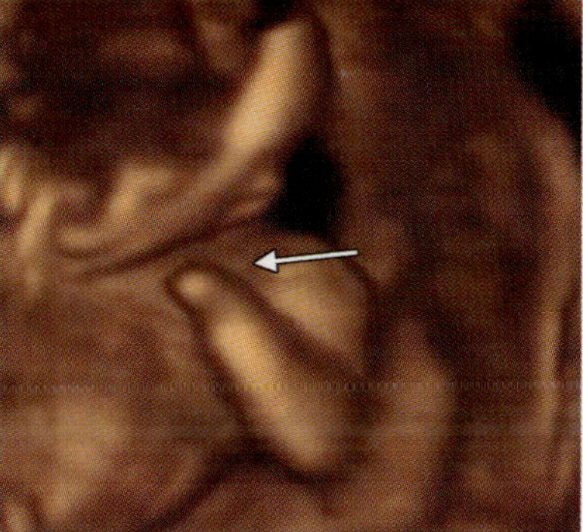

1. **Identify the defect shown in the image.**
2. **Name the abortifacient agent which causes this defect.**
3. **What is the mechanism of action?**
4. **What are other drugs used in pregnancy which result in a similar condition?**

Ans.

1. Terminal transverse defect in the upper limb.
2. Misoprostol
3. Use of Misoprostol leads to hypoperfusion of the fetus, and ischemia and infarction in tenuously perfused areas served by end arteries (limbs, brainstem, spinal cord, intestine, and tongue). The resulting vascular

disruption defects include cranial nerve hypoplasia and terminal transverse defects in the arms and legs (and other limb abnormalities). This combination of abnormalities has been referred to as the Mobius sequence.

4. Teratogen-induced limb defects can be either the result of limb dysmorphogenesis (thalidomide, warfarin, and phenytoin), or vascular disruption of a limb that had formed normally [chorionic villus sampling (CVS)].

SUGGESTED READING

1. Auffret M, Bernard-Phalippon N, Dekemp J, Carlier P, Gervoise Boyer M, Vial T, et al. Misoprostol exposure during the first trimester of pregnancy: Is the malformation risk varying depending on the indication? Eur J Obstet Gynecol Reprod Biol. 2016;207:188-92.

STATION 7.

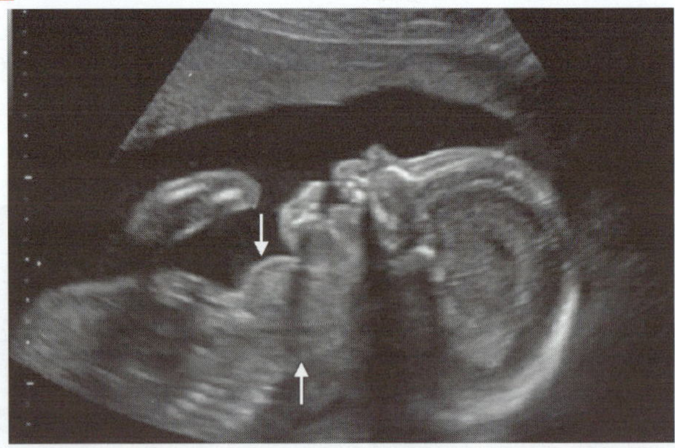

1. **Identify the condition and detail the ultrasound findings.**
2. **What drugs can be associated with this condition?**
3. **How would you further investigate the case?**
4. **What should be the plan for management?**
5. **How should the case be followed-up?**

Ans.

1. *Fetal thyroid goiter ultrasound findings:* Anterior cervical echogenic mass of variable size. The fetal head is hyperextended.
2. Methimazole, carbimazole, and propythiouracil (PTU) can cause fetal goiter and hypothyroidism if used after 10 weeks of gestation when the fetal thyroid begins to concentrate iodide.
3. In most cases, assessment of the maternal condition can help decide whether the cause is fetal hypothyroidism or hyperthyroidism. In uncertain cases, cordocentesis and measurement of fetal blood thyroid hormones and thyroid stimulating hormone (TSH) can help

distinguish between hypothyroidism, with low thyroid hormones and high TSH, due to antithyroid drugs or congenital dyshormonogenesis, and hyperthyroidism, with high thyroid hormones and low TSH, due to thyroid-stimulating immunoglobulins.

4. - *Fetal hypothyroid goiter:* Reduce or even discontinue maternal antithyroid medication aiming to maintain maternal blood thyroxine levels in the upper level of the normal range. The second-line of treatment is intra-amniotic injection of levothyroxine (100 μg/kg) every 1–2 weeks until delivery at term.
   - *Fetal hyperthyroid goiter:* Administration of antithyroid drugs to the mother.
5. Every 4 weeks to monitor fetal growth, size of the tumor, fetal heart rate, amniotic fluid volume, and cervical length.

SUGGESTED READING

1. Figueiredo CM, Falcão I, Vilaverde J, Freitas J, Oliveira MJ, Godinho C, et al. Prenatal diagnosis and management of a fetal goiter hypothyroidism due to dyshormonogenesis. Case Rep Endocrinol. 2018;2018:9564737.

STATION 8.

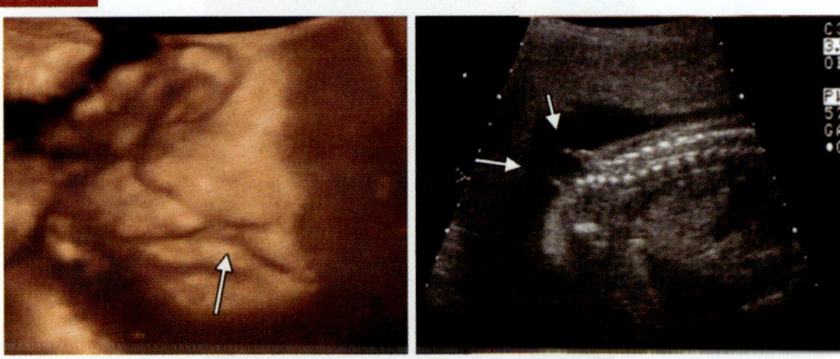

1. **Identify the conditions shown in the images above.**
2. **Name the anticonvulsant drugs associated with these conditions.**
3. **What are the spectrum of conditions seen with use of these drugs. Name four other abnormalities.**

Ans.

1. Cleft lip and palate, neural tube defect—myelomeningocele, facial dysmorphism.
2. Phenytoin, trimethadione, valproic acid, primidone, and carbamazepine.
3. There is a wide clinical spectrum which includes:
   - Scoliosis
   - Intellectual disability
   - *Craniofacial anomalies:* Hypertelorism, long flattened philtrum, micrognathia, microphthalmia, strabismus, midfacial hypoplasia, low-set ears

- *Limb anomalies:* Radial ray anomalies, polydactyly, arachnodactyly, overlapping digits
- Congenital cardiac anomalies
- *Thoracic:* Tracheomalacia
- *Abdominal defects:* Omphalocele, inguinal hernia, duodenal atresia
- *Genitourinary anomalies:* Hypospadias
- *Fetal growth restriction (FGR):* Hyperbilirubinemia, hepatotoxicity, transient hyperglycemia, afibrinogenemia

SUGGESTED READING

1. RCOG green top Guideline No. 68. Epilepsy in pregnancy. [online] Available from https://www.rcog.org.uk/globalassets/documents/guidelines/greentop guidelines/gtg68_epilepsy.pdf [Last accessed May, 2025].

STATION 9.

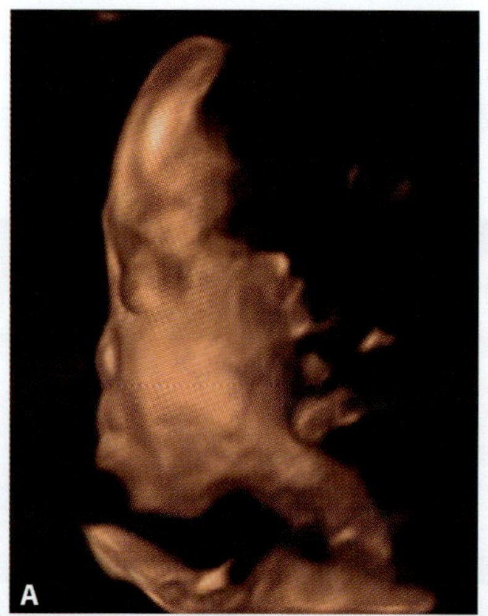

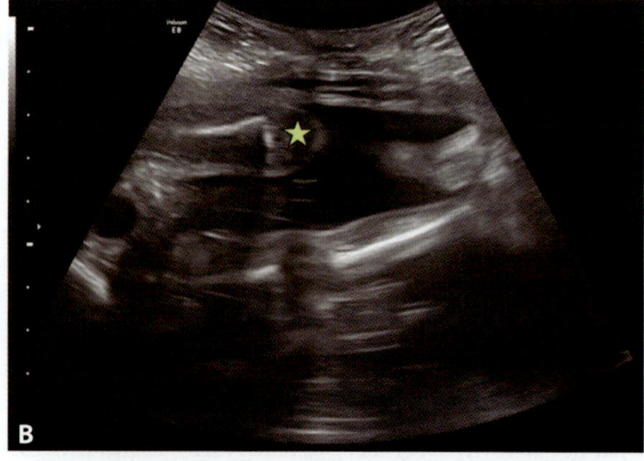

(A) Flat facial profile; (B) Stippling of long bones.
Courtesy: Dr K Aparna Sharma.

1. **Identify the anticoagulant use which causes these changes.**
2. **Write ultrasound findings seen with this condition.**
3. **What dose of this drug is less likely to be associated with fetal teratogenicity?**
4. **Give one differential diagnosis of this condition.**

Ans.

1. Vitamin K antagonists such as Warfarin
2. *Ultrasound features:*
   - Stippled epiphysis
   - Shortened fingers
   - Nasal hypoplasia
   - Limb hypoplasia
   - Choanal atresia
   - Fetal growth retardation
3. *Central nervous system (CNS) malformations:* Dandy Walker malformation, microcephaly, eye defects, agenesis of the corpus callosum
4. *Congenital cardiac defects:* The defects are dose-dependent with less risk at doses <5 mg per day

SUGGESTED READING

1. Regitz-Zagrosek V, Roos-Hesselink JW, Bauersachs J, Blomström-Lundqvist C, Cífková R, De Bonis M, et al. 2018 ESC Guidelines for the management of cardiovascular diseases during pregnancy. Eur Heart J. 2018;39(34):3165-241.

STATION 10.

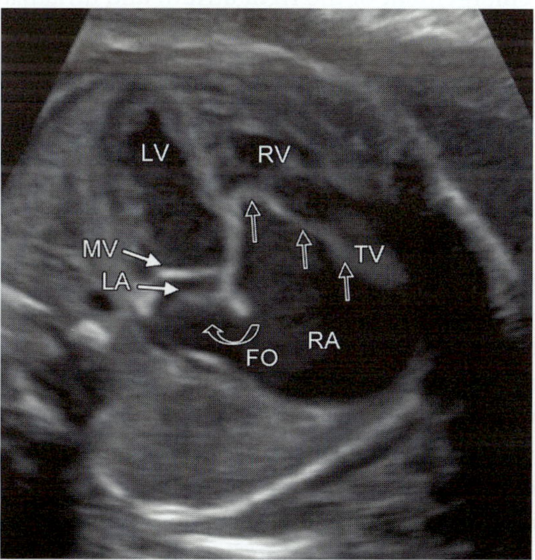

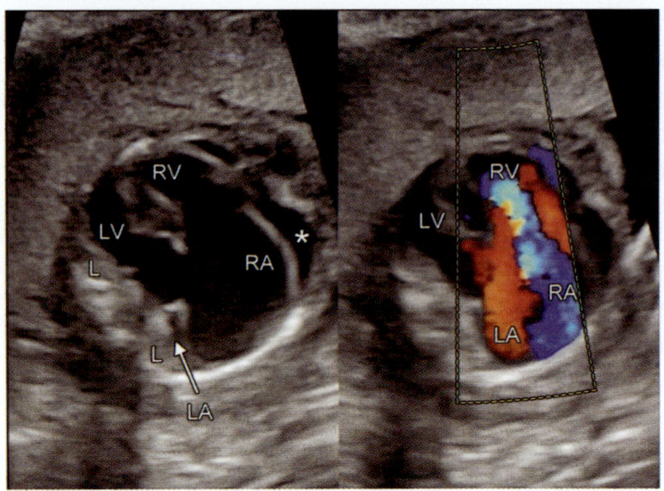

1. **Identify the cardiac anomaly.**
2. **Which drug caused this condition?**
3. **What are the ultrasound diagnosis findings in this condition?**
4. **What are the complications?**
5. **What is the management?**

Ans.

1. Ebstein anomaly
2. Lithium
3. Sonographic findings of Ebstein's anomaly include:
   - Apical displacement of the septal leaflet of the tricuspid valve, which is the principal feature of the anomaly.
   - Marked enlargement of the right atrium and atrialization of the right ventricle are seen.
   - Due to the malformation of the valve, tricuspid valve regurgitation is often noted.
4. Complications include:
   - Cardiomegaly
   - Hydrops fetalis
   - Tachyarrhythmia
5. Management includes:
   - When the diagnosis of Ebstein's anomaly is made in utero, the fetus should be monitored closely for progression of cardiac dysfunction with resultant cardiomegaly, hydrops fetalis, and tachyarrhythmia.
   - Delivery at an appropriate center with a neonatal intensive care unit, pediatric cardiologist, and pediatric anesthesiologist should be arranged.
   - A treatment plan including resuscitation, medical therapy, and the options for surgical intervention should be discussed before delivery.

SUGGESTED READING

1. Patorno E, Huybrechts KF, Bateman BT, Cohen JM, Desai RJ, Mogun H, Cohen LS, et al. Lithium use in pregnancy and the risk of cardiac malformations. N Engl J Med. 2017;376(23):2245-54.

STATION 11.

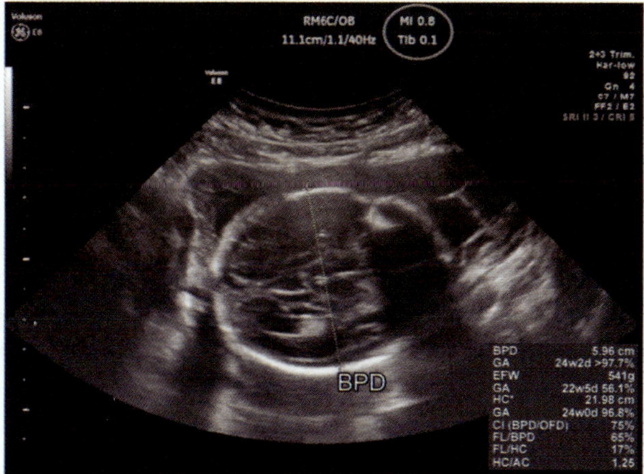

1. **What is depicted in the encircled portion in the ultrasound image?**
2. **What are the main effects of radiation exposure in fetus?**
3. **What is the safe dose and safe period of gestation with radiation exposure?**
4. **What are the diagnostic imaging modalities of choice during pregnancy and what are their irradiation exposure risks?**
5. **What principles should be followed during ultrasound use to keep it safe for fetus?**

Ans.

1. Two safety indices—thermal index and mechanical index-related to likelihood of thermal and nonthermal effects of ultrasound.
2. The main effects include microcephaly, fetal growth retardation, mental retardation, and eye malformations, but spina bifida cystica, cleft palate and skeletal, and visceral abnormalities have also been described.
3. *Dose related:* Risks to the embryo are negligible at doses of diagnostic X-ray studies, usually, ≤5 rads. Microcephaly and mental retardation are associated with doses of 50 rad or greater. 0.05–0.5 Gy is considered safe during the second and third trimesters, less so during the first.
   Gestation related: 2–18 weeks—most sensitive to radiation as period of organogenesis. After 20–25 weeks—less sensitive.
4. Ultrasound and magnetic resonance imaging (MRI) considered safe in pregnancy.

Single plain radiograph does not contribute to a significant radiation dose to the fetus. The estimated radiation dose to the fetus varies and ranges from 0.001–10 mGy depending on the type of study. The highest radiation dose is the lumbar spine radiograph, which has a maximal fetal radiation dose of 10 mGy. Nonetheless, even fetus radiation exposure for the lumbar spine radiograph is significantly lower than the threshold limit of the safe radiation exposure dose of 50 mGy, radiation level that is considered safe and without significant harm.

On the other hand, computed tomography (CT) contributes to a significant amount of fetal radiation. The amount of fetus radiation exposure again varies by the type of study with CT pelvis contributing the highest amount of fetal radiation of 50 mGy. This dose is right at the limit, above which there is a documented negative impact to the fetus.

The plain film, CT, nuclear medicine studies, and fluoroscopy use ionizing radiation to obtain diagnostic images. A high level of radiation has adverse effects on the fetus; therefore, referring clinicians should consider alternative imaging modalities for pregnancy patients.

5. There are a few major rules needed in order to keep the fetal ultrasound safe.
   - TI must be kept below 1. If TI ranges from 0.7 to 1, recommended maximum scanning time for obstetrical scanning may even last up to 60 minutes, which should usually be long enough to obtain relevant clinical information, even in complicated fetal anomalies. However, increasing TI to 2–2.5 decreases recommended maximum time of scanning to <4 minutes.
   - Secondly, exposure time must be limited to be as short as possible, according to the As Low As Reasonably Achievable (ALARA) principle.

SUGGESTED READING

1. Kim E, Boyd B. Diagnostic imaging of pregnant women and fetuses: literature review. Bioengineering (Basel) 2022;9(6):236.
2. Varthaliti A, Fasoulakis Z, Lygizos V, Zolota V, Chatziioannou MI, Daskalaki MA, et al. Safety of Obstetric Ultrasound: Mechanical and Thermal Indexes—A Systematic Review. J Clin Med. 2024;13(21):6588.

CHAPTER 24

Fetal Autopsy

Manisha Kumar

STATION 1. **The case below came as G2P1L0A0, consanguineous marriage, previous baby also had post axial polydactyly, polycystic kidney, and short limbs.**

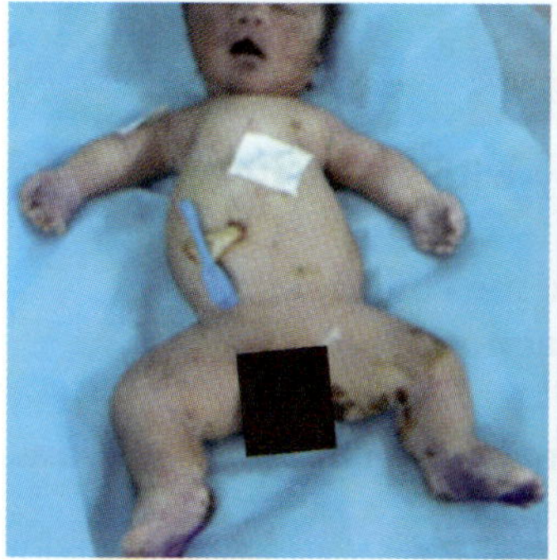
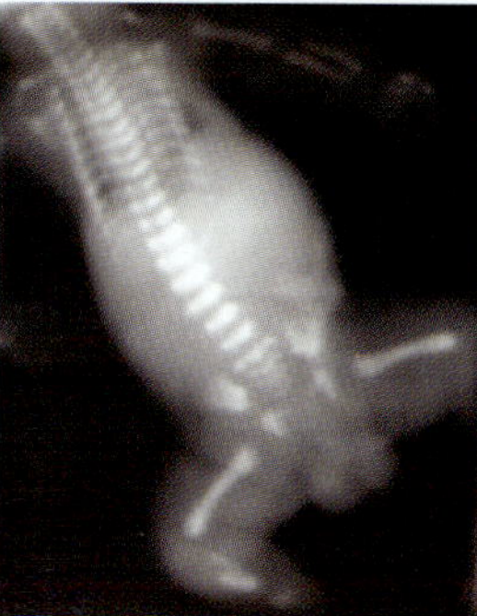
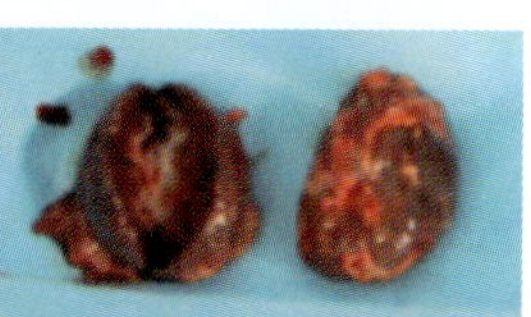
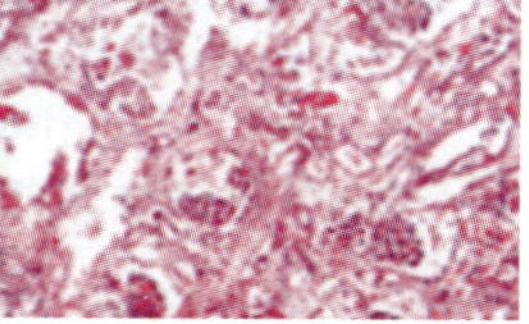

Baby with polydactyly, cleft lip, and narrow thorax, infantogram showing oval tibia, polycystic kidneys, histopathology showing corticomedullary cysts.

1. **What comment can be given regarding thorax of baby on X-ray?**
2. **What could be the probable mode of inheritance?**
3. **What would be the recurrence risk?**
4. **What genetic test can be done to confirm the diagnosis?**

Ans.

1. Narrow thorax/short ribs
2. Autosomal recessive
3. Recurrence risk is 25%.
4. Molecular test for gene mutation—whole exome sequencing

SUGGESTED READING

1. Kumar M, Anand R, Jain R, Shukla S, Bhatt C. Prenatal Diagnosis of Short Rib-Polydactyly Type II by Ultrasound in Three Consecutive Pregnancies. J Obstet Gynaecol India. 2016;66(Suppl 2):620-2.

STATION 2.

The ultrasound of this primigravida at 13 weeks shows cystic hygroma and hydrops. Medical termination of pregnancy (MTP) was done, the baby on external examination was female.

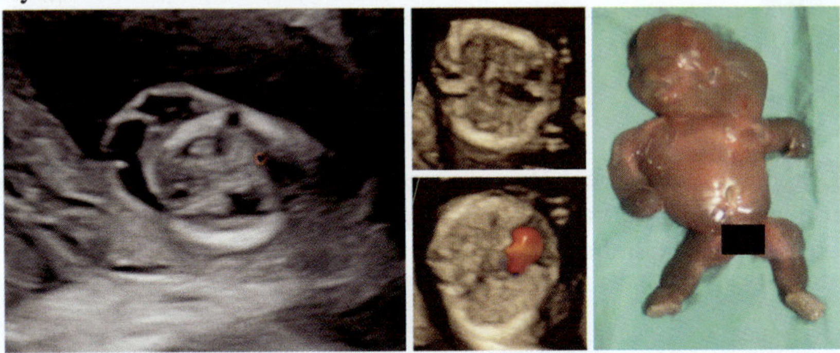

The ultrasound and photograph of the baby with cystic hygroma and hydrops.

1. **What is the most probable cause leading to the condition?**
2. **What test will be advised to confirm the diagnosis?**
3. **What would be the chance of recurrence?**
4. **Anomaly is expected in which organ system on internal examination.**

Ans.

1. Chromosomal anomaly, most commonly, Turner syndrome followed by Down.
2. Chorionic villous sampling for prenatal diagnosis; chromosomal microarray analysis (CMA) on product of conceptions (POCs) for post-termination analysis.
3. No increase in recurrence risk
4. Heart and kidneys

SUGGESTED READING

1. Kumar M, Jha V, Singh A. Nonimmune Hydrops Fetalis: Factors Which Predict Outcome. J Obstet Gynaecol India. 2018;68(3):197-203.

STATION 3.

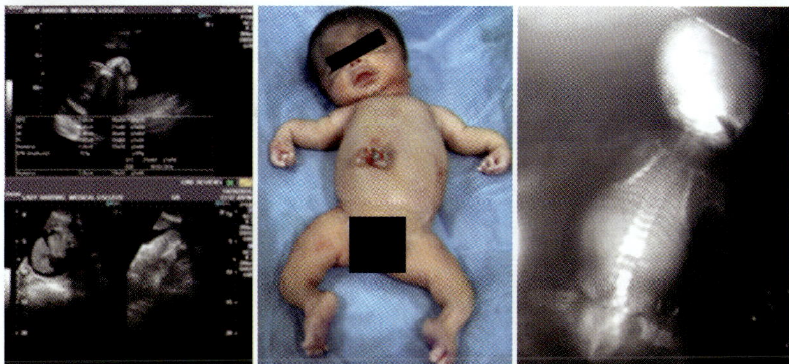

The ultrasound of the antenatal woman at 20 weeks showed short and long bones with fractures and nibbling. There was hydrops also. MTP was advised as the condition was found to be lethal on ultrasound.

1. **What test will confirm that the hydrops are non-immune?**
2. **What are the criteria for lethality on ultrasound?**
3. **Infantogram of the baby shows fractures and rehealing, what is the most probable diagnosis and type?**
4. **What associated anomaly can be present in the eyes?**

Ans.

1. Indirect Coomb's test
2. TC/AC <0.6 or FL/AC <0.16
3. Osteogenesis imperfecta type II
4. Blue sclera

SUGGESTED READING

1. Forlino A, Cabral WA, Barnes AM, Marini JC. New perspectives on osteogenesis imperfecta. Nat Rev Endocrinol. 2011;7(9):540-57.
2. Subramanian S, Anastasopoulou C, Viswanathan VK. Osteogenesis Imperfecta. [Updated 2023 Feb 6]. In: StatPearls. Treasure Island (FL): StatPearls Publishing; 2025.

STATION 4. **A 23-year-old G2P1L1, 20 weeks, with antenatal ultrasound showing small dysplastic kidney. After MTP, fetus was brought for autopsy. Acro-renal-mandibular syndrome was diagnosed.**

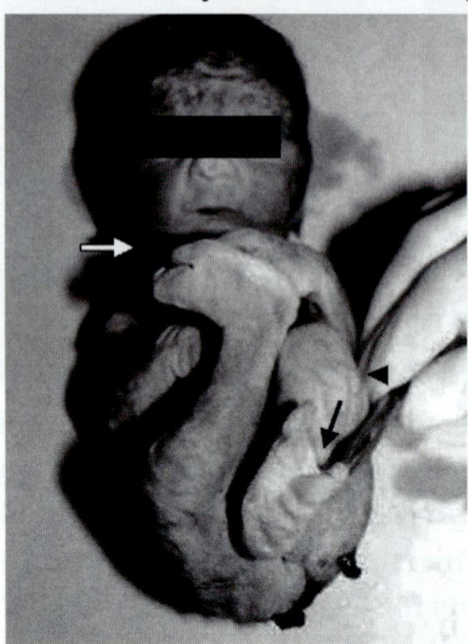

1. **What are the typical facies seen in fetus with non-functioning kidneys?**
2. **What will be the associated ultrasound finding if kidneys are absent or dysplastic?**
3. **How will the presence of dysplastic kidneys be confirmed?**
4. **What is the additional finding in the foot is observed on external examination?**
5. **What would be the risk of recurrence?**

Ans.

1. Potter's facies
2. Severely decreased liquor/absent bladder
3. By histopathological examination of kidneys
4. Split foot or ectrodactyly
5. Since the mode of inheritance is autosomal recessive, 25%.

SUGGESTED READING

1. Phadke SR, Manisha. Further delineation of acro-renal-mandibular syndrome. Clin Dysmorphol. 2006;15:119-20.

STATION 5. **Primigravida with 17 weeks' gestation. Ultrasound showed huge cystic mass in abdomen with absent liquor, MTP was done and among other findings the baby was found to have ambiguous genitalia.**

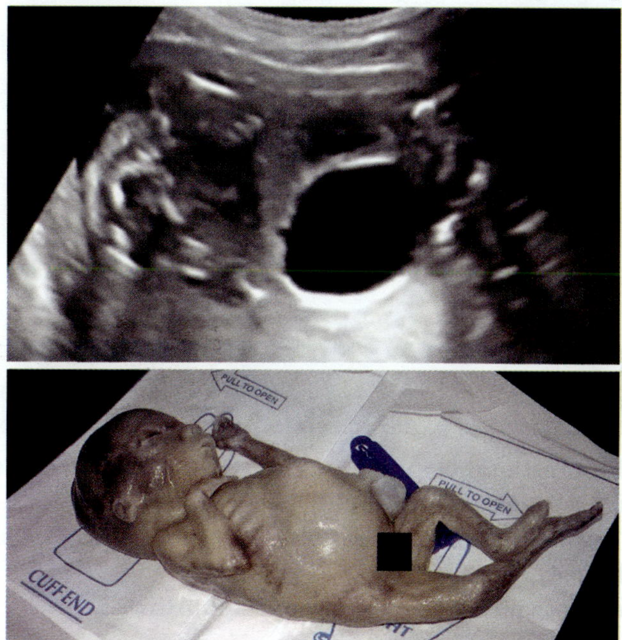

1. **What is the most probable diagnosis of the above case?**
2. **Name three distinct features of this syndrome.**
3. **What is the common mode of inheritance?**
4. **What percent of cases are males?**

Ans.

1. Prune belly syndrome
2. Thin abdominal wall, urethral atresia, and ambiguous genitalia
3. Multifactorial and sporadic occurrence
4. Approximately 95% in males

SUGGESTED READING

1. Lopes RI, Baker LA, Dénes FT. Modern management of and update on prune belly syndrome. J Pediatr Urol. 2021;17(4):548-54.

STATION 6.

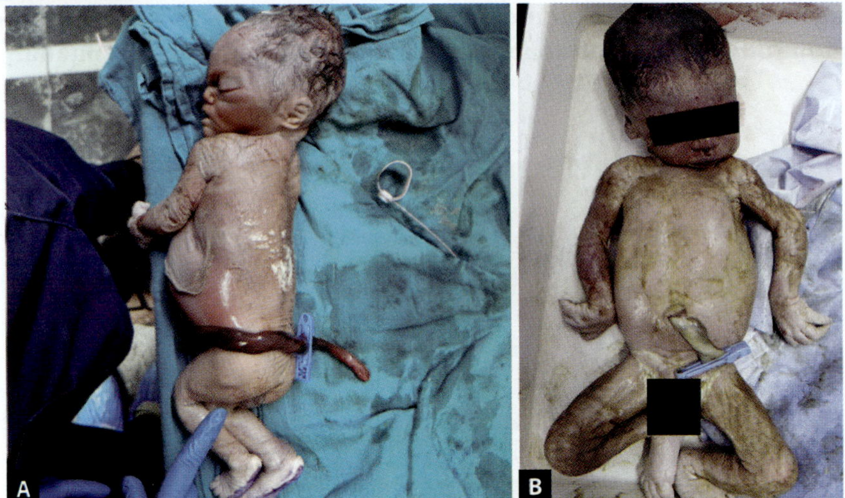

1. **In which one of the above images (A) or (B) the stillbirth is antepartum?**
2. **Mention two signs of maceration.**
3. **If signs of maceration are present minimum how many hours have elapsed since death?**
4. **Is fetal autopsy possible in macerated stillbirth?**

Ans.

1. In image (A)
2. Bullous edema, skin slippage, brown color of cord, and skin peeling
3. Minimum 8 hours
4. Yes, autopsy is possible.

SUGGESTED READING

1. Gold KJ, Abdul-Mumin AR, Boggs ME, Opare-Addo HS, Lieberman RW. Assessment of "fresh" versus "macerated" as accurate markers of time since intrauterine fetal demise in low-income countries. Int J Gynaecol Obstet. 2014;125(3):223-7.

STATION 7. **An antenatal woman, G2P1L1, is found to have large omphalocele at 22 weeks, MTP was done. On external examination on baby omphalocele was found to involve the lower abdominal wall, there was absence of anterior wall of bladder resulting on ectopia vesicae.**

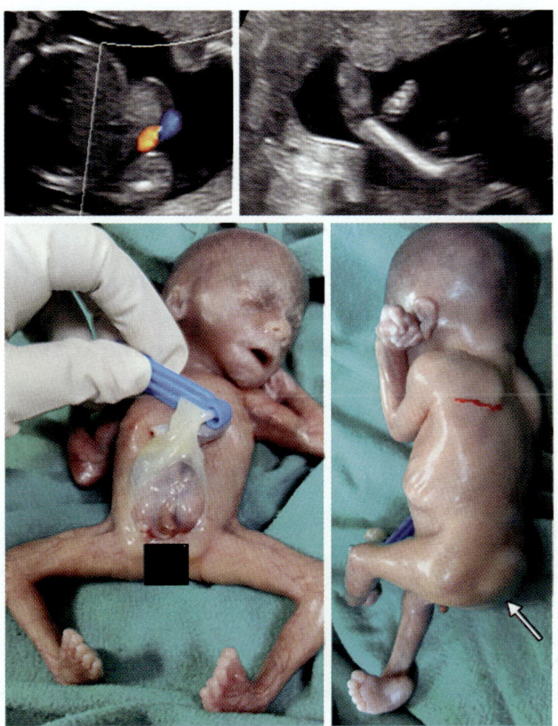

1. **What are the other two features of omphalocele-exstrophy-imperforate anus-spinal defects (OEIS) complex?**
2. **What finding on ultrasound can suggest presence of ectopia vesicae?**
3. **What is the probable reason for bilateral congenital talipes equinovarus (CTEV)?**
4. **What is the chance of chromosomal abnormality in:**
   (a) Isolated omphalocele and
   (b) OEIS complex

Ans.

1. Anal atresia and spinal defect
2. Absent bladder with adequate liquor
3. Spinal defect
4. *Chromosomal abnormality*
   (a) In omphalocele—up to 30%
   (b) OEIS—rare

SUGGESTED READING

1. Advanced Life Support Group (ALSG), Burns R, Dent K. Managing Medical and Obstetric Emergencies and Trauma: A Practical Approach, 4th edition. Wiley; 2022.
2. Nurani KM, Abdalla W, Ayub KM. Understanding and managing a case of the omphalocele-exstrophy-imperforate anus-spinal defect complex. J Surg Case Rep. 2024;2024(3):rjae166.

STATION 8. A 25-year-old G2P1L1, with screen positive for Down syndrome, had an invasive procedure done, which showed trisomy 21 with Robertsonian translocation 21. MTP was done at 21 weeks.

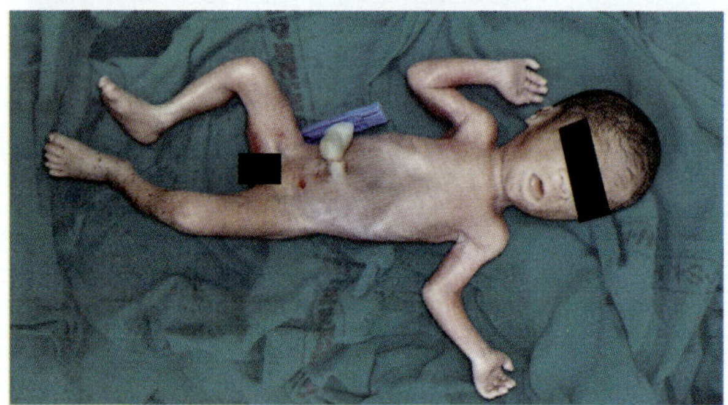

1. **Mention three external features suggestive of Down syndrome.**
2. **What are the chances of Down syndrome if the mother is 40 years old?**
3. **What further testing needs to be done if baby has Robertsonian translocation?**
4. **What is the major reason for trisomy 21 in fetus among women with advanced maternal age?**

Ans.

1. Hypertelorism, up slant in eyes, depressed nose, protruding tongue, short neck, clinodactyly, simian crease, and sandal gap
2. 1:100
3. Parental karyotyping—to know whether coming from parent or de novo
4. Non-disjunction during meiosis

SUGGESTED READING

1. Centers for Disease Control and Prevention (CDC). (2023). Down syndrome. [online] Available from https://www.cdc.gov/birth-defects/about/down-syndrome.html [Last accessed May, 2025].

STATION 9. **This is a case of twin pregnancy with hydrops at term and delivery of stillborn twins.**

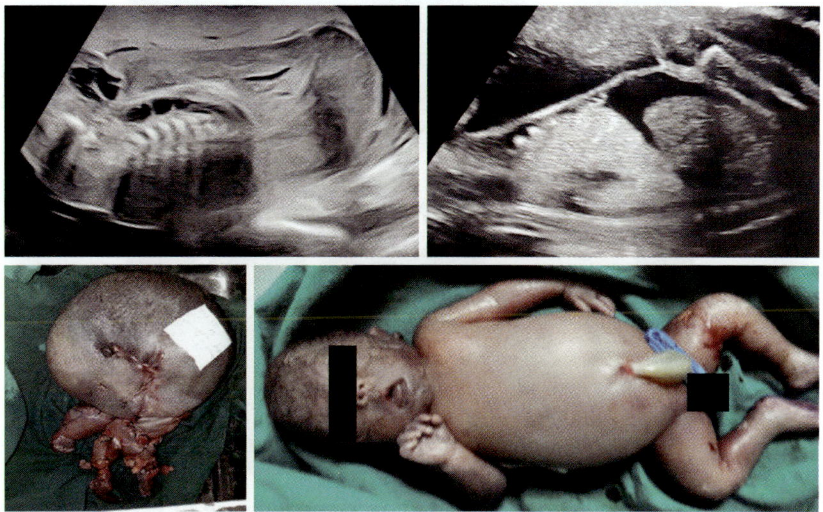

1. **What is the diagnosis in the above case?**
2. **What is chorionicity?**
3. **What are the chances of mortality in pump twins?**
4. **What could have been done in early pregnancy to avoid this outcome?**

Ans.

1. Twin reversed arterial perfusion (TRAP) sequence leading to hydrops and stillbirth
2. Monochorionic
3. 50%
4. Radiofrequency ablation or bipolar ablation of the acardiac twin

SUGGESTED READING

1. Buyukkaya A, Tekbas G, Buyukkaya R. Twin Reversed Arterial Perfusion (TRAP) Sequence; Characteristic Gray-Scale and Doppler Ultrasonography Findings. Iran J Radiol. 2015;12(3):e14979.

STATION 10. **A 22-year-old G2PILI, low risk, presented at 30 weeks' gestation with intrauterine fetal death on admission. Baby was 700 g, placenta 300 g. Baby was diagnosed with fetal growth restriction (FGR). Cord examination showed four coils/10 cm of umbilical cord.**

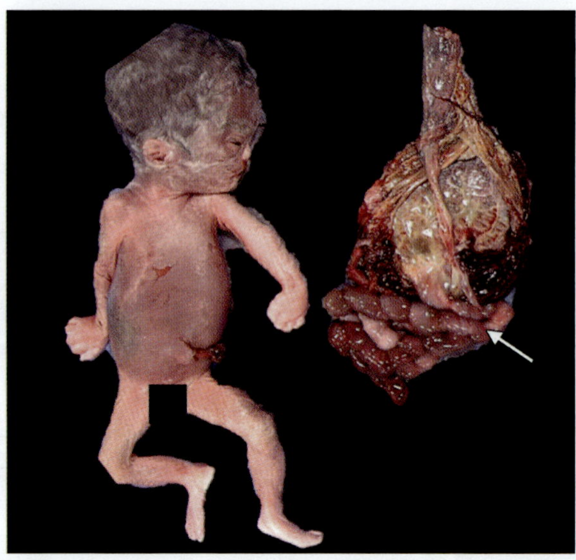

1. **What finding in the cord can explain the presence of FGR in this low-risk woman?**
2. **Enumerate three cord events related to leading to stillbirth.**
3. **Cord abnormalities can be seen in what percentage of stillbirth?**
4. **Mention what added test is necessary to confirm the cord event leading to stillbirth.**

Ans.

1. Hypercoiling of umbilical cord
2. Cord entrapment, knots, torsions, or strictures, cord prolapse, vasa previa, and compromised fetal microcirculation.
3. In 2.5–30% of stillbirth
4. Histopathological examination of cord

SUGGESTED READING

1. Hammad IA, Blue NR, Allshouse AA, Silver RM, Gibbins KJ, Page JM, et al. NICHD Stillbirth Collaborative Research Network Group. Umbilical Cord Abnormalities and Stillbirth. Obstet Gynecol. 2020;135(3):644-52.
2. Maslovich MM, Burke LM. Intrauterine Fetal Demise. In: StatPearls. Treasure Island (FL): StatPearls Publishing; 2025.

STATION 11.

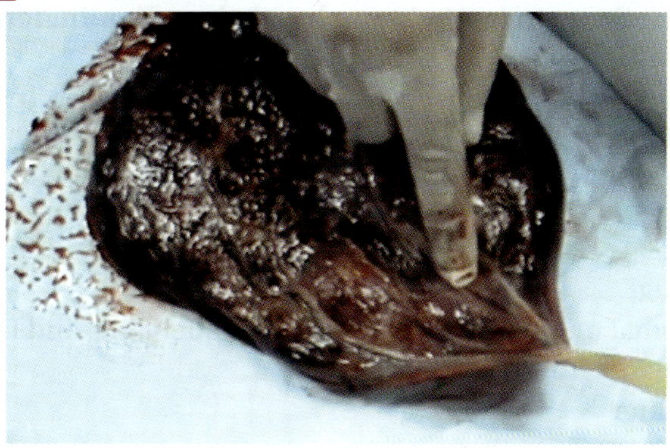

This is the placenta of antepartum stillbirth at 36 weeks' gestation with hydrops. Patient gave history of bleeding off and on. The CBC of cord blood showed Hb of 5 g/dL.

1. **What is the pathology found on placental examination?**
2. **What problem could it have led to?**
3. **What are the morphological types of cord insertion?**
4. **In what medium will you send placenta for histopathology?**

Ans.

1. Membranous or velamentous insertion
2. Vasa previa
3. The umbilical cord insertion site to the placenta can be described as central, eccentric, marginal (battledore), and velamentous (membranous) insertions.
4. In 10% formalin

SUGGESTED READING

1. Ismail KI, Hannigan A, O'Donoghue K, Cotter A. Abnormal placental cord insertion and adverse pregnancy outcomes: a systematic review and meta-analysis. Syst Rev. 2017;6(1):242.

STATION 12.

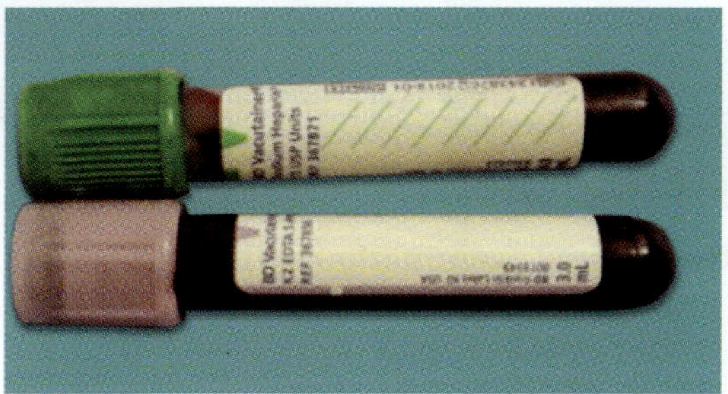

1. **For what genetic test will you send cord blood in green cap vial?**
2. **Which genetic tests can be done in ethylenediaminetetraacetic acid (EDTA) vial, mention two of them?**
3. **What other tissue can be sent for genetic testing if blood is not available?**
4. **In what medium will you send the tissue?**

Ans.

1. Karyotyping
2. Chromosomal microarray, whole exome sequencing, and DNA storage
3. Placenta, tissue from fetal thigh
4. Normal saline

SUGGESTED READING

1. Dolanc Merc M, Peterlin B, Lovrecic L. The genetic approach to stillbirth: a systematic review. Prenat Diagn. 2023;43(9):1220-8.

STATION 13. Mrs S, G2P0L0A1, 18 weeks has bilateral echogenic lungs, almost absent liquor, bilateral absent kidneys, on antenatal ultrasound. MTP was done due to poor fetal prognosis. The fetus had cryptophthalmos, mitten hands, and bilateral renal agenesis. There is history of similar affection in previous baby.

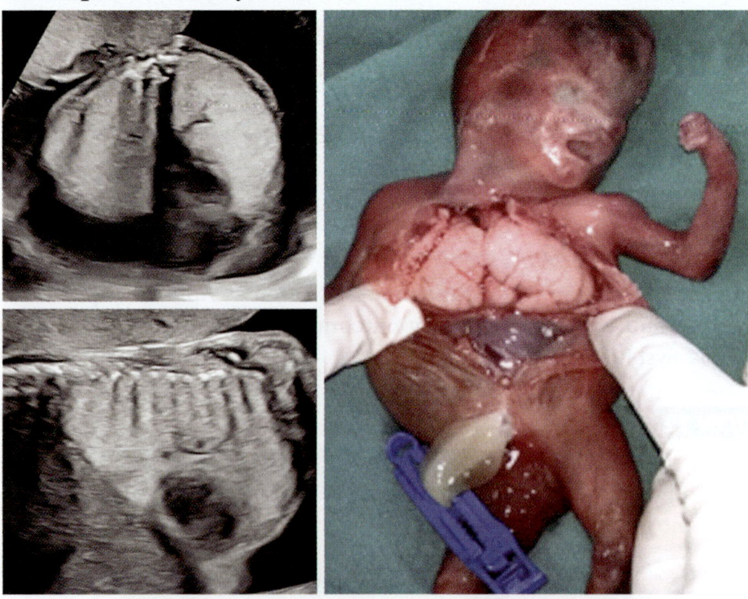

1. **What does the internal examination of thorax suggest?**
2. **What is the probable cause of this abnormality?**

3. **What can be the associated syndrome?**
4. **What is the mode of inheritance?**

Ans.

1. Hyperinflated and fluid filled lungs
2. Congenital high airway obstruction
3. Fraser syndrome
4. Autosomal recessive inheritance

SUGGESTED READING

1. Madan J, Shetty M, Ramamurthy BS, Managoli S. A multidisciplinary approach for prenatal diagnosis of FRASER SYNDROME-report of a novel variant in FRAS1. Taiwan J Obstet Gynecol. 2022;61(1):129-31.

STATION 14.

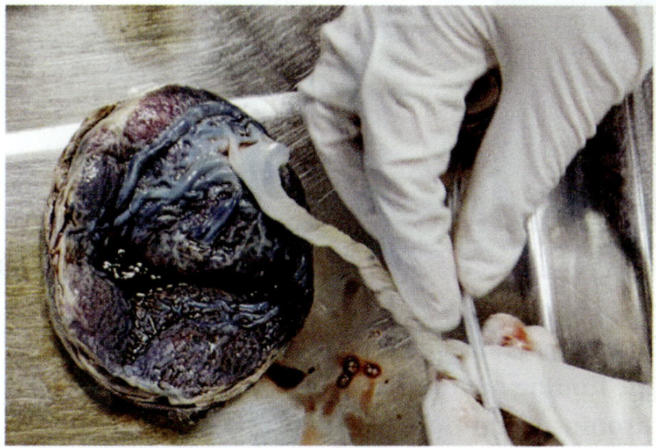

The placenta of the stillborn fetus was examined. The placenta was found to be small, with marginal insertion of cord.

1. **When is the insertion of umbilical cord considered marginal?**
2. **What problems are expected in fetus if the placental insertion is marginal?**
3. **What is the normal length and thickness of umbilical cord?**
4. **What is the process that leads to marginal insertion of cord?**

Ans.

1. When cord insertion is within 2 cm from placental edge
2. Fetal growth restriction, small for gestational age (SGA), preterm birth, and intrapartum hypoxia
3. Umbilical cord is about 45–50 cm in length and 1–2 cm in diameter.
4. Trophotropism

SUGGESTED READING

1. Aragie H, Oumer M. Marginal cord insertion among singleton births at the University of Gondar Comprehensive Specialized Hospital, Northwest Ethiopia. BMC Pregnancy Childbirth. 2021;21(1):211.

STATION 15. The following case came with ultrasound suggestive of holoprosencephaly. MTP was advised and baby was examined after birth.

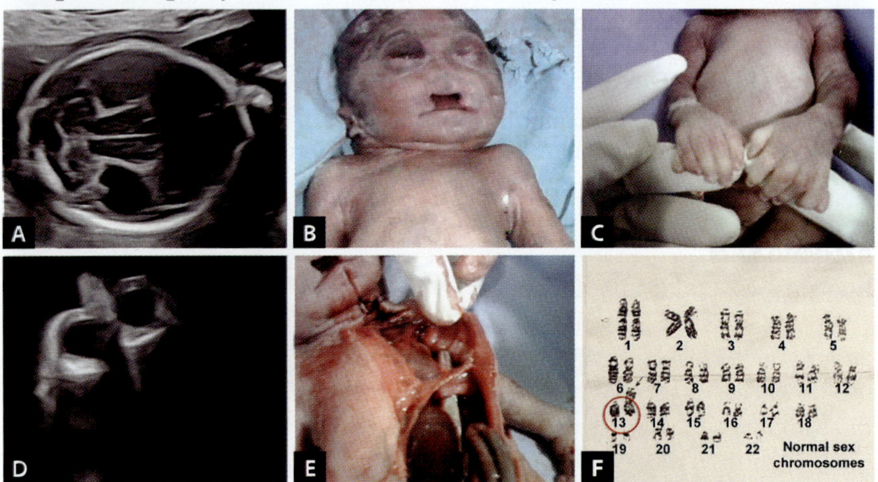

1. **What are the characteristic facial findings in the examination of baby after birth in image (B)?**
2. **What is the typical finding in the hands in image (C)?**
3. **What is the finding on internal examination in image (E)?**
4. **Which chromosome number is abnormal in image (F)?**

Ans.

1. Hypotelorism, median cleft lip and palate, and depressed nose
2. Postaxial polydactyly
3. Left-sided congenital diaphragmatic hernia
4. Trisomy 13

SUGGESTED READING

1. Williams GM, Brady R. Patau Syndrome. In: StatPearls. Treasure Island (FL): StatPearls Publishing; 2025.
2. Wyllie JP, Wright MJ, Burn J, Hunter S. Natural history of trisomy 13. Arch Dis Child. 1994;71(4):343-5.

STATION 16.

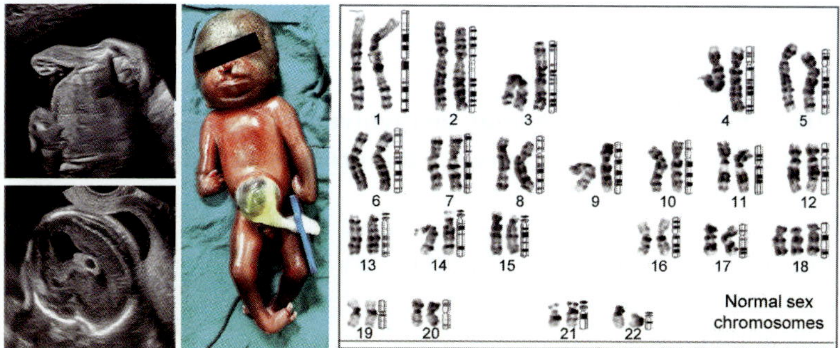

1. **What is the other name for this trisomy?**
2. **What abnormality can be seen in face?**
3. **What defect is observed in the upper limb?**
4. **Which soft marker is found to be associated in 50% cases with this abnormality?**

Ans.

1. Trisomy 18
2. Median cleft lip and palate
3. Radial aplasia
4. Choroid plexus cyst

SUGGESTED READING

1. Cereda A, Carey JC. The Trisomy 18 syndrome. Orphanet J Rare Dis. 2012;7(1):81.
2. Shravya MS, Girisha KM, Nayak SS. Comprehensive phenotyping of fetuses with trisomy 18: a perinatal center experience. Clin Dysmorphol. 2024;33(1):16-26.

STATION 17. **In the case below, the antenatal ultrasound showed abnormal four chambers and three vessels view at 22 weeks. MTP was done, baby was sent for autopsy for the confirmation.**

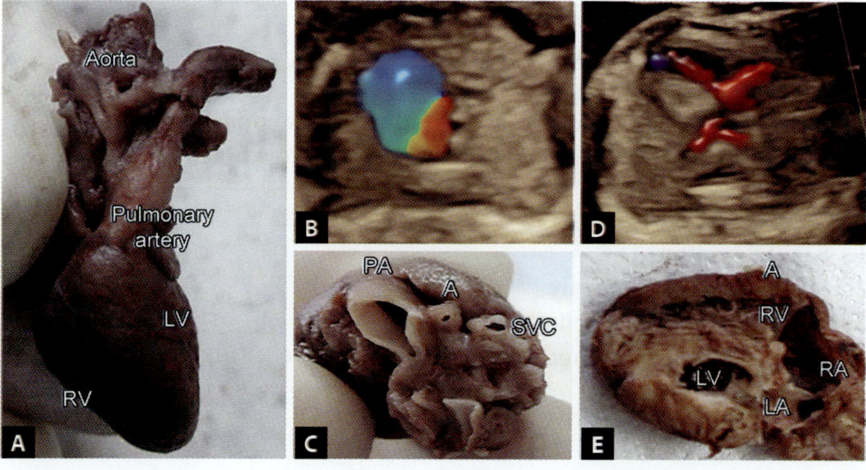

1. **What is the finding on examination of aorta in comparison to pulmonary artery in image (C)?**
2. **What is the condition of left atria and ventricle in comparison to right side of heart [image (E)]?**
3. **What other organ system may be involved?**
4. **What is the chance of recurrence if there was associated trisomy 21?**

Ans.

1. Thin atretic aorta and normal pulmonary trunk
2. Hypoplastic left side of heart
3. Brain and kidneys
4. 1:100 risk of recurrence of trisomy 21 in the next pregnancy

SUGGESTED READING

1. Kritzmire SM, Cossu AE. Hypoplastic Left Heart Syndrome. In: StatPearls. Treasure Island (FL): StatPearls Publishing; 2024.

STATION 18. **The below image is formalin-fixed brain autopsy specimen.**

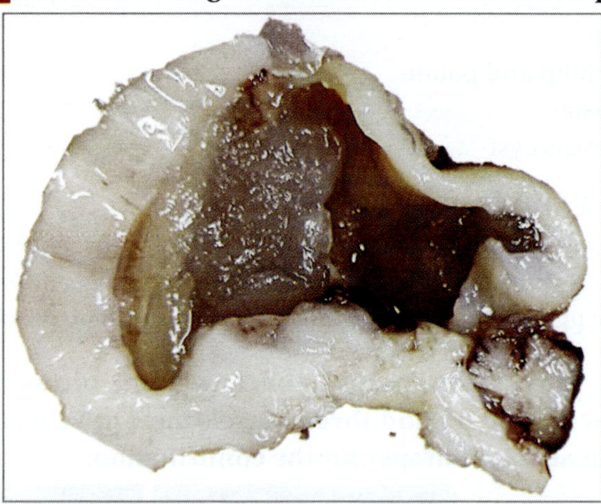

1. **What is the plane of brain section?**
2. **What is the pathology seen?**
3. **Name one infective cause associated with this condition.**
4. **What will be the antenatal confirmatory test for this infection?**

Ans.

1. Sagittal section
2. Severe ventriculomegaly
3. Cytomegalovirus infection/toxoplasmosis
4. Amniotic fluid polymerase chain reaction (PCR) for cytomegalovirus (CMV)/Toxoplasma

SUGGESTED READING

1. Guo D, He D, Shen Q, Lin N, He S, Dai Y, et al. Comprehensive Assessment of Fetal Bilateral Ventriculomegaly Based on Genetic Disorders, Cytomegalovirus Infection, Extra Prenatal Imaging and Pregnancy Outcomes in a Tertiary Referral Center. Int J Gen Med. 2021;14:7719-28.

STATION 19.

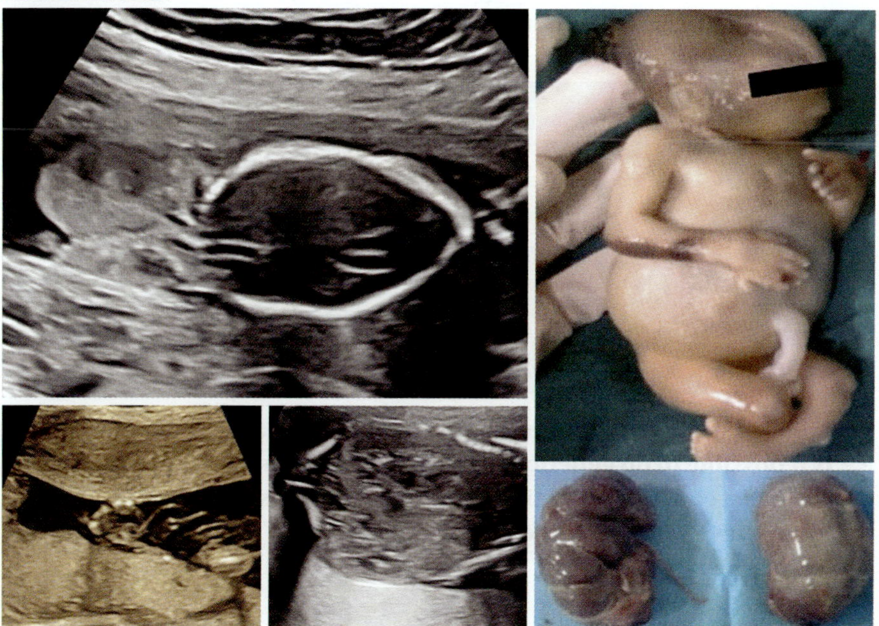

The above baby was a case of Meckel-Gruber syndrome.

1. **What characteristic findings of the syndrome are seen in this baby in external and internal examinations?**
2. **What is the pathology behind the mutation?**
3. **Name two other disorders with which the MGS displays allelism.**
4. **What is the risk of recurrence in next pregnancy?**

Ans.

1. Polydactyly, encephalocele (posterior fossa abnormality), and enlarged cystic kidneys
2. Mutations in ciliary genes—ciliopathy
3. Joubert syndrome (JBTS), COACH syndrome (cerebellar vermis hypo/aplasia, oligophrenia, congenital ataxia, ocular coloboma, and hepatic fibrosis), oro-facio-digital (OFD) syndrome, nephronophthisis (NPHP), and Bardet-Biedl syndrome (BBS).
4. Recurrence risk 25%

SUGGESTED READING

1. Hartill V, Szymanska K, Sharif SM, Wheway G, Johnson CA. Meckel-Gruber Syndrome: An Update on Diagnosis, Clinical Management, and Research Advances. Front Pediatr. 2017;5:244.

STATION 20. A 30-year-old, primigravida, had unexplained intrauterine death. There was no maternal high risk such as hypertension, diabetes, or cholestasis of pregnancy. The couple were counselled for fetal autopsy but were not willing.

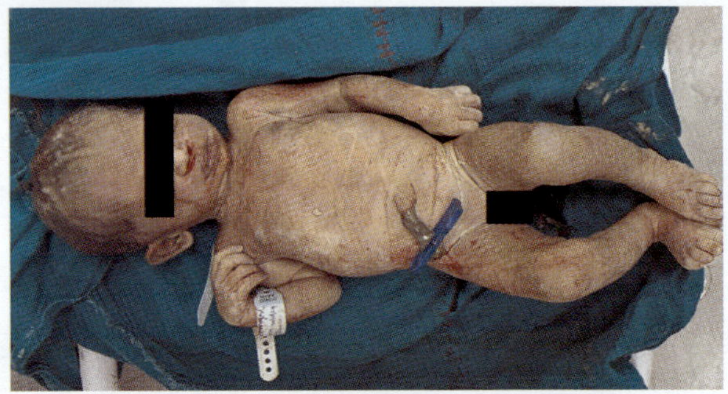

1. **Name two options for noninvasive fetal autopsy.**
2. **Is it possible to do genetic testing later, if yes, how?**
3. **What test can be done if single gene disorder is suspected?**
4. **If you have fetal tissue for testing, would you prefer microarray or karyotype and why?**

Ans.

1. Magnetic resonance imaging (MRI) (virtuopsy), minimally invasive tissue sampling
2. Yes, by DNA extraction and storage at –20°C
3. Whole exome sequencing
4. Chromosomal microarray, CMA report will give additional information in approximately 2–4% more cases in which the karyotype will be normal.

SUGGESTED READING

1. McPherson E, Nestoridi E, Heinke D, Roberts DJ, Fretts R, Yazdy MM, et al. Alternatives to Autopsy for Fetal and Early Neonatal (Perinatal) Deaths: Insights from the Wisconsin Stillbirth Service Program. Birth Defects Res. 2017;109(18):1430-41.
2. The American College of Obstetricians and Gynecologists. Microarrays and Next-Generation Sequencing Technology: The Use of Advanced Genetic Diagnostic Tools in Obstetrics and Gynecology, 2016.

Index

A

Abdomen 391
Abdominal circumference 213, 256
Abdominal wall 391
  defect 44
    midline ventral 167
  edema 248
Aberrant right subclavian artery 109, 137, 314
Abortifacient agent 379
Abruption 342
Acardiac twin 342, 347, 395
  weight to pump twin weight ratio 347
Achondroplasia 218
Acrania 40, 168
  incidence of 40
  twin with signs of 91
Acro-renal-mandibular syndrome 390
Adrenal mass, left-sided 125
Advanced maternal age 72, 394
Aedes mosquito 252
Agyria 203, 252
Aicardi syndrome 197
Aicardi-Goutières syndrome 204
Alobar holoprosencephaly 39, 195
Alpha fetoprotein 6, 10
  raised 259
Alpha-thalassemia 38, 281, 299, 300, 325
  coinheritance of 278, 280
  genes 284
Altman classification 297
Ambiguous genitalia 351, 391
  recurrence of 351
Amelia 378
Amino acid 279
Amiodarone 269, 294
Amnio drainage 345
Amniocentesis 197, 204, 216, 228, 242, 273, 288, 289, 304, 308, 315, 335
  gestation for 6
  maternal contamination in 349
Amniotic fluid 281, 340
  disorder 248
  leakage 307
  polymerase chain reaction 242, 245, 402
  volume 379
Anal atresia 393
Anemia 161, 280, 288
  polycythemia syndrome 274
  severity of 280
Anencephaly 40
Aneuploid placenta 20
Aneuploidy 9, 13, 73, 77, 79, 104, 183, 197, 235, 291, 340
  biochemical screening for 3
  detection of 36
  for pregnancy, baseline risk of 225
  increased risk of 85
  low risk for 8, 14, 187
  posterior risk of 73
  risk of 232
  screening 7
    method for 93
    negative 226
    test 3, 16
  tests for 9
Angioma 322
Angiomatous 302
Angiotensin receptor blockers 379
Angiotensin-converting enzyme inhibitors 379
Anisocytosis 279, 284
Anorectal atresia 175
Anorectal malformation 171
Antenatal complications 253
Antenatal test 372
Antenatal ultrasound 401
Anterior diaphragm, deficiency of 150
Antibody titer 267
Anticoagulants, use of 201
Anticonvulsants and retinoic acids 158
Anti-double-stranded DNA antibodies 159
Anti-human platelet antigen 283
Antihypertensive drugs 379
Anti-inflammatory drug 160
Anti-La antibodies 295
Antinuclear antibody test 159
Antiphospholipid syndrome 23
Antiribonucleoprotein antibodies 114
Aorta 130, 145
  coarctation of 136, 137, 146
  cross-section of descending 138
Aortic arch
  reversed flow in 146
  transverse 139
Aortic coarctation 140
Aortic stenosis 139, 144
Aplastic crisis 248
Arnold-Chiari malformation 199, 362
Arrhinia 108
Arrhythmia 136, 352
Arterial switch operation 154
Arteriovenous shunting 319

Arthrogryposis 104
Ascites 174, 240, 241, 248, 350
Ascitic tap 300
  and analysis 300
Aspirin 28, 30
  effect of 369
  prophylaxis 29
Assisted reproductive technology 32
Atracurium 274
Atria 138
Atrial contractions 358
Atrial flutter 294, 354
Atrial rate 354
Atrial septal defect 139, 378
Atrial systole 138
Atrioventricular heart block, high-degree 157
Atrioventricular septal defect 158, 150
Atrioventricular valve 141
Audiometry assessment 364
Autologous hematopoietic stem cells 288
Autosomal dominant 151, 209, 214, 219, 286
Autosomal recessive 102, 216, 286, 352, 387, 390
  condition 185, 378
  genetic syndrome 113
  inheritance 198, 399
  pattern 184, 279
  syndrome 127

B

Baby, infantogram of 389
Baby's blood group 273
Banana sign 199, 369
Barcelona staging 265
Bardet-Biedl syndrome 403
Basophilic stippling 279
Beckwith-Wiedemann syndrome 45, 174
Beta 2 microglobulin 192
Beta-blockers 294
Beta-gene 280
Beta-globin genes 282
Beta-human chorionic gonadotropin 36, 76
  injections 21
  value 7
Betamethasone 159, 350, 358, 370
Beta-sympathomimetic drugs 159
Beta-thalassemia 280, 281
Betibeglogene autotemcel 288
Biallelic pathogenic variants 285
Biochemical component 5
Biochemical marker 28
Biochemical results 6
Bipolar ablation 395
Bipolar cord coagulation 309, 347
Biventricular echogenic foci 313
Bladder
  absent 390
  function 328
Blake's pouch cyst 197, 212
Blocked atrial bigeminy 157
Blood
  clot 302
  group 267, 270
    RhD positive 271
  pressure 30
    diastolic 26
    systolic 26
  stained sample, risk for 315
  test 245
  transfusions, repeated 287
Blue sclera 214, 389
Body mass index 3, 26, 266
Brachiocephalic vein, left 132
Bradycardia needing emergency cesarean section 275
Brain
  abnormalities 249
    higher chance of 94
  malformations 217
  section, plane of 402
  sparing effect 258
  tubers 209
Brainstem 35
  dorsal aspect of 212
  occipital bone 35
  tentorium angles 212
  vermis, measurement of 212
Brilliant cresyl blue 285
Bronchopulmonary anomaly 124
Bronchopulmonary sequestration 122
Bullous edema 392

C

Calcium 192
Calculate cardiac performance 138
Calyceal dilation 186
Carbamazepine 381
Carbimazole 356, 380
Cardiac abnormalities 38
  higher chance of 94
Cardiac anomaly 384
Cardiac apex 151
Cardiac axis deviation 135
Cardiac chamber 140, 143
Cardiac cycle, part of 138
Cardiac defects 141
Cardiac disorders 38
Cardiac failure, high output 162, 163
Cardiac lesion
  diagnosis of 352
  in utero 352

Cardiac malformations 269, 298
Cardiac rhabdomyoma 352
Cardiac rhythm
 abnormalities 269
 appears intermittently irregular 154
 assessment of 154
Cardiac system 248
Cardiac type 148
Cardiac walls 151
Cardiomegaly 240
Cardiomyopathy
 cause of 287
 prevent 287
Cardiovascular disorders 206
Cardiovascular malformation 306
Cardioversion 294
Cavum septum pellucidum 39
Celermajer index 152
Celiac trunk 165
Cell, type of 287
Central nervous system 246
 abnormalities 194
 malformations 383
Cerebellar atrophy 252
Cerebellar malformations 42, 113
Cerebral atrophy 252
Cerebral calcifications 241, 252
Cerebrospinal fluid shunting 328
Cerebrovascular thromboembolism 162, 163
Cervical
 length assessment 349
 rib malformation 206
Cesarean births 298
Chiari II malformation 362
Child developed intracerebral hemorrhage 283
Chloride 192
Chloroquine 286
Cholangitis, risk of recurrent 170
Chondrodysplasia punctata 114
Chorioamnionitis 328, 342
Chorioamniotic separation 328
Chorioangioma 274, 302, 319, 325
Chorionic villous
 minimum amount of 318
 sampling 38, 88, 184, 220, 282, 288, 289, 290, 291, 299, 317, 332, 333, 352, 372, 388
Chorioretinitis 246
Choroid plexus cyst 222, 252, 401
 report containing 227
Chromosomal abnormality 72, 74, 107, 120, 124, 173, 177, 298, 393
 chance of 393
 risk of 167
Chromosomal anomaly 170, 388
Chromosomal defects 39, 41
Chromosomal microarray 38, 228, 292, 308, 328, 404
 analysis 196, 292, 388
Chromosome 71, 372
 22Q11.2, microdeletion of 149
 tested 77, 79
Chylous ascites fetal paracentesis 180
Ciliary genes, mutations in 403
Ciliopathy 185
Cingulate sulcus 207
Circle of Willis 300
Circulating maternal antibodies cross 160
Cleft lip 106, 118, 206, 381
 bilateral 107, 112
 cases of unilateral 117
 complete bilateral 105
 median 401
Cleft palate 106, 118, 168, 206, 381, 385
 bilateral 107
 complete bilateral 105
 median 401
Clinodactyly 394
Cloacal exstrophy 45
Cloverleaf skull 215
Clubfeet 378
Coach syndrome 403
Coagulopathy 201
Coinherited delta-thalassemia 278
Combined first trimester screening 34, 36, 68, 82, 83
Combined screening, false-positive rate of 36
Common arterial trunk 150
Complete atrioventricular block 358
Complete blood count 283, 364
Completing jigsaw 373
Compound heterozygous thalassemia, type of 281
Conception, type of 68
Congenital adrenal hyperplasia 38, 351
 detecting 372
 mutation of 352
Congenital anomalies, absence of 257
Congenital atrioventricular block 158, 295, 357
Congenital cardiac
 anomalies 378
 conditions 142, 150
Congenital cardiac defects 383
Congenital cystic adenomatoid malformation 121
Congenital cytomegalovirus infection 363
Congenital diaphragmatic hernia 119, 179, 308, 329
Congenital facial palsy 378
Congenital heart block 296, 357, 366
 risk of 366

Congenital high airway obstruction syndrome 127, 293
Congenital infections 239, 298
  causes of 239
Congenital pulmonary
  adenomatoid malformation 121
  airway malformation 306, 350
  stenosis 141
Congenital rubella triad 250
Congenital talipes equinovarus, bilateral 393
Congenital toxoplasmosis
  neonatal sequelae of 245
  risk of 244
Congenital zika syndrome 252
Congestive heart failure 174
Conotruncal defects 378
Consanguineous marriage 173
Contingent screening 15
Contralateral lung dimensions 308
Contralateral renal artery 181
Convulsions 254
Coomb's test
  direct 271
  indirect 267, 325, 389
Coomb's titer, maternal indirect 325
Cord
  blood 398
  entrapment 396
  free loop of 260
  hematoma 275
  histopathological examination of 396
  insertion 270
    morphological types of 397
  intravascular in 327
  marginal insertion of 399
  occlusion
    interrupts 347
    technique 347
  prolapse 396
Cordocentesis 322, 380
Coronary sinus 144
Corpus callosal agenesis 240
  pointer of 208
Corpus callosum 39
  abnormalities 252
  agenesis of 196, 241
  normal 208
Cortical abnormalities 241, 252
Cortical development, malformation of 207
Corticosteroids 370
Co-twin
  demise 342
  survival with morbidity 342
Cranial nerve hypoplasia 380
Craniofacial anomalies 381
Craniofacial disproportion 254
Craniorachischisis 206
Cri du chat syndrome 293
CRISPR Cas 9 technology 288
Critical aortic stenosis 146
Critical titers 325
Crossed fused ectopia 193
Crown-rump length 34, 37, 75, 97
Cryptophthalmos 398
Culture failure, risk for 316
CYP11B2 gene 372
CYP21A2 gene 372
Cyst 130
  adrenal 165
  bronchogenic 128, 131
  connatal 210
  echolucent 227
  enteric duplication 169, 178
  esophageal duplication 131
  fetal
    choledochal 169
    gonadal 178
  germinolytic 204, 241
  hepatic 169
  laryngeal 293
  mesenteric 178
  neurogenic 131
  ovarian 169
  pancreatic 165
  pericardial 128
  periventricular 240, 241, 252
  splenic 165
  subependymal 240, 241
  thymic 128
  volume ratio 320
Cystic biliary atresia 169
Cystic fibrosis, mutation analysis for 230
Cystic hygroma 10, 44, 103, 104, 105, 127, 291, 322, 388
Cystic mass 391
  diagnosis of 178
Cystic spaces 305
Cytomegalovirus 177, 239, 300, 321, 325
  infection 204, 254, 402
  serology tested 363
  suspected 240

D

Dacryocystocele 101
Dandy-Walker malformation 197, 211, 212, 216, 383
Deepest vertical pocket 97
Deferoxamine 287
Delayed brain development in utero 154
Delayed sulcations 204
Delta gene 280
Delta-globin genes 282
Deltoid muscle 267, 271
Deoxyribonucleic acid 244-246
Depressed nose 400

Dexamethasone 159, 352, 355, 358, 370
 low-dose 372
Dextrocardia 140
Dextroversion 150
Diabetes mellitus 23, 221
 type 2 158
 uncontrolled 376
Diagnostic invasive testing 331
Diamond-Blackfan anemia 38
Diaphragm 293
Diaphragmatic hernia 206, 306
 left-sided 150
  congenital 119, 135, 400
Diastematomyelia 200
Dichorionic diamniotic
 placentation 83
 twin 17, 85, 86, 90, 338
  gestation 68
  set of 332
Dichorionic twins 20
Dichorionic vs. monochorionic pairs, termination techniques in 341
Digeorge syndrome 149
Digitalis 354
Digoxin 163, 269, 294, 353
Dilated coronary sinus 148
Dilated fetal cardiomyopathy 141
Diode laser ablation 342
Discordant anomalous 333
Discordant nuchal translucency, implications of 85
Discrepant hemispheres 203
Discrepant ventricles 203
Disease, severity of 284
Disseminated intravascular coagulation 339
Dizygotic twins 93
Donor twin 309
Doppler velocimetry parameter 25
Doppler waveform 138, 346
Double bubble sign 164, 165
Double marker test 3
 report, final risk in 5
Down syndrome, risk for 19
Down's syndrome 5, 6, 38, 44, 164, 222, 291, 340, 394
Drugs 375
Dual marker test 36
Ductus arteriosus 139
 right 149
Ductus venosus 3
 Doppler 264
  measurement 264
 extrahepatic agenesis of 173
 measurement of 260
 wave reversal in 292
Duodenal atresia 10, 164, 165
Dysgenesis 252, 306
Dysplastic corpus callosum 197

E

Early hydrops, besides features of 309
Early-onset fetal growth restriction 80, 364
Ebstein's anomaly 150, 152, 384
Echocardiography, left axis deviation on 139
Echogenic bowel 109, 174, 204, 230, 240
Echogenic choroid 227
Echogenic foci 313
Echogenic intracardiac focus, adverse effect of 226
Echogenic kidney
 approach for 188
 bilateral 219
Echogenic mass 122, 124
Ectopia vesicae 392
 presence of 393
Ectopic kidney 187
Ectrodactyly 390
Edward's syndrome 6
Electrolytes 354
Encephalocele 41, 42
 anterior 101
 posterior 113
End-diastolic velocity, absent 346
Endocardial cushion defects 296
Endocardial fibroelastosis 296, 358
Enzymes, hepatic induction of 361
Epsilon gene 280
Erythrocyte enzymopathies 300
Esophageal atresia, types of 178
Estimated fetal weight 96, 255, 358
Estriol 9
 levels 9
Ethmocephaly 109
Ethylenediaminetetraacetic acid 398
Euploid fetuses 226
Evolving skeletal dysplasia 236
Ex utero intrapartum treatment 293
Exagamglogene autotemcel 288
Exome sequencing 120
Exomphalos 44, 45
Extracorporeal membrane oxygenation 324
Extrahepatic umbilical venous drainage 173
Extralobar sequestration 306
Extralobar-bronchopulmonary sequestration 125
Extramedullary hematopoiesis 242, 249

F

Facial abnormalities 101, 378
Facial clefts 179
Facial dysmorphism 381
Fallot's tetralogy 168
Fanconi's anemia 38, 325
Feeding vessel
 endoscopic laser coagulation of 319
 laser photocoagulation of 302

Femur 222
- bowing of 220
- in infantogram, shape of 215

Fetal abdomen 134
- structural abnormalities 179

Fetal akinesia 38
- deformation sequence 179, 304

Fetal alcohol spectrum disorders 376
Fetal alloimmune thrombocytopenia 283, 360
Fetal anemia 133, 248, 249, 269, 270, 371
- causes of 249
- diagnose 276

Fetal anomalies
- scan 73
- targeted imaging for 187

Fetal ascites 179, 273
Fetal autoimmune congenital heart block 296
Fetal autopsy 387
- counselled for 404

Fetal bladder 183, 191
Fetal blood
- sampling 356
- thyroid hormones, measurement of 380
- transfusion, indications of 274

Fetal bradycardia 157, 345
- causes for 157

Fetal brain, lateral ventricles of 227
Fetal cardiac
- diagnosis 357
- rhythm
  - irregularities 155
  - M-mode tracing of 161

Fetal condition, stage of 358
Fetal cord ablation procedure 348
Fetal demise 10, 76, 353
Fetal development
- assessment of 340
- critical period of 375

Fetal echocardiography 44, 94, 157, 301
- examination 154, 155

Fetal endoscopic tracheal occlusion 329
Fetal evaluation, preoperative 328
Fetal face 179
Fetal fluorescence in situ hybridization, invasive testing for 120
Fetal fraction 74, 77, 79
Fetal goiter 322
- treatment of 323

Fetal growth 179, 379
- normal 187
- restriction 30, 141, 171, 174, 204, 240, 253, 255, 261, 355, 378, 379, 382, 395
  - fetuses, long-term risks for 266
  - screening for 96
- velocity 262

Fetal heart rate 269
- deceleration, persistent unprovoked 261
- normal 161

Fetal hemoglobin, level of 278
Fetal hemolytic disease with anemia 371
Fetal hepatic tumors 174
Fetal hydrops 241, 269
- development of 296
- frequency of 319

Fetal hyperthyroidism 356
Fetal indication 367
- administration for 367

Fetal infection 133, 174, 239, 250
- detect 244
- draws 301
- sonographic markers of 241

Fetal interventions 311, 344
Fetal intrauterine
- death 271
- transfusion 248

Fetal karyotype 107, 110, 182
Fetal liver calcification 249
Fetal loss, risk of 89
Fetal malformations 377
Fetal malpresentation, development of 40
Fetal mediastinal cysts, prognostic factors of 128
Fetal medicine
- foundation software 26
- outpatient department 68

Fetal movements 179
Fetal neck
- mass 324
- occipitocervical region of 104

Fetal nuchal translucency thickness 87
Fetal oliguria 379
Fetal paracentesis 179
Fetal prognosis 190
Fetal pyelectasis
- bilateral 231
- pathological causes of 231

Fetal reduction procedure 339
Fetal renal
- artery 181
- pelvis 182

Fetal right upper quadrant cystic lesion, differential diagnosis of 169
Fetal skull 40
Fetal stomach 138
Fetal structural anomalies 316
Fetal supraventricular tachycardia 162
Fetal thorax 122, 127, 134, 179
Fetal thyroid goiter ultrasound 380
Fetal thyrotoxicosis 161
Fetal trauma 307
Fetal treatment 353
Feticide, twins for selective 342
Fetomaternal hemorrhage 300
Fetoplacental Doppler, normal 265
Fetoplacental volume 327

Fetoscopy 330
  endotracheal occlusion 308
  laser surgery 98
Fetus 93, 174
  hypoperfusion of 379
  specific risk 16, 17
  swallows amniotic fluid 323
  upper limb of 378
FGFR3 gene mutation 218
Fibroma 129
First trimester 19, 183
  evaluation 1
  scan 34
  screen 3
    test 331, 332
  skeletal dysplasia in 214
Flat facial profile 382
Flecainide 269, 294, 353
Fluorescence in situ hybridization 38, 228, 291, 313, 332
Fluorinated corticosteroids 358
Fluorinated steroids 159
Folic acid deficiency 377
Folinic acid 246
  rescue 301
Foramen ovale 138, 143
  flap 143
Formalin-fixed brain autopsy specimen 402
Fossa, posterior 211
Fraser's syndrome 127, 399
Fresh blood smears 285
Frontal bones, scalloping of 199
Frontal horn, angle of 210
Fryns syndrome 105
Fused cerebral lobes 195
Fused frontal horns 194
Fused globin chain comprising 282

G

Gallbladder duplication 169
Gamma gene 280
Gamma-globin chain production 288
Gastrointestinal malformations 206
Gastrointestinal system 249
Gastrointestinal tract 234
  and abdominal wall, congenital abnormalities of 164
Gastroschisis 45, 166
Gene
  addition 288
  and transcript 216, 219
  modified 288
  mutation, molecular test for 387
Genetic abnormalities 38, 44, 229
  detection rate of 196
Genetic association 149
Genetic disorder, common associated 126
Genetic malformation 164
Genetic syndromes 106, 124, 131, 197, 202, 235
Genetic test 219, 333, 398
Genitalia, developing female 372
Genitourinary anomalies 382
Genitourinary conundrum 193
Genitourinary defects 217
Genotype 284
Gestation 385
  period of 22
  specific reference charts 367
Gestational age 298, 399
  diagnosing small for 255
  small for 265
Gestational hypertension, induction for 360
Glaucoma 250
Global developmental delay 6
Globoside 249
Glossoptosis 115
Glucose-6-phosphate dehydrogenase
  deficiency 246, 286, 290, 300
    inheritance pattern of 286
    neonatal complication of 286
  enzyme assay 290
  gene, mutation analysis of 290
Glutamic acid 279
Glycoprotein 7
Goiters 323
Grandmother phenomenon 268
Graves' disease 322
Great arteries
  dextro-transposition of 154
  transposition of 141
Great vessels, transposition of 147
Growth assessment 257
Gut malrotations 164

H

Hamartomas 151
HBB gene 282
  mutation of 281, 288
  sanger sequencing of 290
Head circumference 6
Healthy cotwin 91
Heart 130
  apex of 143, 146
  chamber of 143
  congenital abnormalities of 136
  defect 216, 217
  failure 287
  left axis deviation of 150
  right axis deviation of 150
  right side of 402
  right ventricle of 140
Heart block
  complete 355
  first-degree 355

risk of recurrent 365
screening for 160
third-degree 355, 358
Hemangioma 129, 174
Hematocrit
high 327
volume 327
Hematological disorders 277
Hematopoietic stem cell therapy 287
Hemimegalencephaly 203
Hemodynamic burden 347
Hemodynamic changes 341
Hemodynamic redistribution 174
Hemoglobin 284
Bart syndrome 284
E 280
Hemoglobinopathy 284, 300
type of 282
Hemolysis 300
Hepatic calcification 177
Hepatic carcinoma 287
Hepatic fibrosis 287
Hepatic vessels, thromboembolism of 177
Hepatoblastoma 174
Hepatomegaly 174, 240, 241, 273, 360
Hepatosplenomegaly 177, 204, 242, 246
Hereditary hematological conditions 38
Hereditary spherocytosis 286
Herpes simplex virus 2 177
High tumor volume index 297
Higher order pregnancy 17
Hirschsprung's disease 175
Holoprosencephaly 107, 208, 400
spectrum 106
types of 110
Horseshoe kidney 193
Human chorionic gonadotropin 7
Human fetal risk, evidence of 376
Human leukocyte antigen 287
Human parvovirus B19 infection 247
Hydramnios 273
Hydroceles, bilateral 248
Hydrocephalus 113, 246, 249, 306
Hydrometrocolpos 178
Hydronephrosis 186
mild 109
Hydrops 10, 162, 163, 273, 308, 319, 353, 358, 388
fetalis 121, 350, 384
causes 248
presence of 273
Hydro-uretero-nephrosis, bilateral 192
Hydroxychloroquine 160, 296, 357, 366
Hyperechogenic bowel 241
Hyperreflexia 254
Hypertelorism 394
Hypertension, chronic 23, 29
Hypervolemia 343
Hypoechoic mass 302
Hypoplasia 143
cerebellar 241
vermis 212
nasomaxillary 114
ventricular 141
Hypoplastic left heart 402
syndrome 140, 146
Hypoplastic right
lung 125
pulmonary artery 125
Hypotelorism 107, 400
Hypotonia 183

I

Iatrogenic preterm births 94
Immune
complexes containing 366
hydrops 247
Immunoglobulin G test result 245
Immunomodulatory drug 160
In utero
demise 162, 163
repair, pregnancy complications of 328, 329
In vitro fertilization 23, 31, 37, 68
conception 74
Inborn errors 300
Indirect antiglobulin test 325
Infection, recurrent 280
Inheritance 184
mode of 399
of disorder, mode of 214
pattern 279
Inhibin
decrease in 13
source of 13
Intact posterior palatal line 111
Intellectual disability 304
Interhemispheric fissure 195
Interventricular septum 151
Intrabdominal vascular cystic mass 171
Intracardiac echogenic focus 109
Intracardiac segmental anatomy 357
normal 353, 354
Intracranial calcifications 240, 241, 249
Intracranial hemorrhage 239-241
Intracranial translucency 35
Intrafetal laser 309
ablation 91
Intrahepatic umbilical vein 327
drainage 173
Intramuscular digoxin 294
Intramuscular injections 267
Intrapartum
hypoxia 399
stillbirth 350

Intrapulmonary cystic mass 321
Intrauterine blood transfusion 98
Intrauterine embolization 319
Intrauterine fetal
    blood transfusion 272
    death 171, 307
    demise 254
    infections 177
Intrauterine fetus, single live 187
Intrauterine growth restriction 249
Intrauterine neuronal injury, halting progressive 328
Intrauterine transfusion 272, 299, 371
Intrauterine viral infection 247
Intravenous immunoglobulin 360
Intravenous transfusion, formula for 327
Intraventricular adhesions 240, 241
Intraventricular synechia 241
Invasive testing 333
Iodine deficiency 322
Ipsilateral alae nasi, flattening of 117
Iron
    chelators 279
    deficiency anemia 278, 279
Isoimmunization, cause of 325
Isoimmunized mother 247
Isolated fetal ascites developing 179
Isolated septal agenesis 194
Isomerism 150

J

Jaundice 246
    episode of 289
    neonatal period for 286
Jejunal atresia 306
Joubert syndrome 197, 403

K

Kartagener syndrome 141
Karyotyping 398
    amniocentesis for 230
    invasive testing for 39
    sample sent for 221
Kernicterus 286
Kidney
    congenital abnormalities of 181, 193
    histopathological examination of 390
Kinked Z-shaped brainstem 113
Klippel-Trenaunay syndromes 203

L

Labeling twins, method of 333
Labio-alveolar cleft, unilateral 117
Labor, induction of 265
Lacrimation, abnormal 378
Large white lung, differentials of 319
Laryngeal atresia 127, 293
Laryngeal web 293
Laser ablation 345
    preferred over amnioreduction 344
    technique employed for 344
Laser photocoagulation 347
Last menstrual period 351
Late-onset bowel dilatation, causes of 175
Lateral ventricle
    frontal horn of 208
    posterior horn of 208
Left atrioventricular groove, posterior 144
Left ventricular
    cardiomyopathy, late-onset 158
    outflow tract 138
Leiomyoma 302
Lemon sign 199, 369
Lentivirus 288
Lethal multiple pterygium syndrome 105
Lethal skeletal dysplasia 214, 305
Levorotation 129
Levo-transposition 150
Lifestyle modification 266
Lignocaine 90
Limb
    abnormalities 378
    anomalies 382
    dysmorphogenesis 380
    reduction defects 317
Liquid chromatography, high-performance 278
Liquor amount 179
Lissencephaly 240, 241, 252
    type 2 113
Lithium 384
Live birth rate 298
Liver 173
    biopsy 360
    bypass 173
    cirrhosis 170
    function tests 364
Lobar holoprosencephaly, diagnosis of 39
Local anesthesia infiltration 342
Long bones
    appendicular 236
    stippling of 382
Long philtrum thin upper lip 221
Low beta-human chorionic gonadotropin value 7
Low placental growth factor 262
Lower abdominal wall 392
Lower urinary tract obstruction 193
Lowest false-positive rates 68
Lumbar puncture needle, gauge of 348
Lung 130
    hypoplasia, severe 188
    right 125

Lymphangioma 101, 131, 206, 322
Lymphocytes, pleural fluid analysis for 321
Lysosomal storage
disease 325
disorders 300

M

Macerated stillbirth 392
Maceration, signs of 392
Macrocystic congenital cystic adenomatoid malformation 321
Main pulmonary artery 139
Massive parallel shotgun sequencing 71
Maternal age 68
Maternal anti-Rho 295
Maternal autoimmune disorders 114
Maternal bleed 342
Maternal body weight 352
Maternal cell contamination 349
risk for 315, 318
Maternal characters 22
Maternal corticosteroid 350
Maternal drug toxicity 353
Maternal hyperthyroidism 161
Maternal infection 244
Maternal isoimmunization 325
Maternal salbutamol 296
Maternal serology 301
Maternal serum
alpha-fetoprotein 10
screening tests 340
Maternal stimulants 161
Maxilla, frontal process of 112
Maxillary gap sign 168
Maxillary line, absence of 108
Mean arterial pressure 12
Mean uterine artery pulsatility index 12, 25
Meaning arterial pressure 22
Meckel–Gruber syndrome 185, 198, 197, 403
Meconium
peritonitis 177, 249
plug syndrome 175
Mediastinal shift 121
Mediastinal tumor 129
Mediastinum
anterior 129
posterior 131
Medical fetal reduction 339
Medical termination of pregnancy 388
Medical transplacental therapy 350
Medulla oblongata 113
Mega cisterna magna 197, 240, 241, 252
Megacystis 183
Membrane
premature rupture of 342
preterm
prelabor rupture of 328, 345
premature rupture of 91
rupture, high risk of 329
stabilization 359
Mesenteric ischemia 174
Mesocardia 293
Metabolic disorders 269
Methimazole 356, 380
Microcephaly 204, 242, 243, 246, 249, 252, 385
Microcirculation, vaso-occlusion of 280
Microcytic hypochromic
anemia 279
blood picture 299
Micrognathia 115, 206, 221
Micromelia 215, 378
Microphthalmia 127, 250, 378
bilateral 107
Microretrognathia 179
Microtia 378
Middle cerebral artery 299
Doppler 270
peak systolic velocity 268, 326
signify 258
waveform 263
Middle interhemispheric variant 39
Minimally invasive tissue sampling 404
Misoprostol 379
Mitral valve
dysplastic syndrome 146
opens 156
Mixed bag 237
M-mode echocardiography 155
Monitor growth velocity 255
Monoamniotic pregnancy 347
Monochorionic diamniotic twins 77, 82, 91, 98, 333
Monochorionic twin 342
complications of 201, 247
disorder in 343
modality for fetal reduction in 341
pregnancy 98, 274
selective reduction of 344
sequelae of 347
Monosomy X 120
Multicystic dysplastic kidney 193
unilateral 190
Multifetal gestation 32, 337, 349
fetal interventions in 331
screening in 81
Multifetal pregnancy reduction 337
Multiple gestation 336
Multiple organ systems 151
Multiple pregnancy 10, 84, 88, 173
invasives in 89
risk of preterm births in 94
Multiple pterygium syndrome 303
Multiple septated cystic structures 104
Multiplex ligation-dependent probe amplification 282
Munich classification 303

Mutations 281
Myasthenia gravis 304
Myelomeningocele 381
Myocardial performance index 138
Myocarditis 161, 248, 357
Myotonic dystrophy 304
Myxoma 129

N

Narrow with short ribs 217
Nasal bones 35, 112
  verticalization of 114
National Institute for Health and Clinical Excellence 22
Natural demise 347
Neck
  abnormalities 101
  of fetus, uniform echogenicity in 322
Negative predictive value 12
Neonatal abdomen ultrasound revealed ascites 360
Neonatal alloimmune thrombocytopenia 201, 283, 360
Neonatal clinical charts 351
Neonatal hemochromatosis 360
Neonatal intensive care unit 42, 289, 351
Neonatal jaundice, developed 286
Nephronophthisis 403
Neu-Laxova syndrome 105, 197
Neural tube defects 239, 339, 381
Neurodevelopmental delays, risk of 209
Neurodevelopmental dysfunctions 154
Neurodevelopmental sequelae 242
Neuromuscular involvement 304
Neuroprotection 367
Neurosonogram 39, 254
Nociceptive nerve fibers, stimulation of 280
Non-communicable diseases, increased risk of 266
Nonimmune hydrops 105, 130, 142, 247, 307
  fetalis 247, 248, 291
Nonimmunological hydrops 319
Noninvasive fetal autopsy 404
Noninvasive prenatal
  diagnostic tests 340
  screening 66, 84, 271
    low-risk 232
    methods of 71
    technique 75
  testing 20, 85, 272
    low risk 13
Nonpresenting twin 333
Noonan's syndrome 38, 104, 105, 120, 173, 292
Normal vaginal delivery 273
Nuchal fold thickness 103
Nuchal translucency 35
  discordance 85
  increased 167, 214, 317
  scan 3, 36
Nucleated red cells, circulating 279
Nucleotide polymorphism, single 71

O

Obstructive uropathy, initial stages of 183
Occipital encephalocele 41, 198, 206
Ocular abnormalities 250
Oligohydramnios 10, 186, 204, 219, 240, 343, 344, 379
Omphalocele 166, 167, 393
  exstrophy-imperforate anus-spinal defects 167
  exstrophy-imperforate anus-spinal defects complex 393
  large 167
Open neural tube defect 199, 362
Open spina bifida 369
Optic chiasma 194
Optimal gestational age 35
Organ specific anomalies 99
Organogenesis 375
Orofacial clefts 378
Osmolality 192
Osteogenesis imperfecta 214, 389
Outflow conus 151
Outflow tract obstruction 352
Ovulation induction 19

P

Pacemaker implantation 159
Pachygyria 203, 252
Palatal line, posterior 111
Pancreatic insufficiency 287
Pancreatitis 170
Papillary muscles, microcalcification of 226
Pappenheimer bodies 279
Paramedian defects, bilateral 113
Paraumbilical defect 166
Parenchymal appearance and thickness 231
Parenchymal calcifications 204
Parental karyotyping 394
Parieto-occipital sulcus, level of 233
Partial pulmonary venous drainage 125
Parvovirus 177, 247, 300, 325
  B19 247, 249
    infection 247, 274
    main receptor for 249
Patau's syndrome 6
Pathognomonic sign 146
Peak systolic velocity 299
Pelvic kidneys, renal cysts of 178
Pelvicalyceal dilatation 186

Pelvicalyceal system 231
Pelviureteric junction obstruction 186
Pentalogy of Cantrell 45, 150, 168
Perianal muscular complex 176
Pericardial cavity, collection of fluid in 142
Pericardial effusion 128, 129, 133, 142, 240, 241, 248, 273
Pericardiocentesis 129
Peripheral blood film 284
Peripheral calyceal dilatation 231
Peripheral edema 287
Peripheral nervous system abnormalities 194
Peripheral smear 279, 285
  type of 279
Periventricular cystic changes 241
Permanent pacemaker 296
Persistent pulmonary hypertension 125
Persistent right umbilical vein 172
Petechial rash 242
Phenytoin 380, 381
Phocomelia 378
Phototherapy 286
Physiological midgut herniation 169
Pierre Robin
  sequence 115
  syndrome 306
Placenta 266, 302
  cross 323
  leading to bloody tap 349
  syncytiotrophoblasts of 66
Placental abnormalities 10
Placental abruption 345
Placental calcifications 240
Placental chorioangioma 302
Placental dysfunction 259
Placental edge 399
Placental examination 397
Placental growth factor 22, 28
Placental mosaicism 21, 68
  risk for confined 315, 318
Placental pathology 302
Placental position 333
Placental teratoma 302
Placental vascular tumor 319
Placentation, type of 82, 83
Placentomegaly 240, 273, 297
Plasma protein-A 8
  placenta-associated 8
  pregnancy-associated 76, 87
    low 259
Pleural effusion 120, 128, 177, 248, 321
  unilateral 321
Pleurocentesis, time of 321
Pleurodesis 120
Pneumococcal vaccination 290
Pneumonitis 246
Pneumothorax 125
Poikilocytosis 284
Polycystic dysplastic kidney 193
Polycystic kidney 184, 387
  disease, fetal-onset bilateral 184
Polydactyly 216, 378
Polyhydramnios 10, 175, 179, 240, 297, 304, 306, 307, 309, 316, 326, 344, 347
  risk of 40
Polymalformative syndromes 167, 170
Polymerase chain reaction 363
Polymicrogyria 203
Portal hypertension 170
Positive predictive value 12
Postaxial polydactyly 387, 400
Postnatal repair 328
Postpartum hemorrhage, traumatic 298
Post-termination analysis, product of conceptions for 388
Postural limb abnormalities 188
Potential cardiac pathology 357
Potential maternal complications 337
Potter's facies 188, 390
Power Doppler image signify 124
Preconceptional counseling 282, 290
Prednisone 360
Pre-eclampsia 12, 22
  assessment of risk of 11
  prediction of 32
  prevention 369
  risk of 11, 259
  screen for 11, 22, 369
Preferred technique 333
Pregnancy
  continuation of 90
  develop 29
  high risk 25
  loss 309
  prevent in 369
  previous affected 37
  specific risk 16, 17
Premature atrial contraction 157
Premature infant 359
Premature sulcations 203
Premaxilla, absence of 108
Premaxillary protrusion 108, 112
Premaxillary triangle intact 117
Preterm birth 253, 307, 309, 399
  develops 348
  high risk of 370
  in twins, prevention of 94
Preterm delivery 162, 163
Preterm labor 275, 298, 328, 342
  risk for 316
Preterm premature rupture of membranes, risk of 309
Primaquine 286
Primary cesarean delivery, proceed with 261
Primary intestinal loop, degree of rotation of 169

Primary maternal infection 301
Primidone 381
Primigravida 32, 86, 267
  management of 260
Prophylactic interventions 365
Propythiouracil 380
Proteinuria 30
Protruding tongue 394
Proximal diaphysis 218
Proximal femoral focal deficiency 221
Prune belly syndrome 391
Pseudocyst
  meconium 176, 178
  periventricular 210
Pseudothalidomide syndrome 378
Psychomotor developmental delay 212
Pterygoid processes marks 111
Pulmonary artery 402
Pulmonary atresia 139, 141
Pulmonary embolism, large bilateral 307
Pulmonary hypoplasia 191, 306, 307
  primary 125
  right 125
Pulmonary stenosis 152
Pulmonary trunk, normal 402
Pulmonary valve, absent 139
Pulmonary vein 138
  obstruction 141
Pulsatility index 258
Pulse-wave Doppler echocardiography 155
  supplement m-mode 155
Pulse-wave echocardiography 157
Pump twin 347
Pyrimethamine 246, 301
Pyruvate kinase deficiency 300
Polyhydramnios sequence 343

Q

Quadruple
  marker 6, 14
  test 19
Quantitative fluorescent polymerase chain reaction 89, 120, 313, 332
Quintero stage 2, optimal therapy for 344
Quintero staging 343

R

Radial aplasia 401
Radial ray anomalies 378
Radiation 375
Radiofrequency ablation 91, 309, 342, 347, 395
Recipient twin 343
Recurrent congenital heart block, prevention of 365
Red blood cell 279
  supravital stain 285
Red cell 284
  aplasia 300
  isoimmunization 267
  precursors, immature 284
Reflect inadequate trophoblastic invasion 258
Renal agenesis 127, 193
  bilateral 188, 306, 398
Renal dysgenesis 379
Renal ectopia 193
Renal parenchyma 186
Renal pelviectasis 182
Renal vessels, bilateral 191
Resistance index 25
Respiratory distress 287
  syndrome, prevent 370
Respiratory failure, acute 125
Respiratory tract infection, developed recurrent 288
Reticulocyte count 271
Retinopathy 250
Retronasal triangle 111
Reverse end-diastolic
  flow 96, 261
  velocity 346
Rh blood group alloimmunization: 300
Rh isoimmunization 274
  pregnancy 270
Rh negative pregnancy 353
Rhabdomyomas 129, 142, 151, 209, 352
Rhythm abnormality 156, 158
Right atrial isomerism 141
Right atrium 137, 144
Right ventricle
  double-outlet 147, 150
  enlargement in utero, causes of 140
Right ventricular outflow-tract 139
Roberts syndrome 378
Robertsonian translocation 394
Rubella 177, 250, 254, 325

S

Sacral agenesis 377
Sacrococcygeal teratoma 297
Salbutamol 159
Sampling gate 24
Sandal gap 394
Sanger sequencing 282, 288
Scimitar syndrome 125
Second trimester 19, 314, 368
  aneuploidy markers 13
  serum screening 6
Selective fetal
  growth restriction, classification of 96
  reduction 91
Selective feticide 338, 342
  critical aspect of 338
  technique offered for 338

Selective termination 338
Sensorineural hearing loss 242
Sepsis 307
Septal agenesis 194
Septo-optic dysplasia 194, 208
Septum
  pellucidum 39
  transversum 168
Sequential stepwise screening 15
Serial fetal
  echocardiograms 160
  sonograms 379
Serositis 204
Serum
  analytes 26
  ferritin levels 287
  free beta-human chorionic gonadotropin 7, 87
  marker levels 5
  screening test 13
Severe acute graft vs. host disease 287
Severe cyanotic heart disease in infancy 141
Severe early onset fetal growth restriction 316
Severe shortening 213
Severely decreased liquor 390
Sex chromosomal
  abnormalities 78
  aneuploidies 69, 77, 78
Short humerus 222
Short-rib polydactyly syndrome 217, 293
Shunt occlusion 307
Sickle cell 281
  disease 279, 288, 290
Sildenafil
  effects of 261
  maternal use of 262
Simian crease 394
Single base-pair point mutation 279
Single deepest pocket 261
Single gene disorders 38, 195, 404
Single ventricle physiology 141
Single-needle technique in twins, disadvantage of 333
Singleton pregnancy 18
  fetal interventions in 313
Sinus bradycardia 157, 161
Sirolimus 209, 352
Situs
  inversus 150
  solitus 139, 140
Sjogren's syndrome 158, 159, 160
Skeletal dysplasia 180, 213, 235
  diagnosis of 213
  type of 305
Skeletal malformation 306
Skull defects 379
Slapped-cheek appearance 247
Small dysplastic kidney 390
Small stomach bubble 178
Smith-Lemli-Opitz syndrome 109
Sodium 192
Sonographic sign 164
Sotalol 294, 353, 354
Spina bifida
  cystica 385
  occulta 200
  utero repair of 328
Spinal defect 393
Spinal dysraphism 297
  type of 200
Spine 130, 138
Spiral artery 258
Spiramycin 246
Spleen enlargement 177
Splenomegaly 174, 240, 273
Split foot 390
Spontaneous conception 4, 77
Sporadic defect 199
Static growth 257
Stillbirth 254
  percentage of 396
Stillborn
  fetus, placenta of 399
  hydropic infant 284
Stomach bubble, persistent nonvisualization of 179
Storage diseases 174
Structural brain anomalies 239
Subcutaneous edema 127, 350
Sulfadiazine 246, 301
Sylvian sulcus 207
Symphysio fundal height 257
Systemic lupus erythematosus 23, 158, 159, 295

T

Tachyarrhythmia 142, 156
Tachycardia, supraventricular 353, 354
Tandem mass spectrometry 286
Tei index 138
Teratogen 375
  induced limb defects 380
Teratogenic effects 375
Teratoma 10, 129, 206, 322
Terbutaline 159
Termination, best method of 91
Tetralogy of Fallot 139, 142, 145, 147, 150
Thalassemia
  gene therapy used for 288
  major 278, 281, 286, 288
  minor 278
  prenatal testing of 280
Thalidomide 378, 380
  exposure 378
Thanatophoric dysplasia 215

Theoretical concerns 334
Thin atretic aorta 402
Third trimester 236
Thoracic circumference 213, 305
Thoracoamniotic shunt 120, 307, 321
Thoracocentesis 307
Thorax 217
  abnormalities of 119
  of baby on X-ray 387
Thrombocytopenia 201, 283
Thrombophilia, testing for 266
Thrombus formation 171
Thymic-thoracic ratio 132, 133
Thymus gland 149
Thyroid disorders 287
Thyroid-stimulating hormone 380
  receptor antibodies 356
Thyrotropin 356
Tocolysis maintains 324
TORCH
  group 239
  immunoglobulin 133
Total anomalous pulmonary venous connection 148
Toxoplasma 244-246, 301
  gondii 243
  infection 244
  polymerase chain reaction 204
Toxoplasmosis 239, 243, 254, 300, 325, 402
Trachea, three-vessel 137
Tracheal atresia 293
Tracheal occlusion 329
Tracheomalacia 125, 382
Transcerebellar plane 103
Transient bradycardia 275
  in fetus, cause of 157
Transplacental therapy 351
  drugs for 354
Transvaginal sonography 94
Tri radiant hand 219
Trichorionic triamniotic triplets 94
Tricuspid regurgitation 3, 152, 273
  degree of 296
Tricuspid valve 144
  posterior leaflet of 152
  septal of 152
Trimester nuchal translucency scan 34
Trimethadione 381
Triplets, type of 81
Trisomy 7, 13, 104, 120, 137, 220, 394, 400, 401
  first-trimester screening for 87
  high risk for 18 79
  low risk for 75
  part of 39
Trisomy 21, intermediate risk for 16
  posterior risk for 73
  recurrence of 402
Trophotropism 399
Tuberous sclerosis 151, 209
Tubulinopathy 203
Tumor, rate of growth of 297
Turner's syndrome 38, 44, 104, 105, 173, 291
Twin
  anemia-polycythemia sequence 98
  chorionic villus sampling 334
  chorionicity of 331, 332
  interventions 333
  invasives in 89
  late amniocentesis in 336
  low-risk asymptomatic 94
  quadruple screening in 93
  screening structural anomalies in 93
Twin gestation
  in first trimester 16
  risk of sampling error in 336
Twin pregnancy 32, 337
  with hydrops 395
Twin reversed arterial perfusion 395
  sequence 87, 308, 346
Twin-specific reference ranges 32
Twin-to-twin transfusion syndrome 85, 97, 343, 345
  severe 342
  treatment of 344

U

Ultrasound examination 259
Ultrasound-guided
  laser coagulation 123
  puncture 330
Umbilical artery 346
  Doppler 256, 261
    velocimetry of 343
  pulse-wave Doppler examination 156
  signify 258
  single 234, 259
Umbilical cord 395, 399
  hypercoiling of 396
  thickness of 399
Umbilical vein 172, 343
  intrahepatic portion of 274
Unconjugated estriol 6
Underlying genetic disorder 292
Unilateral renal agenesis 181, 187
  prevalence of 181
Unossified nasal bone 108
Upper abdomen, level of 138
Upper limb, terminal transverse defect in 379
Upper lip, bilateral paramedian cleft of 106
Upper urinary tract obstruction 193
Ureterocele, presence of 186
Urethral atresia 391
Urinary bladder, enlarged 178

Urinary tract
  congenital abnormalities of 181, 193
  dilatation classification 186
Urine electrolytes 192
Urogenital sinus 171
Uropathy, developing 186
Uterine 261
  bleeding 328
  tone 324
  trauma 307
Uterine artery 30
  notching 25
  pulsatility index 22, 26
    measurement 25
  waveform 24
Utero spina bifida repair 328
Uteroplacental blood flow 324

V

Vacuolated lymphocytes 300
Valacyclovir 363
Valine 279
Valproate 376
Valproic acid 381
Vanishing twin 17, 87
  pregnancy 75
Variant nomenclature 216
Varicella-zoster virus 177
Vasa previa 396, 397
Vascular communication 347
Vascular equator 344
Vascular malformations 201
Vascularization index 297
Vecuronium 274
Velamentous insertion 397
Velocardiofacial defect 293
Velocardiofacial syndrome 106
Vena cava
  inferior 125, 138, 141, 172
  left superior 148
    persistent 137, 144
  superior 139
    connecting 140
Venous congestion 174
Ventricles, inversion of 150
Ventricular contractions 358
Ventricular ejection, beginning of 355
Ventricular halo 204
Ventricular septal defect 141, 146, 168, 378
Ventricular tachycardia 287
Ventriculomegaly 109, 241, 243, 246, 252
  mild 239
  severe 197, 200, 234, 402
Vermian agenesis 252
Vermian hypoplasia 197, 198, 212
Vesicoureteric reflux 186
Vessel drain blood 136
Viral infections 158
Viral polymerase chain reaction 230
Viral vector 288
Virilization, prevent 372
Visceral abnormalities 385
Vitamin K antagonists 383
Vomer 113
V-wave signifies blood flow 156

W

Walker-Warburg syndrome 42, 113, 197
Warfarin 380, 383
Waveform 24
White matter abnormalities 252
Whole exome 321
  sequencing 196, 220, 289, 293, 300, 387

X

X-linked recessive 286

Z

Zellweger syndrome 174
Zika virus 241, 243, 252
  infection 252
    maternal 254
Z-score 68, 74, 75
  denote 67
Zygosity 216, 219